THE MATTER OF THE TEXT

The Bible in the Modern World, 37

# The Matter of the Text

## Material Engagements between Luke and the Five Senses

Anne F. Elvey

Sheffield Phoenix Press

2011

Published by Sheffield Phoenix Press
Department of Biblical Studies, University of Sheffield
45 Victoria Street, Sheffield S3 7QB

www.sheffieldphoenix.com



A CIP catalogue record for this book
is available from the British Library

Typeset by the HK Scriptorium
Printed by Lightning Source

ISBN 978-1-907534-16-4 (hbk)

ISSN 1747-9630

*For my parents,*
*Honor and Joe Elvey,*
*with love and appreciation,*
*for all that you have made possible*

# Contents

# List of Illustrations

# Acknowledgments

At the heart of this book is an idea that has been with me for some years, that the texts we read as biblical scholars are underscored by a materiality we have mostly ignored. What an awareness of this materiality means for reading biblical texts is the question I circle around, approaching it but never quite unravelling it in a weaving and unweaving that includes several critical theorists, the Gospel of Luke and the five senses. Many have contributed to the warp and weft of this book. I acknowledge first the country in which the book in large part has taken shape: the lands of the Wurundjeri and the Bunurong, in what is now suburban Melbourne, Australia. I honour the peoples of the Kulin nation, who maintain their connection to the places where I live and work, and the country that sustains my writing. People and country, Aboriginal and Torres Strait Islander peoples and those who have arrived in Australia more recently, local and international colleagues are part of a more-than-human community that acts together in the production of a work such as this book. Amid that community, I want to thank particularly those who have given permission for their words or artwork to inform and enhance my exploration of a material intertextuality.

- Michelle Boisseau for permission to include her wonderful poem 'Parchment' as an epigraph to the book; Michelle Boisseau, 'Parchment', from *Trembling Air*. Copyright © 2003 by Michelle Boisseau. Reprinted with permission of the University of Arkansas Press, www.uapress.com.
- The British Library for permission to quote from Thomas Pattie, 'The Creation of the Great Codices', in *The Bible as Book: The Manuscript Tradition* (ed. John L. Sharpe III and Kimberly Van Kampen; London: British Library, 1998) © The British Library Board 98/04805 DSC.
- Friends of the Earth UK for permission to quote from 'The Environmental Consequences of Pulp and Paper Manufacture' by Friends of the Earth (England, Wales and Northern Ireland), 1996.
- Continuum International Publishing Group for permission to quote from Michel Serres, *The Five Senses: A Philosophy of Mingled Bodies* I (trans. Margaret Sankey and Peter Cowley; London:

Continuum, 2008). By kind permission of Continuum International Publishing Group.

- Austrian National Library, Vienna, for permission to reproduce *Bible moralisée,* Cod. 2554, fol. 16r. Copyright Austrian National Library, Vienna, Picture Archiv+Signature.
- Michael Riley Foundation, National Gallery of Australia, Canberra, and Viscopy for permission to reproduce Michael Riley, *untitled [bible]* from the *cloud* series. Copyright © Michael Riley Foundation / Licensed by Viscopy, 2010.
- Anne Brewster to quote from her article 'Oodgeroo: Orator, Poet, Storyteller', *Australian Literary Studies* 16.4 (1994), pp. 92-104.
- Friends of the Earth Australia for permission to quote from Monica Morgan, 'Colonising Religion', *Chain Reaction* (Summer 2005/2006), pp. 36-37.
- Victor Majzner and Viscopy for permission to reproduce *Vayeitzei* (Jacob's Dream). Copyright © Victor Majzner / Licensed by Viscopy, 2010.
- Robert Gray for permission to quote from his poem 'On a Forestry Trail', in *Certain Things* (Port Melbourne: William Heinemann Australia, 1993).
- Tom Thomson and ETT Imprint for permission to quote from Judith Wright, 'Gum Trees Stripping', in *A Human Pattern: Selected Poems* (Sydney: ETT Imprint, 1996).
- New Directions Publishing Corporation and Bloodaxe Books for permission to include at the head of Chapter 8 Denise Levertov's poem 'O Taste and See'. By Denise Levertov, from *POEMS 1960–1967*, copyright © 1964 by Denise Levertov. Reprinted by permission of New Directions Publishing Corp. Denise Levertov, *New & Selected Poems* (Bloodaxe Books, 2003).

Several parts of this book appeared in earlier versions. Chapter 1 draws from 'The Bible and the Earth: Toward a Materialist Ecological Hermeneutics', *Colloquium: The Australian and New Zealand Theological Review* 42.2 (2010), pp. 131-50; used here with permission. Short sections in Chapters 1 and 3 appeared originally in 'Can There Be a Forgiveness That Makes a Difference Ecologically? An Eco-Materialist Account of Forgiveness as Freedom (Ἄφεσις) in the Gospel of Luke', *Pacifica* 22 (2009), pp. 148-70. A short excerpt from 'Ashes and Dust: On (Not) Speaking about God Ecologically', *Concilium* 3 (2009), pp. 33-42, appears in Chapter 1; used here with permission. Parts of Chapter 4 appeared in an earlier version as 'Touching (on) Death: On "Being Toward" the Other in the Gospel of Luke', *The Bible and Critical Theory* 2.2 (2006), pp. 15.1-15.17; used here with permission. The latter part of Chapter 6 appeared in an earlier version as 'Earth as Intertext: " ... the stones would shout out ..." (Luke 19:40)', *The Council of Societies for the Study of Religion Bulletin* 35.2 (April 2006), pp. 27-29. A version of Chapter 2 is appearing in 2011 as 'The Matter of Texts: A Material Intertextuality and Ecocritical Engagements with the Bible', in *Ecocritical Theory: New European Approaches* (ed. Axel Goodbody and Kate Rigby; Charlottesville: University of Virginia Press, 2011), pp. 341-66. Chapter 8 draws in part on material to be published in 2011 as 'Living One for the Other: Eucharistic Hospitality as Ecological Hospitality', in *Eucharist: Embodied and Embedded in the Land—Interdisciplinary Perspectives* (ed. Kim Power, Claire Renkin, Anne Elvey and Carol Hogan; London: Equinox Publishing, 2011). Copyright © Equinox Publishing Ltd 2011.

Many people have supported my research and writing. Melbourne College of Divinity assisted the work with generous study-leave provisions during my time there as Director of Research in 2006 and 2007, with a position as an MCD Research Scholar in Semester 2, 2008, and since as an honorary research associate. The Centre for Comparative Literature and Cultural Studies has supported my work as an adjunct research fellow with the School of English, Communication and Performance Studies, Monash University. Trinity College Theological School, Trinity College, Parkville, in particular the former Dean of the School, Dr Tim Gaden, have been generous in their hospitality to my work. I am grateful to colleagues who have entered into conversation about this book, especially Dr Elizabeth Dowling, who took time at the busy end of semester to read and comment on the entire manuscript in draft form. Professors Elaine Wainwright and Mark Brett have been excellent conversation partners, and each read and commented on several chapters. Dr Claire Renkin was encouraging of my engagement with images; I am particularly grateful that she drew my attention to the *Bible moralisée* image I discuss at the start of Chapter 4. With Claire, Drs Carol Hogan and Kim Power have supplied a respite of feminist sanity and support as we worked together on another project. Dr Shane Mackinlay provided many congenial conversations on matters philosophical. The Phenomenology and Theology research group in which he is a participant challenged me to think more critically. Over several years, I discussed the issues at the heart of this book with different groups; I mention in particular the Australian Catholic Biblical Association and a helpful conversation with Dr Mark O'Brien; the supportive environment of the Baptists Today Conference (August 2005), especially Merrill Kitchen and Deborah Storie; and the students of the MCD Research School (July 2009), especially Rabbi Aviva Kipen.

This work would not have taken its place in my consciousness but for the ongoing collegiality and companionship of numbers of eco-friends, especially Kate Rigby, whose generosity, grace and professional expertise in the ecological humanities are exemplary, Norm Habel, Deborah Rose, Jan Morgan, and the participants in the MCD-based cross-institutional Ecological Theology and Spirituality research group. Thanks, too, to Aunty Elizabeth (Betty) Pike for her friendship.

In the time it takes to write a book, many things change in a life, and sometimes the writing occurs in the mode of Derrida's gift as a sacrifice not only of the matter that is transformed into a text but also of the needs of kin. I thank my parents for their forbearance as they wrestled with the demands of aging with a writer–daughter for support. My partner, Greg Price, as always has been generous and sound, especially when unexpectedly we had to move house after sixteen years; Matthew and Andrew Elvey Price, our adult sons, have been staunch in their humour and kindness. Finally, my thanks to Sheffield Phoenix Press, especially Ailsa Parkin for her kind responses to each delay and to editors David Clines and Cheryl Exum, for taking a punt on the idea of *The Matter of the Text*.

# ABBREVIATIONS

| | |
|---|---|
| *3 Macc.* | *3 Maccabees* |
| AB | Anchor Bible |
| AnBib | Analecta Biblica |
| *Andr.* | Demosthenes, *Adversus Androtionem*, *Against Androtion* (trans. A.T. Murray; Cambridge, MA: Harvard University Press, 1939; http://www.perseus.tufts.edu) |
| *AusBR* | *Australian Biblical Review* |
| *AHR* | *Australian Humanities Review* |
| BAGD | Walter Bauer, *A Greek–English Lexicon of the New Testament and Other Early Christian Literature* (trans., revised and augmented by William F. Arndt, F. Wilbur Gingrich and Frederick W. Danker; Chicago: University of Chicago Press, 2nd edn, 1979). |
| *B. Bat.* | *Bava Batra* (*Baba Batra*; *The Last Gate*) (Jewish Virtual Library: A Division of The American–Israeli Cooperative Enterprise, http://www.jewishvirtuallibrary.org/jsource/Talmud/bavabatra1.html) |
| BDB | Francis Brown, S.R. Driver and Charles A. Briggs (eds.), *A Hebrew and English Lexicon of the Old Testament: With an Appendix Containing the Biblical Aramaic* (based on the lexicon of William Genesius; trans. Edward Robinson; Oxford: Clarendon Press, 1951). |
| *BibInt* | *Biblical Interpretation: A Journal of Contemporary Approaches* |
| BNTC | Black's New Testament Commentaries |
| *CBQ* | *Catholic Biblical Quarterly* |
| *CH* | *Church History* |
| *De an.* | Aristotle, *De anima* (*On the Soul*) (trans. Hugh Lawson-Tancred; London: Penguin Books, 1986) |
| *Deipn.* | Athenaeus, *Deipnosophistae*; *The Deipnosophists or Banquet of the Learned* (trans. C.D. Jonge; London: Henry G. Bohn, 1854; http://digicoll.library.wisc.edu/Literature/) |
| *Eupol.* | *Eupolemus* |

| | |
|---|---|
| *Hist.* | Polybius, *Historiae* (ed.Theodorus Büttner-Wobst after L. Dindorf; Leipzig: Teubner, 1893); *Histories* (trans. Evelyn S. Shuckburgh; New York: Macmillan. 1889; reprinted, Bloomington, IN, 1962; http://www.perseus.tufts.edu) |
| *HTR* | *Harvard Theological Review* |
| ICC | International Critical Commentary |
| *Int* | *Interpretation* |
| *JAAR* | *Journal of the American Academy of Religion* |
| *JBL* | *Journal of Biblical Literature* |
| *JFSR* | *Journal of Feminist Studies in Religion* |
| *JSNT* | *Journal for the Study of the New Testament* |
| JSNTSup | Journal for the Study of the New Testament Supplement Series |
| *JSOT* | *Journal for the Study of the Old Testament* |
| JSOTSup | Journal for the Study of the Old Testament Supplement Series |
| *Liv. Proph.* | *Lives of the Prophets* |
| LNTS | Library of New Testament Studies |
| LSJ | Henry George Liddell and Robert Scott, *A Greek–English Lexicon* (revised and augmented throughout by Sir Henry Stuart Jones, with the assistance of Roderick McKenzie; Oxford: Clarendon Press, 1940; http://www.perseus.tufts.edu/hopper/text?doc=Perseus%3Atext%3A1999.04.0057) |
| *Nat.* | Pliny the Elder, *Natural History: A Selection* (trans. John F. Healy; with an introduction and notes; London: Penguin, 1991). |
| NCBC | The New Century Bible Commentary |
| NICNT | New International Commentary on the New Testament |
| NIGTC | The New International Greek Testament Commentary |
| *NovT* | *Novum Testamentum* |
| NRSV | New Revised Standard Version |
| NTL | The New Testament Library |
| NTM | New Testament Monographs |
| *NTS* | *New Testament Studies* |
| *Odes* | *Odes of Solomon* |
| *Pacifica* | *Pacifica: Australasian Theological Studies* |
| *RBL* | *Review of Biblical Literature* |
| SBL | Society of Biblical Literature |
| SNTSMS | Society for New Testament Studies Monograph Series |
| TNTC | Tyndale New Testament Commentaries |
| *T. Sol.* | *Testament of Solomon* |
| *TTod* | *Theology Today* |

| | |
|---|---|
| *Vit. Mos.* | Philo, *De vita Mosis* (*On the Life of Moses*), in *Philo: In Ten Volumes* VI (trans. F.H. Colson; Loeb Classical Library; London: William Heinemann, 1935) |

*Parchment*

I'm holding in my hand the skin of a calf
that lived 600 years ago, translucent
skin that someone stretched on four strong poles,
skin someone scraped with a moon-shaped blade.
Here is the flesh side, it understood true dark.
Here is the hair side that met the day's weather,
the long ago rain. It is all inscribed
with the dark brown ink of prayer,

the acid galls of ancient oaks, though these reds,
deluxe rivulets that brighten the margins,
are cinnabar ground to a paste, another paste
of lapis for these blue medieval skies,
and for flowering meadows or a lady's long braids—
the orpiment—a yellow arsenic—
whose grinding felled the illuminator's
boy assistants like flies, or the insect kermes

whose pregnant bodies gave pigment, and the goose
who supplied quills, the horse its hair, and flax
the fine strong thread that held the folded skins
into a private book stamped with gold for a king.

# 1

# EARTH AND TEXT

> When he came to Nazareth, where he had been brought up, he went to the synagogue on the sabbath day, as was his custom. He stood up to read, and the scroll of the prophet Isaiah was given to him. He unrolled the scroll and found the place where it was written:
>
> The Spirit of the lord is upon me,
> because he has anointed me
> to bring good news to the poor.
> He has sent me to proclaim release to the captives
> and recovery of sight to the blind,
> to let the oppressed go free,
> to proclaim the year of the lord's favor.
>
> And he rolled up the scroll, gave it back to the attendant, and sat down. The eyes of all in the synagogue were fixed on him.
>
> Lk. 4.16-20 (NRSV modified)

What is the Lukan Jesus holding in his hands? Luke tells us it is a scroll of the prophet Isaiah, although the words Jesus reads bring together more than one text from Isaiah as we know it. While Luke's text comes to us in Greek, we do have an extant Hebrew scroll of Isaiah from the Second Temple period, namely the Great Isaiah Scroll from Qumran. C.D. Elledge writes:

> The scroll comprises fifty-four columns of text, written upon seventeen sheets of leather parchment that have been stitched together to form a vast scroll over 7 meters in length and 26 centimeters in height.... At least two scribes originally copied *Great Isaiah*, one who copied the first twenty-seven columns (Isaiah 1–33) and another who completed the scroll.[1]

If the scroll is parchment, the Lukan Jesus is indeed 'holding in his hand' a skin or several skins. But perhaps the scroll Luke has in mind is papyrus, as are several of the Septuagint fragments from the second and first centuries

1. C.D. Elledge, *The Bible and the Dead Sea Scrolls* (SBL Archaeology and Biblical Studies, 14; Atlanta: Society of Biblical Literature, 2005), p. 89.

BCE among the Dead Sea Scrolls. According to Pliny the Elder, the paper we call papyrus is woven:

> First an upright layer is smeared on the table—the whole length of the papyrus is used and both its ends are trimmed; then strips are laid across and complete a criss-cross pattern, which is then squeezed in presses. The sheets are dried in the sun and then joined together (Pliny the Elder, *Nat.* 13.77).

If the scroll is papyrus, then the physical interweaving of the plant matches the interweaving of texts that Luke has Jesus read from the scroll.

At this moment, which most commentators read as programmatic for the Gospel of Luke, the Lukan Jesus holds in his hands animal skin or plant fibre, scraped or woven, sewn or glued, to form a scroll that can be unrolled and read. It has the touch and feel of the thing from which it is shaped. The ink with which the scribes have inscribed its unfolding columns gives to the eye the shape of words that the mouth will form and speak for the ears both of the reader and those assembled in the synagogue. There is a sensual materiality to the act of reading which Luke has inscribed in a text that already, in its own interweaving of texts, is an interpretation, that is, a reading.

## *The Material Text*

When in the process of biblical criticism, I pick up a book, journal or printed article, my senses are engaged as mediators of the materiality of the text. I touch, smell and see paper and ink. I hear the faint rustle of the page. Without too great a leap of the imagination, I know that this matter produced as a volume's leaves was once part of plants with living foliage. When I read this text as I write it on my laptop, as dark marks stand out against the light of a screen, and my fingers and ears are tuned to the touch and tap of the keys, my eyes and ears to the buzz and contrast of the machine, I can know by imagination the myriad transformations of Earth that produced the fossils and minerals that constitute this computer and form the matter of this text.[2]

2. In this writing, I refer to Earth with a capital letter in acknowledgment of its status both as a planet and as the material context for this exploration of the matter of the text. While this is not to imply that Earth is divine, it is to give it a proper name. When referring to the usage in ancient texts, such as the Gospel of Luke, I use 'the earth'; and when referring to Earth more locally as ground or soil, I use 'earth'. In ecological, feminist and postcolonial frameworks, it is difficult to decide what word to use for the divine other and what translations to use for κύριος and for divine names. Allowing a capital for Earth informs my decision to allow a capital for God. When I refer to the divine other, I use God, or where the Hebrew Bible uses a name, I use that name. For the tetragrammaton, I use Yhwh, without vowels, respecting the unspeakable character of the name.

As I engage with these material elements, transformed by human hands, I can imagine the complex interrelationships of more-than-human production and reproduction that underscore the being of a text as matter.[3] As I write and read, and silently report the words to myself, I can imagine the interplay of body and breath, human and machine, producing this text.

My evocation of the text as matter is more than an incidental imaginative exercise. Since Lynn White's now famous essay if not before, biblical scholars have understood that certain traditions of interpretation and uses of the Bible, particularly in the West, have been implicated in harm toward the wider Earth community, in what is now denoted—with an eschatological sense of urgency—an ecological crisis.[4] This understanding parallels those arrived at in relation to the many European projects of colonization in the Americas, Africa, Asia, Australia, Aotearoa New Zealand and the Pacific. In the ensuing postcolonial contexts, the scene of Christian biblical scholarship, while still dominated by the voices of European and settler scholars, has become multiple and increasingly open to, if less often written in, the voices of many human persons, especially those who have inherited its legacies of violence. Since the mid-1990s, the Earth Bible project emerging in Adelaide, South Australia, adopting a framework of ecojustice, has sought to bring the voice of Earth, and of the many more-than-human others who constitute the Earth community, into this scholarly and wider ecclesial conversation by way of the adoption and use of six ecojustice principles articulated from an Earth-centred perspective (intrinsic worth, interconnectedness, voice, purpose, mutual custodianship and resistance).[5] The subsequent Ecological Hermeneutics consultations at the Society of Biblical Literature international and annual meetings and the Uses of the Bible in Environmental Ethics project at the University of Exeter have each furthered the process of developing ecocritical approaches to biblical inter-

For κύριος, it is tempting to use a translation that hides the kyriarchal language of lordship with its underlying imagery of the master/slave relation. I have decided to modify the NRSV translation, retaining the term but using lower case for 'lord'. Where κύριος unambiguously refers to God, I occasionally use 'God'. Rather than translating the difficult term βασιλεία when it refers to the kingdom, reign, rule, or commonweal of God, I leave it untranslated as 'the βασιλεία of God'.

3. The term 'more than human' is not intended to exclude humans; rather, 'more than human' includes humankind as one diverse species among many constituents of an Earth community of which mammals, and animals more generally, are only a part.

4. Lynn White, 'The Historical Roots of our Ecological Crisis', in *This Sacred Earth: Religion, Nature, Environment* (ed. Roger S. Gottlieb; London: Routledge, 1996), pp. 184-93.

5. Norman C. Habel (ed.), *Readings from the Perspective of Earth* (The Earth Bible 1; Sheffield: Sheffield Academic Press, 2000), p. 24.

pretation.[6] The Society of Biblical Literature consultations have brought to the Earth Bible ecojustice principles three further hermeneutics: suspicion (especially of anthropocentrism in texts, readings and readers); identification (with a wider Earth community of which human readers are part and with Earth others as agents within the text); and retrieval (of an Earth perspective and voice in the text).[7] The Uses of the Bible in Environmental Ethics project is developing biblically based doctrinal and ethical lenses for an ecological hermeneutics.[8] In each project, the context of ecological crisis both prompts contemporary ecocritical readings and challenges readers to attend to biblical traditions differently. Nonetheless, to my knowledge, none of these projects attends to the ecocritical implications of the text as material artefact.

Considered against the ecological cost of the production and reproduction of Bibles and the vastness of the contemporary book industry, the question of the ecocritical implications of the text as material artefact is particularly relevant to the context of ecological crisis. Furthermore, the artefactual nature of the text, its being as a physical thing existing within a network of relations, situates the text in the wider material context of the Earth community. My writing that comes to you as a particular material artefact—for example, a printed book, or perhaps a photocopy—asks what conceptions of the biblical text can account for, and open readers to, both the materiality of the text and the material contexts of interpretation.

6. See Habel (ed.), *Readings from the Perspective of Earth*; Norman C. Habel and Shirley Wurst (eds.), *The Earth Story in Genesis* (The Earth Bible, 2; Sheffield: Sheffield Academic Press 2000); Norman C. Habel and Shirley Wurst (eds.), *The Earth Story in Wisdom Traditions* (The Earth Bible, 3; Sheffield: Sheffield Academic Press, 2001); Norman C. Habel (ed.), *The Earth Story in the Psalms and the Prophets* (The Earth Bible, 4; Sheffield: Sheffield Academic Press, 2001); Norman C. Habel and Vicky Balabanski (eds.), *The Earth Story in the New Testament* (The Earth Bible, 5; London: Sheffield Academic Press, 2002); Norman C. Habel and Peter L. Trudinger (eds.), *Exploring Ecological Hermeneutics* (SBL Symposium Series, 46; Atlanta: Society of Biblical Literature, 2008); David G. Horrell, Cherryl Hunt and Christopher Southgate, 'Appeals to the Bible in Ecotheology and Environmental Ethics: A Typology of Hermeneutical Stances', *Studies in Christian Ethics* 21.2 (2008), pp. 219-38. See also the Web sites for the Earth Bible and Uses of the Bible in Environmental Ethics projects: http://www.flinders.edu.au/ehlt/theology/ctsc/projects/earthbible/earthbible_home.cfm and http://huss.exeter.ac.uk/theology/research/ubee.php respectively. In being positively focused as ecohermeneutic projects in their own right, each of these approaches differs from earlier apologetic and critical responses by biblical scholars, to White, 'Historical Roots'.

7. Norman C. Habel, 'Introducing Ecological Hermeneutics', in *Exploring Ecological Hermeneutics* (ed. Norman C. Habel and Peter L. Trudinger; SBL Symposium Series, 46; Atlanta: Society of Biblical Literature, 2008), pp. 1-8 (3-8).

8. Horrell, Hunt and Southgate, 'Appeals to the Bible'.

For postcolonial, feminist and other approaches focused on inter-human social justice and ethics, a consonance exists between texts as human artefacts written in human languages, handed down over centuries in human cultures however different from one's own, and their contemporary human interpreters. In contrast, although an ecojustice approach emphasizes the interconnectedness of social and environmental justice, the more-than-human *Earthy* context of the text, without which there would be no text, appears less readily in its readings. Mark Brett asks:

> In what sense does 'the earth' have a voice? ... Who speaks on behalf of the earth? ... This sort of eco-ideology clearly has strategic value, but one wonders (on analogy with postcolonial hermeneutics) whether the earth is thereby reduced, all too often, to a cipher.[9]

Moreover, at what seems something of a remove from a more-than-human context, but perhaps only *seems* so, the Bible as text, as a collection of texts, has already been received within most Jewish and Christian scholarly and liturgical contexts as originating in, communicating, or mediating another more-than-human context of divinely initiated relationship with humankind. The biblical creation stories, the Deuteronomic connection of land and justice, the Prophets, Psalms, the other Wisdom literature, the Christian Second Testament and later theologies of sacrament and incarnation point in their various ways to a necessary interrelationship between God, Earth, cosmos and human beings. We might speak, therefore, of *one* more-than-human context for the text that is materially spiritual and spiritually material, if the terms spiritual and material remain useful at all.[10]

To date, however, Christian interpreters seem more at home with the divine and human elements of this more-than-human context for the text than with the multiple other-than-human members of the Earth community. The extent to which we emphasize the divine or human side of this depends on our scholarly and ecclesial contexts and experiences of such. But whether the focus is on the divine or the human as context for the text, readers generally approach the text as word, words, or, in a post-modern return to the meaning of *Scripture*: writing or writings. However sophisticated our approaches, when, as biblical interpreters, we approach the text as word or words, writing or writings, human or divine, we seem already at a remove from the Earth matter on which the text depends and toward which our ecological sensitivities impel us to attend. This presses me to

9. Mark G. Brett, 'Earthing the Human in Genesis 1–3', in *The Earth Story in Genesis* (ed. Norman C. Habel and Shirley Wurst; The Earth Bible, 2; Sheffield: Sheffield Academic Press, 2000), p. 73.

10. Cf. Val Plumwood, *Environmental Culture: The Ecological Crisis of Reason* (Environmental Philosophies; London: Routledge, 2002), pp. 222-23.

ask whether there is a model or a mode of biblical interpretation that might account for, and be open to, the material embeddedness of the text in its more-than-human contexts.

### *The Material Given*

Underlying my concern with the Bible as material artefact is the notion of the material given, a term referring to the givenness of material phenomena.[11] Earth, bodies and pregnant bodies are paradigms of a material givenness that is necessary to produce and sustain human species-life. This necessity has the character of (1) a gift that cannot be defined wholly in terms of exchange, property or what is proper; (2) a space, like the body in pregnancy, in which self and other are interconnected in ways that 'can be reduced neither to a *prior* givenness nor to economics'.[12] Both human sociality (hereafter, the social) and a wider more-than-human sociality (hereafter, sociality) are aspects of the material given.

The Bible has a relation of dependence on, and indebtedness to, the material given. Because Bibles are material artefacts, of certain human cultures, the Bible is plural. Not only is there a variety of canonical collections that are called Bibles (e.g. the Hebrew Bible, the Roman Catholic Bible), but any one of these collections is a site of interconnectedness between plants, minerals, fossils; habitats and climates; bodies, breath, languages; oral and written traditions; societies and their stories; and the convergences and dissonances among these. Moreover, since the production, reproduction and transmission of Bibles require plants, animals and human labour and since biblical texts have been interpreted to support both destruction of and care for Earth, the Bible affects the unfolding of the material given over time.[13] Thus, the Bible's dependence on the material given is also an interrelatedness that is inter-influential.

11. I develop the notion of the material given in Anne Elvey, *An Ecological Feminist Reading of the Gospel of Luke: A Gestational Paradigm* (Studies in Women and Religion, 45; Lewiston, NY: Edwin Mellen Press, 2005), esp. Chapter 3.

12. Elvey, *Ecological Feminist Reading*, p. 100; Anne Elvey, 'The Material Given: Bodies, Pregnant Bodies and Earth', *Australian Feminist Studies* 18.4 (2003), pp. 199-209 (205-206). The term 'aneconomic' is borrowed from Jacques Derrida, *Given Time.* I. *Counterfeit Money* (trans. Peggy Kamuf; Chicago: University of Chicago Press, 1992), p. 7. Cf. Rosalyn Diprose, *The Bodies of Women: Ethics, Embodiment and Sexual Difference* (London: Routledge, 1994), p. 118; and Luce Irigaray, *Sexes and Genealogies* (trans. Gillian C. Gill; New York: Columbia University Press, 1993), pp. 15, 32.

13. Norman C. Habel, 'Introducing the Earth Bible', in *Readings from the Perspective of Earth* (ed. Norman C. Habel; The Earth Bible, 1; Sheffield: Sheffield Academic Press, 2000), pp. 25-37 (27-33).

### *Materiality and More-than-Human Agency*

As a starting point for conceptualizing the inter-influence of the materiality of the text, the Bible, its interpreters and interpretations, I turn to the concept of agency within the framework of Val Plumwood's critique of a logic of colonization. The logic of colonization Plumwood describes parallels the framework of hierarchical dualism set out by Elisabeth Schüssler Fiorenza as situating agency with the kyriarchal polis of elite freeborn males.[14] When she describes a system of dualisms as the structure of a logic of colonization Plumwood argues that the definition of higher in terms of lower categories follows a pattern of relationship between master and slave, as follows: master/slave; man/woman; human/animal; culture/nature; spirit/matter; soul/body; self/other; and so on.[15] Defined in terms of their second elements, the first elements also form a metonymy so that master, man, human, culture, spirit, soul and the self are identified with reason as superior to and exclusive of slave, woman, animal, nature, matter, body and the other.[16] Mapped onto this structure of hierarchical dualism is the pair freedom/necessity, such that members of the first class possess the quality of freedom and are therefore understood to have agency and members of the second class are characterized by necessity. Thus, in this dualistic framework, women, slaves, bodies and Earth are marked by a material necessity or givenness associated with nature. This association occludes their capacity for agency, at the same time implying that what is denoted nature is without agency.

As Plumwood writes:

> Colonizing perspectives find the category of nature serviceable both to suppress resistance and to hide certain kinds of (human and non-human) inputs they wish to appropriate, refusing to recognize the suppressed oth-

14. Elisabeth Schüssler Fiorenza, *But She Said: Feminist Practices of Biblical Interpretation* (Boston: Beacon Press, 1992), pp. 8, 114-20. A political kyriarchal framework extends a notion of patriarchy focused solely in definitions and relations of sex and gender by describing relations of interlocking oppression based on sex, gender, class, race, sexuality and so forth. Insofar as this framework informs not only the socio-cultural and political, but also the individual imagination and unconscious, we can speak of a kyriarchal imaginary. Psychoanalytic theorists such as Luce Irigaray and Julia Kristeva have dealt carefully with this aspect of the corporeal and material force of the imaginary. See, for example, Luce Irigaray, *Divine Women* (trans. S. Muecke; Local Consumption Papers, 8; Sydney: Local Consumption, 1986); Luce Irigaray, *Je, Tu, Nous: Toward a Culture of Difference* (trans. Alison Martin; London: Routledge, 1993); Julia Kristeva, *Revolution in Poetic Language* (trans. Margaret Waller; New York: Columbia University Press, 1984).

15. Val Plumwood, *Feminism and the Mastery of Nature* (Feminism for Today; London: Routledge, 1993), p. 43.

16. Plumwood, *Feminism and the Mastery of Nature*, pp. 41-68.

> er's agency and creation of value, and assimilating relevant cases to that of nature. Usually this is possible because within the dominant narrative, *nature's agency as such* is denied, so that to be included within the category of nature is to be deprived of recognition as an agent. Indeed, to the extent that nonhuman species have their own forms of culture, agencies and autonomy, the opposition between nature and culture is simply invalid, and depends on an oppressively reductionist and instrumentalist view of nonhuman animals (which may then be read back into selected human cases, to oppress them also).[17]

On occasion Earth appears as agent in the Bible (see, in particular, Lev. 18.28; 20.22). Moreover, the ecojustice principles of voice, mutual custodianship and resistance, and many of the Earth-oriented readings in the Earth Bible volumes and the SBL Ecological Hermeneutics consultations affirm the agency of Earth.[18] Such readings focus on Earth as a character in the text; what is said of Earth's agency by an authorized voice in the text, be it that of the narrator, a prophet, or God; or what can be imagined of Earth's perspective on the narrative. This book asks a different question concerning if, and in what ways, the material artefact through which a text presents itself to be read has agency in relation to our reading of the text. The usual working assumption of biblical scholars, that a text to be interpreted remains the *same* text no matter the material form in which it presents itself, parallels the colonizing assumption that nature is without agency.

The assumption that Earth is without agency is frequently duplicitous. For example, the same person or group can both deny nature's agency, valuing nature only in terms of its use for human purposes, and fear nature as outside human control, for example, in bushfires, tsunamis, earthquakes and hurricanes. In the system of hierarchical dualism, the experience of nature as not under human control does not necessarily unsettle the framework; rather, this experience reinforces the desire for control that underpins the impulses and structures of domination. Plumwood focuses on the dualistic underpinnings of this framework, which she maintains inform a particularly problematic trajectory of Western thought, attitude and practice toward the subordinated other of the elite. She describes five ways in which this system of dualism operates and reinforces itself: backgrounding or denial; radical

17. Val Plumwood, 'Nature as Agency and the Prospects for a Progressive Naturalism', *Capitalism Nature Socialism* 12.4 (2001), pp. 3-32 (6-7).

18. See, for example, Norman C. Habel, 'Geophany: The Earth Story in Genesis 1', in *The Earth Story in Genesis* (ed. Norman C. Habel and Shirley Wurst; The Earth Bible, 1; Sheffield: Sheffield Academic Press, 2000), pp. 34-48; Melissa Tubbs Loya, '"Therefore the Earth Mourns": The Grievance of Earth in Hosea 4:1-3', in *Exploring Ecological Hermeneutics* (ed. Norman C. Habel and Peter Trudinger; SBL Symposium Series, 46; Atlanta: Society of Biblical Literature, 2008), pp. 53-62.

exclusion or hyperseparation; incorporation or relational definition; instrumentalism or objectification; and homogenization or stereotyping.[19]

Of backgrounding, Plumwood writes:

> The view of the other as inessential is the master's perspective. The master's view is set up as universal, and it is part of the mechanism of backgrounding that it never occurs to him that there might be other perspectives from which he is the background. Yet this inessentialness which he believes the slave to have in relation to his own essentialness is an illusion. First, the master more than the slave requires the other in order to define his boundaries and identity, since these are defined against the inferiorised other...; it is the slave who makes the master a master, the colonised who makes the coloniser, the periphery which makes the centre. Second, the master also requires the other materially, in order to survive, for the relation of complementation has made the master dependent on the slave for fulfilment of his needs. But this dependency is also hated and feared by the master, for it subtly challenges his dominance, and is denied in a variety of indirect and direct ways, with all the consequences of repression.[20]

In her commentary on Luke, Sharon Ringe recounts an experience of a seminary class when one of her students prompted her to notice the slaves whose presence and labour forms part of the background in the parable of the Lost Son (15.11-32).[21] From this perspective, the divine hospitality that the father enacts relies on the slaves whom he commands as master: 'But the father said to his slaves, "Quick, bring out a robe—the best one—and put it on him; put a ring on his finger and sandals on his feet. And get the fatted calf and kill it, and let us eat and celebrate"' (15.22-23).

By radical exclusion or hyperseparation, the master not only forgets his or her dependence on the slave but also actively construes the slave as other in kind. A hyperseparation is a relation in which the difference between two terms is rendered in an exclusive and oppositional mode.[22] As Plumwood explains, 'the master defines himself by exclusion against the other'.[23] In its depiction of faithful response to the divine purpose, the Lukan Gospel tends to cast not slaves but the Pharisees and scribes as other (see esp. 7.30).[24] This depiction also operates in the mode of what Plumwood describes as

19. Plumwood, *Feminism and the Mastery of Nature*, pp. 47-55; see also Plumwood, *Environmental Culture*, pp. 100-111.

20. Plumwood, *Feminism and the Mastery of Nature*, pp. 48-49.

21. Sharon H. Ringe, *Luke* (Westminster Bible Companion; Louisville, KY: Westminster John Knox, 1995), pp. 8-9.

22. See Plumwood, *Environmental Culture*, p. 101.

23. Plumwood, *Feminism and the Mastery of Nature*, p. 51.

24. See Robert C. Tannehill, *The Narrative Unity of Luke–Acts: A Literary Interpretation*. I. *The Gospel according to Luke* (Foundations and Facets: New Testament; Philadelphia: Fortress Press, 1986), p. 171; David A. Neale, *'None but the Sinners':*

relational definition (or incorporation), where the other is construed as lacking the qualities desired by the self or central group (e.g. faithfulness of response to the divine purpose).[25]

Instrumentalism refers to the way in which the other is defined solely in terms of its use. The slave must put aside her or his needs in favour of the needs, desires or purposes of the master, becoming his or her instrument or resource.[26] Luke 17.7-9 seems to reflect this attitude: 'Who among you would say to your slave who has just come in from ploughing or tending sheep in the field, "Come here at once and take your place at the table?" Would you not rather say to him, "Prepare supper for me, put on your apron and serve me while I eat and drink; later you may eat and drink"? Do you thank the slave for doing what was commanded?'

Finally, homogenization functions to elide the differences between those construed as other; slaves become a class of people with stereotypical characteristics. Plumwood writes: 'To the master, residing at what he takes to be the centre, differences among those of lesser status at the periphery are of little interest or importance, and might undermine comfortable stereotypes of superiority. To the master, all the rest are just that: "the rest", the Others, the background to his achievements and the resources for his needs.'[27] In the Lukan context, the variety of characterizations of the Pharisees, highlighted by several scholars, may unsettle any homogenizing tendency in their depiction in particular passages or groups of passages.[28] In quoting Isa. 40.4, Luke offers a different image of homogenization, this time of other than humans, namely valleys and hills, in the service of a divine visitation (Lk. 3.4-6).

The examples I have offered from the Lukan narrative to demonstrate features of hierarchical dualism suggest that something of the master/slave dynamic Plumwood critiques is operative in the imagery Luke employs. But these indications by example are not exhaustive either of the outlook of the Lukan Gospel itself or of the particular episodes cited. Moreover, the dualistic framework Plumwood describes represents a boundary situation, where difference is understood as governed by opposition and mutual

*Religious Categories in the Gospel of Luke* (JSNTSup, 58; Sheffield: JSOT Press, 1991), pp. 136-37. See discussion in Elvey, *Ecological Feminist Reading*, pp. 211-17.

25. See Plumwood, *Feminism and the Mastery of Nature*, p. 52.

26. Plumwood, *Feminism and the Mastery of Nature*, p. 53.

27. Plumwood, *Feminism and the Mastery of Nature*, p. 54.

28. See D.B. Gowler, *Host, Guest, Enemy and Friend: Portraits of the Pharisees in Luke and Acts* (New York: Peter Lang, 1991); Joel Green, *The Gospel of Luke* (NICNT; Grand Rapids: Eerdmans, 1997), pp. 301-302; Jack Dean Kingsbury, *Conflict in Luke: Jesus, Authorities, Disciples* (Minneapolis: Fortress Press, 1991), pp. 104-105, 107; cf. Jack T. Sanders, *The Jews in Luke–Acts* (Philadelphia: Fortress Press, 1987).

exclusion.[29] In practice, elite individuals and corporations may not universally or consistently think and act out of such a dualistic framework. Nevertheless, in global capitalist paradigms and practices of domination (and consumption), the oppressive outcomes of tendencies toward hierarchical dualism and its colonizing outlook are all too evident. Further, the concept of nature is itself an example of a problematic tendency to homogenize the myriad plants, animals, minerals, structures, ecosystems and communities that constitute Earth and cosmos. In this book I prefer to speak of a more-than-human Earth community and of matter, albeit itself a general term, as constitutive of all that is Earthy and cosmic, including humans and their writings. For the current project, the question concerns the way in which a reading focused on the materiality of the text, and the agency of the text as material artefact, might unsettle and offer an alternative to readings that assume and support a logic of mastery inimical to the flourishing of a more-than-human Earth community.

My focus on materiality is not intended as a simple reversal of a spirit/matter dualism. Rather, moving beyond a matter/spirit split, the materiality of Earth is already the locus of its transcendence. I have suggested elsewhere that we think in terms of a material transcendence.[30] This has problems insofar as the concept of a material transcendence seems to reverse the spirit/matter dualism by shifting the focus to the previously devalued term 'matter'. While this may be the case, and ideally I would speak of a materially spiritual, spiritually material transcendence, the shift of focus is important. Generally the material has at worst been represented as non-spiritual, even anti-spiritual, at best as the locus of divine immanence; so to put together material and transcendence is to return a certain respect, for matter's inherent otherness and spiritual non-negotiability, to the material. Rather than romanticizing matter, such an openness to the alterity of the other needs to be understood as an orientation to learning from the other of its being, which may call forth variously welcome, compassion, wonder, solidarity, prudence and resistance. But we need also to remember that this other is of a particular kind; it is another of which we are ourselves part, and that in opening to an Earthly otherness we recognize an otherness in ourselves.[31]

29. Plumwood herself argues that difference need not, and should not, be viewed in this way. Nevertheless, she notes that 'residues of dualism are often remarkably persistent' (*Feminism and the Mastery of Nature*, pp. 59-68, esp. p. 59).

30. Anne Elvey, 'Material Elements: The Matter of Women, the Matter of Earth, the Matter of God', in *Post-Christian Feminisms: A Critical Approach* (ed. Lisa Isherwood and Kathleen McPhillips; Aldershot: Ashgate, 2008), pp. 53-69.

31. Material in this paragraph appears in Anne Elvey, 'Ashes and Dust: On (Not) Speaking about God Ecologically', *Concilium* 3 (2009), pp. 33-53 (37-38).

### *The Text as Material Artefact in a Network of More-than-Human Agency*

The material interconnectedness of other-than-human and human beings in a more-than-human Earth community forms a context for the complex meaning-making activity that is the production of a text. I have at least three layers of textual production in view: the early production of biblical texts by their authors and scribes; the continuing history of reproduction of these texts in many material forms, including the variety of textual versions and translations; the production of interpretations of these texts. While I understand the three to be interconnected, I turn to the question of the complex of agency involved in the last of these.

What processes of enactment are involved in reading a biblical text? Who or what acts to produce an interpretation? The common sense response would seem to be that the interpreter acts, through reading, thinking, and writing or speaking, to produce an interpretation of a particular biblical text. But already this is simplistic. Historical criticism, for example, would add a focus on the author as producer of meaning if only the interpreter can discover his or her intent. Forms of narrative and rhetorical criticism focus on the agency of the text, as words on the page, and the particular use of the capacities of language for plot, characterization, metaphor, persuasion, suspense, genre and so on, to produce meaning. While reader-response approaches might focus more directly on the reader, already there is at least a co-agency between author, text, reader and the socio-cultural worlds and worldviews of each as they interact to influence and produce an interpretation. How are we to situate this co-agency ecologically in relation to the materiality of the text, that is, the text as material artefact and the material embeddedness of its production, reproductions and interpretations?

Considering the case of the making of a pot, Lambros Malafouris asks who or what is causing the act? He suggests that the particular properties of the clay, the technology of the wheel and the potter's embodied interaction with these constitute complex relations of responsiveness that are not the result of a single individual intentional act on the part of the potter.[32] Rather, the making of a pot is called forth in the responsive interaction of the elements necessary to the task (clay, wheel, space, potter, water ...) and human engagement with the possibilities their materiality and material situation afford.[33] Human agency is situated in a more-than-human contextual field of action.

32. Lambros Malafouris, 'At the Potter's Wheel: An Argument for Material Agency', in *Material Agency: Toward a Non-Anthropocentric Approach*, (ed. Carl Knappett and Lambros Malafouris; New York: Springer, 2008), pp. 19-36 (33).

33. Malafouris, 'At the Potter's Wheel', p. 33.

Jane Bennett writes of material agency in terms of an assembly of humanity and nonhumanity interacting both together and on one another: 'Humanity and nonhumanity have always performed an intricate dance with each other. There was never a time when human agency was anything other than an interfolding network of humanity and nonhumanity; today this mingling has become harder to ignore.'[34] Rather than focusing on moral agency with its investment in the intentional acts of human agents, Bennett considers distributive agency in which intentionality is 'less definitive of outcomes'.[35] A unique human subject acting intentionally is not the sole cause of a unique effect. Instead, when humans act they are already in relation to a myriad of more-than-human (including human) others; and this interrelationship in any particular situation, such as the making of a pot, is agential. For Bennett, 'An assemblage owes its agentic capacity to the vitality of the materialities that constitute it'.[36]

The concept of agency finds a focus, then, not in an individual entity that acts but in the process of enactment, distributed in 'collectives of humans and nonhumans'.[37] This is not, however, to argue that the enactment is determined by the material situation apart from the potter's embeddedness in it. Rather, the enactment that is the making of a pot is a dynamic process of more-than-human co-agency in which the human potter is agential precisely because she or he consents to being embedded responsively in the more-than-human situation of pot making. This responsive embedding to which the potter consents occurs against the background that is the material givenness not only of the matter and tools of pot making, but of the history of potting and the potter's prior experience and skill.[38]

Can we make a parallel with the work of biblical interpretation? First, we need to consider ways in which the matter and material tools of interpreta-

34. Jane Bennett, *Vibrant Matter: A Political Ecology of Things* (Durham, NC: Duke University Press, 2010), p. 31.

35. Bennett, *Vibrant Matter*, pp. 31-32.

36. Bennett, *Vibrant Matter*, p. 34.

37. Carl Knappett, 'The Neglected Networks of Material Agency: Artefacts, Pictures and Texts', in *Material Agency: Toward a Non-Anthropocentric Approach* (ed. Carl Knappett and Lambros Malafouris; New York: Springer, 2008), pp. 139-56 (140, 143). See also John Law and Annemarie Mol, 'The Actor-Enacted: Cumbrian Sheep in 2001', in *Material Agency: Toward a Non-Anthropocentric Approach* (ed. Carl Knappett and Lambros Malafouris; New York: Springer, 2008), pp. 57-77; and Owain Jones and Paul Cloke, 'Non-Human Agencies: Trees in Place and Time', in *Material Agency: Toward a Non-Anthropocentric Approach* (ed. Carl Knappett and Lambros Malafouris; New York: Springer, 2008), pp. 79-96. See also Jane Bennett's exploration of the possibility of 'thing power' as a kind of material agency ('The Force of Things: Steps toward an Ecology of Matter', *Political Theory* 32.3 [2004], pp. 347-72 (365-67).

38. Malafouris, 'At the Potter's Wheel'.

tion—texts in papyri, codices, books, journals, and on screen; paper, pencils, pens, ink, typewriters, word processors, computer programmes, and the computers on which to run them; the matter underlying these, such as sheep, trees, fossils, minerals—form part of a more-than-human contextual field of action in which an interpretation is produced. Second, we need to consider the material givenness of not only the matter and material tools of interpretation but also the history of production and reproduction of biblical texts, the history of interpretation and the interpreter's prior experience and skills. Third, we need to consider modes of biblical interpretation in which the interpreter consents to being embedded responsively in the more-than-human situation of biblical interpretation outlined in the previous two points. But to consent to the material embeddedness of biblical interpretation may be to inhabit a gap between matter and word.

### *The Text as Material Artefact: Between Word and Earth*

First, words about matter do not reproduce the matter to which they refer.[39] Second, the text's coming after that to which it refers is complicated by the poststructuralist understanding that 'matter', like any signified, is a 'product of writing'.[40] That the text comes both after and before matter describes a chasm around the mediated matter that gives itself to the text as papyrus, paper, ink, plastic, even light and shade. Third, the relationship between text and matter relies on the emergence of literacy. While oral language emerges, and is embedded, in the materiality of human bodies and is intricately related to human breath, literacy creates a further layer of abstraction between matter and word.[41] For Walter Ong, 'writing ... tends to assimilate other things [bodies, cultures, and the matter on which texts depend] to itself'.[42] Fourth, however, there is also an underlying connectedness between text and matter, exemplified by the figure of the Sumerian goddess–scribe, Nisaba, who links human capacity to grow new life with both the soil's capacity to produce grain and human reaping, storing and recording of the ripened grain.[43] For Kate Rigby, writing emerged under

39. See, for example, Kate Rigby's reflections on nature writing in 'Writing after Nature', *AHR* 39–40 (2006), http://www.australianhumanitiesreview.org/archive/Issue-September-2006/rigby.html.

40. Rigby, 'Writing after Nature'.

41. David Abram, *The Spell of the Sensuous* (New York: Vintage Books, 1997), pp. 95-102; Walter J. Ong, *Orality and Literacy* (London: Routledge, 2002), pp. 12, 28.

42. Ong, *Orality and Literacy,* p. 12.

43. Tikva Frymer-Kensky, *In the Wake of the Goddesses: Women, Culture and the Biblical Transformation of Pagan Myth* (New York: Free Press, 1992), pp. 48-50. See also 'A Hymn to Nisaba', in *The Electronic Text Corpus of Sumerian Literature* http://etcsl.orinst.ox.ac.uk/section4/tr4161.htm; http://etcsl.orinst.ox.ac.uk/cgi-bin/etcsl.cgi.

certain material conditions that allowed for the development of agriculture, and to this extent, writing may be understood as prompted by Earth.[44] Such a history resonates in the biblical conjunction of seed and word (e.g. Isa. 55.10-11; Lk. 8.11). Fifth, moreover, texts are dependent on matter; they are matter. The word we use for Bible reminds us of the materiality of the text, when we recall with Jacques Derrida that *biblos* 'in Greek names the internal bark of the papyrus and thus of paper, like the Latin word *liber*, which first designated the living part of the bark before it meant "book"'.[45] Indeed a long Christian tradition of juxtaposing two revelatory texts—the book of nature and the book of Scripture—contributes to a crossing of Earth-word and God-seed.[46]

Finally, we can imagine a multiplicity of relationships between the words of a text and the matter—mineral, floral and corporeal—that mediates it and the subjects that perform and performatively interpret it.[47] For example, consider some scenes of interrelationship between matter and text:

Scene 1: Telling the text to oneself in memory
Scene 2: Reciting the text aloud from memory
Scene 3: Touching the text on an ancient codex with carefully gloved hands
Scene 4: Reading the text on an ancient papyrus
Scene 5: Reading the text in a contemporary printed Greek New Testament
Scene 6: Reading an English translation in a mass-produced Bible
Scene 7: Reading the text on a computer screen
Scene 8: Reading the text juxtaposed with art works
Scene 9: Reading/reciting the text within a liturgical context
Scene 10: Singing the text

On the association of writing with the divine, see William M. Schniedewind, *How the Bible Became a Book: The Textualization of Ancient Israel* (Cambridge: Cambridge University Press, 2004), esp. pp. 24-27.

44. Rigby, 'Writing after Nature'.

45. Jacques Derrida, *Paper Machine* (trans. Rachel Bowlby; Cultural Memory in the Present; Stanford, CA: Stanford University Press, 2005), p. 6; see also Anne Elvey, 'Earthing the Text? On the Status of the Biblical Text in Ecological Perspective', *AusBR* 52 (2004), pp. 64-79.

46. See, for example, Olaf Pedersen, *The Book of Nature* (Rome: Vatican Observatory Publications, 1992); and Constant J. Mews, 'The World as Text: The Bible and the Book of Nature in Twelfth-Century Theology', in *Scripture and Pluralism: Reading the Bible in the Religiously Plural Worlds of the Middle Ages and Renaissance, Studies in the History of Christian Traditions* (ed. Thomas J. Heffernan and Thomas E. Burman; Leiden: E.J. Brill, 2005), pp. 95-122.

47. I am grateful to Mark O'Brien for this very helpful suggestion.

Scene 11: Reading/reciting/singing the text within a public concert or dramatic performance

In each case the medium of the text (memory, voice, papyrus, paper, digital code) is underscored by complex relationships between text, body, mouth, ear, eye, breath, memory, papyrus, tree, ink, fossils, light, language, persons (ancient or contemporary) who laboured to produce the text and the earth that sustained them.[48] Each medium both precedes and intersects with the social, cultural and symbolic worlds and worldviews that influenced the formation of the text, that the text itself constructs, and from which hearers and readers respond to the text. With this interrelationship between material medium and text in mind, in Chapter 2 I will define a *text* as an interrelationship between the written, proclaimed or remembered text, which I call a *writing*, its readers/hearers/interpreters, and the medium/media in which the writing presents itself.

### *The Material Artefact as Agent*

To underscore the materiality of the text, I turn to a consideration of the way in which Bibles can have agency as material artefacts. Rita Nakashima Brock describes a scene from Amy Tan's *The Joy Luck Club* in which, following the loss of her son, a mother whose will and faith fail to bring him back 'places the church's gift Bible on the floor, under the leg of a kitchen table, to steady it', yet is careful to keep it dusted.[49] Considering South African biblical hermeneutics, Gerald West relates an early encounter between European missionaries and the Tlhaping people; he writes: 'Biblical interpretation among this southern African people begins with the Bible as *bola*, an object of power [like divining dice], whether for good or ill, with the Tlhaping uncertain as to which of these will predominate'.[50] In both cases the Bible is a thing—paper, binding, ink—a book with both physical and cultural weight which occasions a kind of respect, and is both more and less than the texts that are the subject of biblical studies.[51]

48. See, for example, Thomas Pattie's description of the lives and labours of animals and humans required for the production of Codex Sinaiticus ('The Creation of the Great Codices', in *The Bible as Book: The Manuscript Tradition* [ed. John L. Sharpe III and Kimberly Van Kampen; London: British Library, 1998], pp. 61-72 [64-65]).

49. Rita Nakashima Brock, 'Dusting the Bible on the Floor: A Hermeneutics of Wisdom', in *Searching the Scriptures: A Feminist Introduction* (ed. Elisabeth Schüssler Fiorenza; North Blackburn, Victoria: Collins Dove, 1993), pp. 64-75 (64).

50. Gerald West, 'Redirecting the Direction of Travel: Discerning Signs of a Neo-Indigenous Southern African Biblical Hermeneutics', in *Redirected Travel: Alternative Journeys and Places in Biblical Studies* (ed. Roland Boer and Edgar W. Conrad, JSOTSup, 382; London: T. & T. Clark International, 2003), pp. 201-25 (208-209).

51. See also Knappett, 'The Neglected Networks', on approaching the text as a thing.

For George Aichele the materiality of the text calls into question any assumptions about its theological or spiritual transparency. Aichele recalls that 'The text is the specific, material product of a concrete act of production.'[52] He contrasts an idealist tradition with a materialist one. In the former, 'the materiality of language is only the temporary and ultimately transparent medium for the spirituality of meaning'.[53] For the latter, 'marks on the surface of the page are not merely the vehicle or channel of a fundamentally independent meaning'; rather, being 'opaque' and 'inert', they are 'resistant to the desire for meaning'.[54] This material resistance suggests a 'concrete theology' open to the tension between 'the desire for, and the resistance to, meaning'.[55] The materiality of language is inseparable from the concrete products in which it presents itself.[56]

Focusing on the printed book, Jean-Luc Nancy understands the book as a thing that materially delivers the idea, the ideality of which is inseparable from its materiality.[57] The idea is not only the idea to which the content of the book addresses itself, and for which the book is a dialogue around the idea, but also the idea of thinking for which books, and their production and reproduction, provide both form and promise. In this respect the book has, and is, a character—being the character of the idea—and this character is its 'voice'.[58] As such, no less than oral performance, a book *speaks* to its readers; it is an *address* to a reader.[59] The medium that is the book, and its relation to booksellers, produces a particular relation to the commerce or trade in thinking that is embedded in, and in excess of, capitalist consumption of books. As will be further noted in Chapter 2, the Bible, especially through the Christian dissemination of the codex, stands in a particular relation to the trade in ideas that has been carried by both the idea and the matter of the book. One key aspect of the Bible's influence in the history of the book is the idea of canon.

52. George Aichele, 'Reading beyond Meaning', *Postmodern Culture* 3.3 (1993), http://muse.jhu.edu/.

53. Aichele, 'Reading beyond Meaning'.

54. Aichele, 'Reading beyond Meaning'.

55. Aichele, 'Reading beyond Meaning'.

56. See also George Aichele, *Sign, Text, Scripture: Semiotics and the Bible* (Sheffield: Sheffield Academic Press, 1997); and George Aichele, 'Electronic Culture and the Future of the Canon of Scripture or: The Hyperreal Bible', in *Redirected Travel: Alternative Journeys and Places in Biblical Studies* (ed. Roland Boer and Edgar W. Conrad; JSOTSup, 382; London: T. & T. Clark International, 2003), pp. 8-23.

57. Jean-Luc Nancy, *On the Commerce of Thinking: Of Books and Bookstores* (trans. David Wills; New York: Fordham University Press, 2009), esp. pp. 9-10.

58. Nancy, *Commerce of Thinking*, p. 9.

59. Nancy, *Commerce of Thinking*, p. 10.

The materials and technologies of textual production have enabled the development of the meta-textual authority of biblical canons that can limit or fix meaning.[60] George Aichele argues:

> The Christian canon of the scriptures is a semiotic mechanism designed to control the meaning of its component texts. It is a list of books that is understood by Christian churches to be an unchanging and complete repository of truths and values, an intertextual network that provides a reading context through which its component texts can be understood correctly—that is, in terms of Christian 'right belief'. The canon is a product of both technological innovation and ideological demand. The technology includes the mechanisms of writing and publication. The ideology arises from the desire for a self-explanatory, authoritative text, the 'word of God'.[61]

For Aichele, shifts in the primary medium of texts—from oral performance to handwritten texts, from papyrus scrolls to codices, to the introduction of print, mass-produced books, and more recently electronic versions—accompany and prompt:

1. anxieties about the authority of the word/text; for example, early writings in the primarily oral cultures of ancient Israel and Greece were received with suspicion;[62]
2. alterations in reading practice; for example, the introduction of print culture was accompanied by more widespread silent, personal reading;[63]
3. different social needs; for example, the exile prompted the need for written texts;[64]
4. changed relationships to canon; for example, the introduction of the codex shaped the Christian canon.[65]

The changing media of scriptural production and reproduction arose both through new technologies and in relation to social necessities.

60. See, for example, Regina Schwartz's analysis of Christian typological readings (*The Curse of Cain: The Violent Legacy of Monotheism* [Chicago: University of Chicago Press, 1997], esp. p. 174) and Jill Robbins's analysis of figurative interpretation (*Prodigal Son/Elder Brother: Interpretation and Alterity in Augustine, Petrarch, Kafka, Levinas* [Chicago: University of Chicago Press, 1991], esp. pp. 2-9).

61. Aichele, 'Electronic Culture', p. 8.

62. Aichele, 'Electronic Culture', p. 9.

63. Aichele, 'Electronic Culture', p. 12.

64. Aichele, 'Electronic Culture', p. 9.

65. Aichele, 'Electronic Culture', pp. 10-11; Larry W. Hurtado, *The Earliest Christian Artifacts: Manuscripts and Christian Origins* (Grand Rapids: Eerdmans, 2006), pp. 69-83.

In the interplay between circumstance and medium, the material artefact situated in a network of more-than-human social relations has agency, for example, in relation to reading and notions of canon. This agency is not singular but exists within the networks, including structures of power, in which the material artefact, as Earth stuff and product of human technologies and ideologies, is situated. Of the codex, Aichele comments:

> The codex itself signifies something about the texts collected in it; it is an intertext produced by the canon, permitting the various texts to comment on each other and thus to control each other.... The codex assembles a complete intertextual network in a format than can be easily used as such—that is, as a text that explains itself. [66]

The advent of electronic reproductions of Scripture produces different intertextual possibilities of readerly performance, where meaning is far less fixed by the medium and intertextuality is fluid.[67] For Aichele, while the rise of individual interpretation especially in Protestant traditions accompanying print culture unsettled the power of a fixed canon, electronic culture unsettles the very fixity of canons themselves. Moreover, this unsettling occurs as 'The hermeneutic tension between signified and signifier collapses and the medium as such disappears, because everything has become medium'.[68] Nancy considers the advent of electronic culture as unsettling not so much the fixity of canons but the matter and the ideas of medium, reader and reading themselves in ways that remain undecidable yet nevertheless have their own relations to the materiality of light, music, exchange, and the pace of writing–reading performance.[69]

The idea of the book, and the commerce of thinking it purveys, resonates with the idea of canon as that which binds together certain sets of mutually interpreting texts. Further, despite the different, and arguably more democratic, capacities to produce electronic texts and linkages, the materiality of the book as an object that is simultaneously an idea underwrites the electronic encoding of texts, not only in the way we refer to 'pages' on screen but also in the way we relate to ideas, including the idea of canon. Because the religious hierarchies that ensure canons and are supported by canonical structures will not easily let go of their power, I am less sanguine than Aichele that biblical canons will disappear into the electronic ether. The question of canonicity is of interest for my project, however, not so much

66. Aichele, 'Electronic Culture', p. 10.

67. Aichele, 'Electronic Culture', p. 17.

68. Aichele, 'Electronic Culture', p. 17.

69. Nancy, *Commerce of Thinking*, pp. 49-57. Note, for example, the parallels and contrasts between the scrolling up and down on a computer screen, the virtual turning of pages of Codex Sinaiticus, the virtual unrolling of the Great Isaiah Scroll, and the Lukan Jesus' unrolling the scroll (Lk. 4.17).

because of its relation to power, although this is important, but because it offers one example of the agency of the material artefact within those networks of power. My suspicion is that attention to the materiality underlying the text, even where the text is the medium, may also unsettle the canonical frameworks it supports, particularly where attention to the materiality that supports the biblical text unsettles the notion of a singular text. Aichele's observation that when text and medium are inseparable the medium disappears needs to be reread in this context.

The assumption of scribes and scholars that the text can be reproduced seemingly infinitely as the same text, its finitude subject only to the availability of material resources and human labour or machine time to reproduce it, is flawed. As I will argued in Chapter 2, the text is not wholly separable from the particular medium in which it presents itself. Each instance of the text arrives with a specific and complex relation of dependence on, and embeddedness in, a more-than-human sociality.[70] When the more-than-human-other is allowed ingress in reading, a focus on materiality and the way in which interpreters shape and are shaped by their material contexts, including the materiality of the text, can unsettle both their own subjectivities and the wider social and ideological frameworks in which they are embedded.

For Aichele, one aspect affecting the agency of the text within these social and ideological networks is its perceived 'aura'.[71] The aura of the text is not simply a function of its place in the canon, but accrues from its ritual usage and importance and from the idea of an original true text that lends authority to its copies. This supposed original text in its original language, however, loses something of its aura in being copied. Moreover, for all practical purposes, there is no longer an original text of Lk. 4.16-20, for example. Versions exist from early in the Common Era, but since we do not know the precise manner in which a Gospel writer produced a text we cannot say for certain if there was ever only one original or rather several texts that came to be nearly one, with mostly minor variants. Nevertheless, the notion of an original text implies a necessary relation between the text and its medium, because an original text can only exist in a singular material instance.

The singularity of the supposed original text, as material artefact, lends the copies their aura, an aura borrowed from the imagined, but undiscovered or unrecoverable, original. The notion of discovery, moreover, presumes the uniqueness of the material artefact. The suspicion that an original, if such

70. Both similarities and differences exist between Marxist and ecological approaches to the agency of the material artefact, the authority of the text and wider relations of power.

71. Aichele, 'Electronic Culture', p. 13.

ever existed, is no longer recoverable also testifies to a text's materiality, because it recognizes that its matter is subject to decomposition over time. The aura of the text then is linked both to the material artefact and to its dynamic ritual and social situation. In contemporary Judaism, Torah scrolls made from parchment under strict rules of Kosher preparation continue to be reverenced in a way that invests them with, and from a certain perspective recognizes in them, a sacred character or aura. A project such as the St John's Bible, to produce a fully hand-written and illuminated copy of the NRSV, returns a focus to the material medium of the biblical text and its sacred character or aura.[72]

## *The Text as Icon*

As Dorothy Lee indicates, this sacred character of biblical texts is a feature of devotion to icons.[73] Following Lee's use of the icon as a metaphor for the Bible, I focus briefly on two aspects:

1. the relationship between the icon and the matter from which it is formed; and
2. the effect of the icon on the subjectivity of the viewer.[74]

John Chryssavgis writes that in the icon 'there is no sharp line of demarcation between "material" and "spiritual". The icon constitutes the epiphany of God in the world and the existence of the world in the presence of God.'[75] For the practice of iconography (icon writing) and the theology of the icon, three important aspects of materiality arise: the icon as matter; the materiality of the human person portrayed, in whom God is incarnate;[76] the materiality of the human viewer/reader.[77]

In icon making, the deeper undercolours of flesh, garments, hair, and background are painted first. Then, layers of light and shadow are added.

72. Susan Sink, *The Saint John's Bible: An Introduction* (Collegeville, MN: Liturgical Press, 2007).

73. Dorothy A. Lee, 'Touching the Sacred Text: The Bible as Icon in Feminist Reading', *Pacifica* 11 (1998), pp. 249-64.

74. Lee, 'Touching the Sacred Text', p. 251.

75. John Chryssavgis, 'The World of the Icon and Creation: An Orthodox Perspective on Ecology and Pneumatology', in *Christianity and Ecology: Seeking the Well-Being of Earth and Humans* (ed. Dieter T. Hessel and Rosemary Radford Ruether; Religions of the World and Ecology; Cambridge, MA: Harvard University Press, 2000), pp. 83-96 (84).

76. Nicolas Prevelakis, 'Iconography: Its Historical, Theological and Philosophical Background', *Ekistics* 70.418/419 (2003), pp. 47-51 (50).

77. James R. Payton, Jr, 'John of Damascus on Human Cognition: An Element in his Apologetic for Icons', *CH* 65 (1996), pp. 173-83.

Finally, highlights and gold leaf are applied. Vladislav Andrejev explains, 'The translucent layers of paint produce final colors that are at once ethereal and strong, representing the movement of the soul toward beauty and harmony'.[78] Paints are mixed from natural pigments: ochres and semi-precious metals. The light in the icon emerges from the application of these material elements, these 'bits' of Earth. A quality of matter (rather than a reflected light)—a soft light emerging from the earthen iconic faces[79]—engages the viewer in a dynamic interplay between the prototype (the one represented in the icon), the particular icon itself, and the person revering it.[80] Moreover, in the production of an icon the 'orderly sequence of stages' invites the iconographer beyond her- or himself into relationship with the prototype toward which the materiality of the icon is oriented.[81]

Like an icon, the biblical text is also not a creation *ex nihilo* but a materially grounded thing. At least since the time of Charlemagne and his scribe Godescale in the eighth century CE, the Bible as a sacred 'physical presence' has been understood as an icon.[82] Not only was the physical presence of the Bible an icon, but the words themselves were a 'verbal icon'.[83] These aspects of the Bible as sacred material thing and letter 'iconizing' the word bring together the traditions of the books of nature and Scripture noted above.[84] Moreover, the materiality of the Bible (or Bibles) suggests that biblical interpretation—subtended by matter, where matter is taken in the widest sense as all that makes up the organic and inorganic physicality of Earth and cosmos—is relational and incarnational.[85]

As Chryssavgis explains concerning the icon, this quality of incarnational relationship is 'transfigurative' rather than 'figurative' or 'nonfigurative'; and the biblical paradigm for iconography is the story of the transfigu-

78. Vladislav Andrejev, 'Art and Religion: Creativity and the Meaning of "Image" from the Perspective of the Orthodox Icon', *TTod* 61 (2004), pp. 53-66 (65).

79. Andrejev, 'Art and Religion', p. 65.

80. Anna Kartsonis, 'The Responding Icon', in *Heaven on Earth: Art and the Church in Byzantium* (ed. Linda Safran; University Park: Pennsylvania State University Press, 1998), pp. 58-80 (60).

81. Andrejev, 'Art and Religion', p. 59.

82. Herbert L. Kessler, 'The Book as Icon', in *In the Beginning: Bibles before the Year 1000* (ed. Michelle Brown; Washington, DC: Freer Gallery of Art and Arthur M. Sackler Gallery Smithsonian Institution, 2006), pp. 77-103 (77-82).

83. Jaroslav Pelikan, *Imago Dei: The Byzantine Apologia for Icons* (A.W. Mellon Lectures in the Fine Arts 1987; Princeton, NJ: Princeton University Press, 1990), esp. pp. 180-82.

84. Pelikan, *Imago Dei*, p. 181.

85. Anne Elvey, 'Women, Authority and the Bible: Ecological Feminist Considerations', *Interface* (forthcoming).

ration (Mt. 17.1-9; Mk 9.2-10; Lk. 9.28-36).[86] For Andrew Louth, drawing on St Gregory the Theologian and Maximus the Confessor, the transfiguration points to the theophany of the word made flesh reflected in the words of Scripture and the created order.[87] This interplay between Scripture and a more-than-human Earth community can occasion in the viewer/reader a shift of worldview.[88] Each Synoptic transfiguration account portrays the disciples unsettled by the encounter in which Jesus is revealed as the icon of God dwelling in the materiality of the cosmos.[89] With Jesus' passion and death in view (esp. Lk. 9.31), the accounts express a divine image restored in a humanity embedded in a more-than-human Earth community.[90] Although the disciples do not immediately experience in the narrative context a lasting shift of worldview there and then on the mountain, the accounts invoke the possibility of such a shift.

For Prevelakis, an icon occasions this shift not by way of allegory or mimesis but by an apophasis.[91] While an appeal to unknowing can be employed to maintain power (as can a construction of the Bible as icon),[92] the invitation to respond to the icon, as pointing to more than it can contain, opens to an ethics of a material transcendence that affirms the alterity of a more-than-human materiality that is the 'stuff' of the icon.

This more-than-human materiality addresses humans in particular ways. James Payton argues that, during the Iconoclastic Controversy of 717–787 CE, John of Damascus appealed in his apology for icons to the materiality of human cognition as sensory.[93] The materiality of the icon speaks to the materiality of human beings as *imago Dei*.[94] Payton writes, 'an icon serves as a reminder of the veracity of the Incarnation.... Seen by a human being, an icon is united to the person's intellect.... An icon ... meets the needs of

86. Chryssavgis, 'World of the Icon and Creation', p. 87.

87. Andrew Louth, 'The Theology of the Word Made Flesh', in *The Bible as Book: The Manuscript Tradition* (ed. John L. Sharpe and Kimberly Van Kampen; London: British Library, 1998), pp. 223-38 (226).

88. Chryssavgis, 'World of the Icon and Creation', pp. 83-84.

89. John Gatta, 'The Transfiguration of Christ and Cosmos: A Focal Point of Literary Imagination', *Sewanee Theological Review* 49 (2006), pp. 484-506 (490, 498).

90. Gatta, 'Transfiguration of Christ and Cosmos', pp. 490, 498.

91. Prevelakis, 'Iconography', esp. p. 50.

92. Cf. Karel van der Toorn, 'The Iconic Book: Analogies between the Babylonian Cult of Images and the Veneration of the Torah', in *The Image and the Book: Iconic Cults, Aniconism, and the Rise of Book Religion in Israel and the Ancient near East* (ed. Karel van der Toorn; Leuven: Peeters, 1997), pp. 229-48 (239-48, esp. p. 248).

93. Payton, 'John of Damascus', esp. p. 179.

94. Payton, 'John of Damascus', esp. p. 178.

human beings ... who inescapably find their thought processes bound up with their materiality.'[95] Human subjectivity is oriented toward matter.

In the interplay between the materiality of the icon and the materiality of the human being, the capacity of the icon to shift its viewer's perspective has its parallel in the capacity of the Bible to unsettle the reader's subjectivity.[96] For Julia Kristeva, in reading the Bible one is drawn toward an engagement with an otherness both inscribed in and exceeding not only the text but also the patriarchal imaginaries associated with it, and with certain influential traditions of biblical reception and interpretation.[97] This engagement challenges the reader to confront her or his losses,[98] so that the unsettling of a worldview is not a momentary discomfort but entails instead the possibility for transformation that like the biblical transfiguration accounts does not turn away from the death-dealing that threatens to close off possibility.

### *Aim and Outline of This Book*

This book aims to evoke a possibility for life-affirming transformation that opens to an ecological ethics through consent to the material embeddedness of biblical interpretation. Such interpretation occurs in a more-than-human community of agency and takes account of the Bible as material artefact. The process is somewhat eclectic. I draw selectively on three main sources for this evocation: critical theorists, predominantly Julia Kristeva on intertextuality, Jean-Luc Nancy on touch and listening, Jean-Louis Chrétien on call and response, and Jean-Luc Marion on the saturated phenomenon; selected artworks and poems that present the Bible as a material object; and the Gospel of Luke. There is an aspect of contingency to this selectiveness: the contingency of the material artefacts to which one has access; the contingency of the ideas that seem to speak to one another in a particular here and now; and the contingency of contact with one biblical writing (in this case, the Gospel of Luke) rather than another.[99] Luke engages me because of the self-conscious address to a reader, Theophilus, expressed in the writerly voice of the author/narrator who attempts to bring theological order to a narrative (1.1-4) that will always be in excess of any harmonizing theology.

95. Payton, 'John of Damascus', p. 82.

96. Julia Kristeva, 'Reading the Bible', in *New Maladies of the Soul* (trans. Ross Guberman; European Perspectives; New York: Columbia University Press, 1995), pp. 115-26.

97. Kristeva, 'Reading the Bible', pp. 115-26.

98. Kristeva, 'Reading the Bible', esp. p. 119.

99. Loveday C.A. Alexander, 'What If Luke Had Never Met Theophilus?', *BibInt* 8 (2000), pp. 161-70, writes of contingency in relation to the writing of Luke–Acts itself. Her thoughts on this ancient contingency helped me clarify my thinking on the contingencies of my own project.

Such excess lends to readings of Luke that engage with contextual hermeneutics—such as feminist, liberationist, ecological, postcolonial and my eco-materialist approach—both a critical ambivalence and a transformative potential.

Chapter 2 describes and performs a material intertextuality, derived from Kristeva's concept of intertextuality. I argue that in the context of the history of Bible production, it is insufficient to describe the text as completely separate from the material artefact by which it presents itself to be read. Chapter 3 considers the five senses as modes of engagement with the materiality of the text. Focusing on the materiality of the scroll referred to in Lk. 4.17-20 and taking Jean-Luc Marion's notion of the saturated phenomenon in the direction of a saturated communion, the chapter proposes a mode of reading that consents to the material embeddedness of biblical interpretation as a saturated communion. I suggest that the senses offer a focus for a materially intertextual mode of reading. This reading mode is less a scholarly reading of biblical texts in a traditional sense than a conversation between contemporary readings of the senses, artistic and literary representations of the biblical text as a material object, and appeals to the senses in biblical writings, with a focus on the Gospel of Luke. The conversation is partial, selective, and performative, repeatedly acting out a return to where the Gospel writing shows traces of its Earthy embeddedness as a material artefact.

The succeeding five chapters each focus on one of the five senses. Chapter 4 enacts a conversation between critical theories of touch; the touch of the Bible as a material artefact in the contact of colonization in Australia; a reading of touch as touching (on) death in the Gospel of Luke; and the death inscribed in the matter that supports a writing. Chapter 5 considers smell as an absence in Luke that parallels the absence of the material artefact from our readings. With an ear to the shouting stones of Luke 19, Chapter 6 moves toward understanding the materiality of the voice as a further aspect of the materiality of a text that, in being read, is *sounded* in the body. Focusing on sight, Chapter 7 describes the text as a visible voice and appeals to the witness in which dust participates in Luke 10 to suggest a community of more-than-human agency. In such a community, the visible voice of the material artefact can be understood as a verbal icon. When the readers/hearers stand under the text, they first stand under the matter that is given to the writing. Chapter 8 considers taste in relation to eating in Luke and describes the hospitality and sacrifice of the material artefact as being in the mode of the 'being for the other' of Eucharist, understood as a sacrament of the Earth community. Metaphorical links between eating and speaking, food and scroll, resonate with an understanding of Earth as eucharistic. I ask what kind of hospitality matter gives to the word. What are the ethical implications for writers and readers concerning this givenness?

This mode of reading resonates with what Edith Humphrey calls 'a hermeneutics of welcome', but where Humphrey intends hospitality to the writings that form the Second Testament, I intend hospitality toward the materiality of the text.[100] Readers who take ecological, feminist and post-colonial approaches to biblical interpretation often highlight the damaging effects of biblical writings. They note the places where a writing, such as the Gospel of Luke, works in both its own terms and the later traditions of interpretation to silence women and to homogenize Earth, or where at best it offers a 'double message' for women and Earth.[101] With the damaging effects of writings in mind, such interpreters frequently employ a hermeneutics of suspicion and a mode of reading against the grain of the writing to formulate both deconstructive and reconstructive readings of writings such as the Gospel of Luke. In focusing on the materiality of the text as an issue of concern for ecological hermeneutics, my writing does not offer an ecological reading of the Gospel of Luke as such. Rather, my writing sits *opposite* (or across the table from) the writing that is the Gospel of Luke, mediated in a variety of material artefacts, *before* several images that represent the text as material artefact and *beside* a number of other writings about the senses. With the five senses as starting points, I enact a conversation between selected writings and images in order to locate metaphors—particularly the verbal icon and the visible voice—for describing the trace of the material artefact in writing.

A key theme of the Gospel of Luke is the hospitality of God. My engagement with Luke around the senses suggests that while matter gives itself in a kenotic hospitality to a writing, the writing itself does not unambiguously receive or return hospitality to the more-than-human (including human, particularly Jewish) others that make it possible. Moreover, when Bibles arrive as material artefacts carried by European colonizers to Australia, their materiality matters. They become part of two stories in which hospitality and its

100. Edith M. Humphrey, *And I Turned to See the Voice: The Rhetoric of Vision in the New Testament* (Grand Rapids: Baker Academic, 2007), p. 29.

101. See, for example, Elizabeth V. Dowling, *Taking Away the Pound: Women, Theology and the Parable of the Pounds in the Gospel of Luke* (LNTS, 324; London: T. & T. Clark, 2007); Elvey, *Ecological Feminist Reading;* Brigitte Kahl, 'Reading Luke against Luke: Non-Uniformity of Text, Hermeneutics of Conspiracy and the "Scriptural Principle" in Luke 1', in *A Feminist Companion to Luke* (ed. Amy-Jill Levine with Marianne Blickenstaff; Feminist Companion to the New Testament and Early Christian Writings, 3; London: Sheffield Academic Press, 2002), pp. 70-88; Barbara E. Reid, *Choosing the Better Part? Women in the Gospel of Luke* (Collegeville, MN: Liturgical Press, 1996); Turid Karlsen Seim, *The Double Message: Patterns of Gender in Luke and Acts* (Nashville: Abingdon Press, 1994).

failure are always at issue, and where on one side the material artefact is an instrument of colonization, though not only this, and on the other side the material artefact may be assimilated to Aboriginal cultures in various ways specific to country. This postcolonial aspect of the Bible as material artefact is not the primary focus of my project, but it is an important instance of the way in which the material text carries meaning in excess of its writing.

By suggesting that the materiality of the text intervenes in the way biblical scholars think about the writings they interpret, I aim to enact connections, between materially mediated writings and images, which might later inform ecological approaches to biblical interpretation. I propose, therefore, to bring into reading a respect for the matter that supports a writing, the matter that a writing both is and is not. Thus, my project is in the mode of returning to the text its uncertain material ground. Reading as a saturated communion with this ground is not so much systematic as engaged, selective, attentive and evocative. I hope biblical scholars and ecological critics will accept the invitation to enter and continue this initial conversation. Among other things, the conversation may take us toward a consideration of the ethical implications of respect for the Earthy context of writing and so call into question our love affair with the book. As I will argue in the next chapter, the production of the book in general is influenced deeply by the long history of production and reproduction of Bibles.

# 2

## A Material Intertextuality

Preserved in the British Library, the fourth-century CE Codex Sinaiticus and the fifth-century CE Codex Alexandrinus recall both a colonial history of appropriation and custodianship of ancient artefacts and a long tradition of production and reproduction of Bibles.[1] Along with Codex Vaticanus and major papyri, these codices provide key witnesses for the authenticity and authority of particular textual variants in the Greek New Testament.[2] By their material difference from contemporary mass-produced Bibles, they also remind me of the materiality of the text.

Very early, Christian usage moved from papyrus scrolls to papyrus codices to the codex manufactured from parchment. Thomas Pattie writes,

> The production of a large fine book on parchment required several hundred animal skins. A gathering of eight folios became the norm as one animal skin produced one gathering of eight folios of an average sized book. ... There would be 32 gatherings of eight in a book of 256 average-sized folios, that is, 32 sheep. An average book has many flaws in the parchment when wounds in the skin have expanded when the skin was stretched. Even a fine manuscript like Vaticanus has many flaws of this nature, including a significant number in the text area, that force the scribe to write around the holes. Sinaiticus has many fewer flaws and most were repaired before the text was inscribed. Its pages are very large: even after trimming they measure 380x340mm, and before trimming perhaps 400x360mm. A sheet of two folios would then have measured 400x720mm, and one sheep, smaller than modern domestic sheep, might have produced enough parchment for only one sheet, taking into account the need to trim off the imper-

1. Scot McKendrick and Kathleen Doyle, *Bible Manuscripts: 1400 Years of Scribes and Scripture* (London: British Library, 2007), pp. 20-21.

2. For example, in Lk. 8.5 τοῦ οὐρανοῦ, 'of the skies', is omitted in some manuscripts but is deemed likely to be 'original' because of its appearance in many major codices, such as Sinaiticus, Alexandrinus and Vaticanus. See Bruce M Metzger, *A Textual Commentary on the Greek New Testament* (Stuttgart: United Bible Societies, corrected edn, 1975), p. 144.

> fections at the edges. In that case Sinaiticus, which seems originally to have had 730 folios, would require the perfect skins of 365 sheep or goats. The labour involved in the scraping, washing, stretching, and polishing would have been substantial.[3]

Pattie notes, moreover, that in 331 CE in the wake of the Bible burnings of previous persecutions 'the Emperor Constantine wrote to Eusebius, Bishop of Caesarea, ordering fifty parchment Bibles written by skilled calligraphers for his new foundations in Constantinople'.[4] Three important points emerge. First, the more-than-human others who give themselves, through plant, skin or labour, to the production and reproduction of the text influence the way in which the text presents itself to be read (for example, through an interruption of script by holes in the skin). Second, the lives and deaths of more-than-human others, including humans, are given *to* or *at the command of* members of the ruling elite. Third, these same lives and deaths are given *for* a sacred purpose. Human social relations and their more-than-human contexts form a complex understory for the production, transmission and preservation of Bibles.[5] If we were to read the written text of a Bible in the mode of scholarly criticism or prayer, how would our reading account for, or open itself to, the myriad more-than-human others whose lives, labours and deaths form an understory for the text? In this chapter, I draw on Julia Kristeva's *Revolution in Poetic Language* to suggest a framework for engaging ecocritically with the materiality of biblical texts.

### *Materiality and the Maternal Body*

Only partially at best, and somewhat impossibly, do notions of matter and materiality relate to the underlying 'stuff' to which the concept of the material given points but which language cannot contain. Recalling metaphysical concepts of substance and Marxist concepts of commodity, the terms matter and materiality are unstable.[6] The relation between language and the material given is uncertain. Since the pregnant body offers one paradigm for the material given, this uncertainty resonates with Kristeva's consideration of

3. Pattie, 'The Creation of the Great Codices', pp. 64-65, © The British Library Board. See also David Diringer, *The Book before Printing: Ancient, Medieval and Oriental* (New York: Dover Publications, 1982), esp. pp. 165-66, Hurtado, *Earliest Christian Artifacts*.

4. Pattie, 'The Creation of the Great Codices', p. 63.

5. See Michele Boisseau, 'Parchment', which appears as an epigraph to this book and Kate Rigby's analysis of the poem in Kate Rigby, 'Introduction', *Religion and Literature* 40.1 (2008), pp. 1-8 (7-8); also, Elvey, 'Earthing the Text?', p. 66.

6. See David Ayers, 'Materialism and the Book', *Poetics Today* 24 (2003), pp. 759-80.

the unsettling relationship between the maternal body, language and texts. To explore this relation, two further concepts—embeddedness and embodiment—require comment.

Embeddedness refers to human interdependence with and rootedness in the sociality of Earth.[7] An underlying interrelatedness of self and other unsettles the notion of individual separate selves. Embodiment is the mode of human embeddedness in this sociality. Initially for the child, the pregnant body mediates sociality, so that the sociality of the pregnant body is already more than human. From the interconnectedness of self and other in the pregnant body, child and mother are born separate from each other. The child enters a more-than-human world that for a time remains largely the world of the maternal body (and this term needs to be understood more broadly than the body of the birth mother as that which stands in relation to the infant as maternal).[8]

> Papyrus grows in the swamps of Egypt and in the sluggish waters of the Nile where they have overflowed and form stagnant pools.... Paper is manufactured from papyrus by splitting it with a needle into strips that are very thin but as long as possible. The quality of the papyrus is best at the centre of the plant and decreases progressively towards the outsides. The first quality used to be called 'hieratic' paper and in early times was devoted solely to books connected with religion, but to flatter the emperor, was given the name 'Augustus'; the second quality was called 'Livia' after his wife, and so the term hieratic was relegated to the third category.
>
> Pliny the Elder,
> *Nat.* 13.71, 74

### *Language and the Maternal Body*

Kristeva's consideration of the relationship between the semiotic and the symbolic is useful for my exploration of the relation between the maternal, language, texts and the material given. A number of key terms appear as central to this consideration: the speaking subject, the semiotic and the symbolic, the thetic phase and mimesis. For Kristeva the emergence of the speaking subject occurs as a separation from the maternal body.[9]

7. See, for example, Kevin Hart, 'Forgotten Sociality' [under the heading Personal Well-Being and Social Conscience], in *Discerning the Australian Social Conscience: From the Jesuit Lenten Series* (ed. Frank Brennan; Richmond, Victoria: Jesuit Publications, 1999), pp. 53-71.

8. Julia Kristeva, 'Stabat Mater', trans. Léon S. Roudiez, in *The Kristeva Reader* (ed. Toril Moi; Oxford: Basil Blackwell, 1986), pp. 160-86 (178). Elvey, *Ecological Feminist Reading*, p. 115.

9. Kristeva, *Revolution*, esp. pp. 43-51. Since Kristeva is writing in a Western psychoanalytic framework, the results of her work may not be directly applicable across all cultures.

First, through language the child separates from the mother so that even pre-grammatical language separates 'an object from the subject', self from other, where the mother is the paradigmatic other.[10] Second, the connection with the maternal body (and hence also the other more generally) remains a trace in, and space for, language.[11]

> Bible paper, as the name implies, was developed for lightweight, thin, strong, opaque sheets for such books as bibles, dictionaries, and encyclopaedias. Bible papers are pigmented (loaded) with such pigments as titanium dioxide and barium sulfate and contain long fibres and artificial bonding agents to maintain strength.
>
> 'Bible paper', *Encyclopaedia Britannica*

The semiotic and the symbolic describe 'two modalities' of the signifying process.[12] Language does not exist as an abstraction separate from its human users; rather the semiotic and symbolic functions of the signifying process represent two aspects of the subject her- or himself. The subject is constituted through language, initially through the dynamic of connection with, and separation from, the maternal body.[13] Within this broad framework, the semiotic describes the language of desire, *eros*, the body, and drives, associated in psychoanalytic terms with the pre-linguistic, infant stage.[14] The symbolic describes socially significant language that presupposes reason, logic, and the possibility of unified, singular communication.[15]

Kristeva uses the term *chora* to describe the semiotic modality. The semiotic *chora* is pre-symbolic. Here signification does not rely on the absence of an object.[16] The maternal body orders the *chora*, which is analogous to the rhythms of movement and voice.[17] Through the mother's management of her response to the child, the maternal body represents the regulation of

10. Kristeva, *Revolution*, p. 43.
11. Kristeva, *Revolution*, esp. pp. 57-71.
12. Kristeva, *Revolution*, p. 24.
13. It is beyond the scope of this book, but not irrelevant to ecocriticism, especially one informed by feminist ethics, that Kristeva's subject is cast as masculine. See Elizabeth Grosz, *Jacques Lacan: A Feminist Introduction* (St Leonards, New South Wales: Allen & Unwin, 1990), esp. p. 167.
14. Kristeva, *Revolution*, p. 27; E.A. Grosz, *Sexual Subversions: Three French Feminists* (Sydney: Allen & Unwin, 1989), pp. 42-44; Toril Moi, *Sexual/Textual Politics: Feminist Literary Theory* (London: Routledge, 1985), p. 161.
15. Kristeva, *Revolution*, p. 29; Marilyn Edelstein, 'Metaphor, Meta-Narrative, and Mater-Narrative in Kristeva's "Stabat Mater"', in *Body/Text in Julia Kristeva: Religion, Women, and Psychoanalysis* (ed. David Crownfield; Albany: State University of New York Press, 1992), pp. 27-52 (31).
16. Kristeva, *Revolution*, p. 26.
17. Kristeva, *Revolution*, pp. 26-27.

social relations for the child.[18] Maternal regulation precedes and informs 'the law of the father', and, for this reason, the semiotic both supports the symbolic order and is an essential element in it.[19]

At the threshold of the realms of the semiotic and the symbolic is the thetic phase, which entails a break that enables the process of signification.[20] This break (between subject and object; signifier and signified) occurs through two transitional moments in the relation between child and mother: (i) a moment of identification and difference, denoted as the 'imaginary mirror stage'; (ii) a moment of desire and its (non)fulfilment, denoted as the 'symbolic castration complex'.[21] In the thetic phase, the child recognizes both that the other is other and that the child's interactions with others are socially regulated. Through this recognition, the child experiences a lack that returns as 'the space of language, sociality and identity'.[22] Moreover, the lack 'implies that the child is fundamentally social: it needs the other for its survival'.[23]

As paradigm of that necessary to the child's survival, the maternal body can stand for the material givenness of (more-than-human) sociality. This appeal to the maternal is not an essentialist over-valuation of the mother.[24] Rather, always in a relation of tension with the symbolic order, the maternal body is an instance of the *subject in process* (or *on trial*), where the other is inter-implicated with the self.[25] Any ethics, ecological or otherwise—and I take ecocriticism to be an expression of an ecological ethics—needs to be articulated based on an interrelationship of self and other, which unsettles the self and the social even as it constitutes them. [26]

18. Kelly Oliver, *Reading Kristeva: Unraveling the Double-Bind* (Bloomington: Indiana University Press, 1993), p. 46; Michael Payne, *Reading Theory: An Introduction to Lacan, Derrida, and Kristeva* (Oxford: Basil Blackwell, 1993), p. 169.

19. Oliver, *Reading Kristeva*, pp. 22-23, 47.

20. Kristeva, *Revolution*, p. 43.

21. Kristeva, *Revolution*, pp. 43, 46-51; Grosz, *Sexual Subversions*, pp. 45-47.

22. Grosz, *Sexual Subversions*, p. 47.

23. Grosz, *Sexual Subversions*, p. 47, also p. 45. See also Kristeva, *Revolution*, p. 48.

24. See Oliver, *Reading Kristeva*, pp. 48-49.

25. Oliver, *Reading Kristeva*, pp. 49-50; Kristeva, 'Stabat Mater'; Dawne McCance, '*L'écriture limite*: Kristeva's Postmodern Feminist Ethics', *Hypatia* 11.2 (1996), pp. 141-60. Cf. Grosz, *Jacques Lacan*, pp. 160-67; Miglena Nikolchina, *Matricide in Language: Writing Theory in Kristeva and Woolf* (New York: Other Press, 2004), esp. p. 51.

26. David Fisher, 'Kristeva's Chora and the Subject of Postmodern Ethics', in *Body/Text in Julia Kristeva: Religion, Women, and Psychoanalysis* (ed. David Crownfield; Albany: State University of New York Press, 1992), pp. 91-106 (102-104); McCance, '*L'écriture limite*'.

Kristeva's work is pertinent, therefore, for a critical affirmation of human interrelationship in this sociality, precisely where her work announces the following two factors as central to the processes of signification. They are (i) the continuity and difference between self and other; (ii) the gap between desire and gratification (and an attendant unsettling of an imaginary of human agency as control of the other, particularly the other-than-human). While the focus on castration suggests a founding violence in signification, problematic from both feminist and ecological perspectives, Kristeva's analysis of signification describes a patriarchal social economy and its accompanying imaginary.[27] She offers one understanding of this imaginary's simultaneous resilience and instability.

This interplay of resilience and instability echoes across the boundary between the symbolic and the semiotic. By an invocation of language open to the semiotic and tending toward an imitation of its object, *mimesis* can transgress the thetic break from the *chora*. Mimesis is less a construction of, than a verisimilar approach to, the other.[28] While affirming that the unifying and structuring character of the symbolic is necessary for a text to be a signifying practice, Kristeva signals the transgression of the thetic through poetic language, especially when it departs from grammatical construction.[29] The language of biblical narration also has this transgressive capacity.[30]

## *Intertextuality*

> When a great crowd gathered and people from town after town came to him, he said in a parable: 'A sower went out to sow his seed; and as he sowed, some fell on the path and was trampled on, and the birds of the air ate it up. Some fell on the rock; and as it grew up, it withered for lack of moisture. Some fell among thorns, and the thorns grew with it and choked it. Some fell into good soil, and when it grew, it produced a hundredfold.' As he said this, he called out, 'Let anyone with ears to hear listen!'
>
> 'Now the parable is this: The seed is the word of God' (Lk. 8.4-8, 11 NRSV).

The thetic break from the *chora* necessary for signification is dynamic. A position occurs when previous positions are unsettled, by a semiotic trace

27. For a feminist critique, see Elizabeth Grosz, *Volatile Bodies: Toward a Corporeal Feminism* (St Leonards, NSW: Allen & Unwin, 1994), pp. 56-71. See also George Aichele and Bible and Culture Collective, *The Postmodern Bible* (New Haven: Yale University Press, 1995), pp. 211-12.

28. Kristeva, *Revolution*, p. 57.

29. Kristeva, *Revolution*, p. 57, Julia Kristeva, 'From One Identity to an Other', in *The Portable Kristeva* (ed. Kelly Oliver; New York: Columbia University Press, 2002), pp. 93-115 (101-104).

30. Kristeva, 'Reading the Bible', pp. 115-26.

in the articulation of those positions. For example, a new signifying system, such as a novel, appears as a passage from one or more signifying systems.[31] 'The term inter-textuality', writes Kristeva, 'denotes this transposition of one (or several) sign systems into another', demanding 'a new articulation of the thetic'.[32] Transposition (hence, intertextuality) characterizes any signifying practice.[33] Moreover, Kristeva's understanding of intertextuality reflects her engagement with Mikhail Bakhtin's understanding of the dialogic nature of writing.[34] As Graham Allen explains, 'All utterances are *dialogic*, their meaning and logic dependent upon what has previously been said and on how they will be received by others'.[35] Differing from the Hegelian dialectic, the dialogic nature of language includes the social, ideological, subject-centred and subject-addressed character of language.[36] Intertextuality concerns the way in which a text, embedded in multiple contexts, represents processes of signification that address the subject-in-process.

> The Bible is the best-selling and the most widely distributed book with 50 million copies sold annually and translations in over 2,200 languages and dialects.
>
> The World Bank Environment and Social Development Sector, East Asia and Pacific Region, 'Faiths and the Environment', p. 38.

Working with the textual multiplicity evoked in the concept of intertextuality, four typical usages emerge in biblical interpretation:

1. The least subtle usage, which Kristeva describes as 'banal', understands intertextuality as the 'study of sources', identifying explicit and implicit traces of other texts—both biblical and extra-biblical—within a particular text.[37]

31. Kristeva, *Revolution*, p. 59.
32. Kristeva, *Revolution*, pp. 59-60.
33. Kristeva, *Revolution*, p. 60.
34. Julia Kristeva, 'Word, Dialogue and Novel', trans. Alice Jardine, Thomas Gora and Léon S. Roudiez, in *The Kristeva Reader* (ed. Toril Moi; Oxford: Basil Blackwell, 1986), p. 37; Kristeva, *Revolution*, pp. 59-60; M. M. Bakhtin, *The Dialogic Imagination: Four Essays* (trans. Caryl Emerson and Michael Holquist; Austin: University of Texas Press, 1981).
35. Graham Allen, *Intertextuality* (London: Routledge, 2000), p. 19.
36. Allen, *Intertextuality*, p. 19. Edelstein, 'Metaphor, Meta-Narrative', p. 32.
37. Kristeva, *Revolution*, p. 60. See, for example, Robert L Brawley, *Text to Text Pours Forth Speech: Voices of Scripture in Luke–Acts* (Bloomington: Indiana University Press, 1995). See also Robbins's comments on the essays in volume 80 of *Semeia*: Vernon Robbins, 'Historical, Rhetorical, Literary, Linguistic, Cultural, and Artistic Intertextuality—A Response', *Semeia* 80 (1997), pp. 291-303.

2. A far more subtle usage focuses on the multi-vocality of the text, in particular tracing underlying socio-cultural and communal voices that inform the text.[38]
3. A further usage notices the function of the repressed in the text, and the way in which the forgotten returns as an otherness not wholly suppressed in the text or later interpretations.[39]
4. Sometimes, intertextuality represents a mode of reading performance between later texts—such as literary works, visual arts, film and multimedia—and biblical ones. The focus is less on the influence of the Bible on these works than on a mode of reading that intervenes deconstructively (and perhaps reconstructively) in the inter-influence between texts.[40]

While useful, the first mode remains largely in the frame of the symbolic. Reading Luke's parable of the sower, for example, I note several genres: a parable (Lk. 8.4-8), a brief conversation within the narrative (Lk. 8.9) opening into a saying (Lk. 8.10a), a quotation from Isaiah (Lk. 8.10b; cf. Isa. 6.9) and an allegorical interpretation (Lk. 8.11-15). These shifts suggest a variety of oral and written sources behind Lk. 8.4-15, including, as most biblical scholars maintain, the version found in the Gospel of Mark (4.1-20). A problem arises when one describes this mode of interpretation as intertextual, because it misses, and may be counter to, the focus of intertextuality on 'the anonymous codes, the ruptures and registers of language itself, as it speaks through the text'.[41]

The second mode indicates a wider view of the textual encoding of the sociality of self and other for which the maternal stands. One aspect of this encoding is the relationship between oral and written traditions. Orality is marked by memory and by forms of expression conducive to remembrance (for example, repetition); meanwhile, literacy may give rise to greater pos-

38. See, for example, Elaine M. Wainwright, 'Rachel Weeping for her Children: Intertextuality and the Biblical Testaments—A Feminist Approach', in *A Feminist Companion to Reading the Bible: Approaches, Methods and Strategies* (ed. Athalya Brenner and Carole Fontaine; Sheffield: Sheffield Academic Press, 1997), pp. 452-69, esp. 453-59; Elaine M. Wainwright, *Shall We Look for Another? A Feminist Rereading of the Matthean Jesus* (Maryknoll, NY: Orbis Books, 1998), esp. pp. 35-49. On polysemy, see Kristeva, *Revolution*, p. 60.

39. See, for example, Catherine Keller, *Face of the Deep: A Theology of Becoming* (London: Routledge, 2003), esp. p. 30.

40. See, for example, Ela Nutu, *Incarnate Word, Inscribed Flesh: John's Prologue and the Postmodern* (The Bible in the Modern World, 6; Sheffield: Sheffield Phoenix Press, 2007).

41. Daniel Boyarin, 'A Question of Theory or Experimentality?', *Semeia* 86 (1999), pp. 223-25 (225).

sibilities for abstract thought.[42] In a literate culture, the development of speech in the child occurs within a subculture of orality shaped by writing. Within those same cultures, preceding oral cultures inform written texts. For an ancient text, such as the Bible, traces of orality cannot be discounted; such traces represent points of connection with the myriad layers of the social underlying the text.[43]

For example, at least four ancient versions of the parable of the sower appear, one in each of the three canonical Synoptic Gospels (Mt. 13.1-23; Mk 4.1-20; Lk. 8.4-15), another in the apocryphal Gospel of Thomas. The last has a version of the parable only, without the accompanying interpretation. Although form criticism might suggest a single oral tradition behind the parable, as Werner Kelber notes, 'oral performance enacts multiple original speech acts, a situation that suggests a culture of speech quite different from that represented by the one, original form'.[44] The emphasis on hearing—in the soundscape of the parable, where rhythm and repetition work on the ear (esp. 8.4); the appeal to hearing at its close (8.8); and the allegory (8.12-15)—resonates with a culture of oral performance, where even reading to oneself entailed reading aloud.[45] Such attention becomes particularly pertinent when biblical texts, as written documents, are introduced in primarily oral cultures, such as Australian Aboriginal and Torres Strait Islander ones. As Anne Pattel-Gray explains, Aboriginal exegesis, focused on interpreting the land, encounters in biblical exegesis practices often problematic for both people and land.[46]

In different ways, the first and second approaches suggest an intertextual multiplicity—by way of sources, voices, genres, and reading contexts—to some extent recoverable in reading. The third approach takes a different turn. While the first and second do not rule out the uncanny, the third orients itself toward it. Just as Kristeva suggests that certain forms of writing, for example, the poetry of Mallarmé and the novels of Joyce, are particularly

42. Ong, *Orality and Literacy*, pp. 31-114.

43. See Alan Kirk, review of *Oral and Manuscript Culture in the Bible: Studies on the Media Texture of the New Testament—Explorative Hermeneutics* (Stellenbosch: Sun Press, 2007), by J.A. (Bobby) Loubser, in *RBL* (April 2008), http://www.bookreviews.org/pdf/5924_6288.pdf; Werner H. Kelber, 'Oral Tradition in Bible and New Testament Studies', *Oral Tradition* 18 (2003), pp. 40-42.

44. Kelber, 'Oral Tradition', p. 41. See also Craig L Blomberg, 'Interpreting the Parables of Jesus: Where Are We and Where Do We Go from Here?', *CBQ* 53 (1991), pp. 50-76. Cf. Mary Ann Beavis, 'Parable and Fable', *CBQ* 52 (1990), pp. 473-98.

45. William A. Graham, *Beyond the Written Word: Oral Aspects of Scripture in the History of Religion* (Cambridge: Cambridge University Press, 1987), pp. 6, 32.

46. Anne Pattel-Gray, 'Dreaming: An Aboriginal Interpretation of the Bible', in *Text and Experience: Towards a Cultural Exegesis of the Bible* (ed. Daniel L. Smith-Christopher; Sheffield: Sheffield Academic Press, 1995), pp. 247-59.

expressive of the semiotic, biblical scholars allude to a quality of strangeness in the genre of parable.[47] C.H. Dodd, for example, defines the parable as 'a metaphor or simile drawn from nature or common life arresting the hearer by its vividness or strangeness, leaving the mind in sufficient doubt about its precise application to tease it into active thought'.[48] For Stephen Curkpatrick, a parable's strangeness becomes apparent in its kerygmatic framing, that is, its framing within the theology of the narrative as a proclamation of good news (gospel). While he refers particularly to parables specific to Luke (for example, the Good Samaritan, 10.25-37, and the Lost Son, 15.11-32), he suggests that Gospel parables disclose 'otherness in the very familiar details', gesturing 'towards the elusive ambiguities of life'.[49] Since their 'ambivalence is resistant to theological interpretation', a 'dissonance' may occur 'between any particular parable and its frame'.[50]

While the Gospel frame for a parable may serve to fix meaning, framing can also open the parabolic world to the ingress of the other. For example, although an allegorical interpretation (8.11-15) focusing meaning in obedience to the word accompanies the parable of the sower (8.4-8), the same allegory stands in, and shapes, the theological imaginary of the Lukan Gospel. Here, the metonymy ear/heart/earth crosses with the maternal body to open a wider field of meaning within the symbolic of obedience.[51] Especially in the figure of Mary of Nazareth, the Lukan maternal is both paradigm for, and in tension with, an imaginary of obedience to the word, employing a metonymy—ear/heart/earth/womb—that is also metaphor (2.19, 51; 8.21; 11.27-28).[52]

The agricultural imagery of seeding and the governing metaphor for the interpretation of the parable—'the seed is the word of God' (8.11)—are part of a dense patriarchal imaginary that in an ancient Mediterranean context links plant seed with human seed; field with womb; earth with woman.[53] While alliteration may be neither common nor particularly significant in Greek poetry, the alliterative rhythm Luke brings to the opening of the parable unites sower (σπείρων), sowing (σπεῖραι) and seed (σπόρον) (8.5; cf.

47. Kristeva, *Revolution*, p. 82.

48. C.H. Dodd, *The Parables of the Kingdom* (New York: Charles Scribner's Sons, 1961), p. 4.

49. Stephen Curkpatrick, 'Parable Metonymy and Luke's Kerygmatic Framing', *JSNT* 25 (2003), pp. 289-307 (291).

50. Curkpatrick, 'Parable Metonymy', p. 291.

51. Elvey, *Ecological Feminist Reading*, pp. 154-63.

52. Cf. Edelstein, 'Metaphor, Meta-Narrative', p. 42.

53. See, for example, Page Du Bois, *Sowing the Body: Psychoanalysis and Ancient Representations of Women* (Chicago: University of Chicago Press, 1991).

Mk 4.4; Mt. 13.3).[54] Where both Mark and Matthew begin explicitly with a command, 'Listen', the opening repetition and rhythm of Luke's version engage its hearer. Rhythm interweaves with imagery to suggest the more-than-human labour expressed in seeder/seeding/seed. The tension between the contingencies incumbent on and the purpose of an agricultural practice of broadcast seeding resonate in the repetition of κατά in vv. 5 and 6 (κατεπατήθη, κατέφαγεν, κατέπεσεν)—a further divergence from Mark and Matthew, who each use the prefix only once in the parallel verses.[55] The prefix κατά refers to downward motion and destruction: κατεπατήθη comes from καταπατέω, to 'tread upon' or 'trample'; κατέφαγεν from κατεσθίω, to 'consume, devour, swallow'; κατέπεσεν from καταπίπτω, to 'fall (down)' (BAGD, 415-16, 422). The destructive resonances in the seed's downward motion reinforce the failure of full fruition. The prefix returns in 8.15, with κατέχουσιν, from κατέχω to 'hold back' or 'down', 'hinder' or 'suppress', but also 'hold fast', 'keep in ... memory', 'retain', signifying descent toward a holding that is fruitful (BAGD, 422-23).

The allegory moves from a focus on the word (8.11) to those who hear it (8.12-15). The word (ὁ λόγος) appears in nominative (8.11) then accusative (8.12, 13, 15) forms. A survey of Luke's Gospel suggests that in the nominative the 'word' has authority and power (4.32, 36), going about much (διέρχομαι, 5.15) and going out (ἐξέρχομαι, 7.17) in the *whole* of Judaea and *all* the surrounding area. In the accusative, the 'word' is the object of hearing (5.1; 8.12, 13, 15, 21; 10.39; 11.28), associated with keeping and doing (8.21; 11.28). The ear/heart/earth is locus of receptivity to the word/seed, whose seeder may be God or Jesus. By the time we get to John's Gospel, the word/seed is the word become flesh in Jesus (Jn 1.1-18). An interrelatedness between seed, word, earth and embodiment suggests the inter-implication of *an androcentric worldview*, in which the seed is *his* (8.5), and *a semiotics of receptivity* that is not simply a passive re-inscription of a woman/nature subordination to the agency of the male seed/word. Through its rhythms, alliteration and repetition, especially around ἀκούω (to hear), Lk. 8.4-15 invites the reader to hear differently, as if the body is a sonorous cavity for a Scripture that arrives as parable.[56] How might we hear differently?

54. On alliteration in Greek poetry, see Christos C. Tsagalis, 'Style and Construction, Sound and Rhythm: Thetis' Supplication to Zeus (Iliad 1.493-516)', *Arethusa* 34 (2001), pp. 1-29 (18).

55. I. Howard Marshall, *The Gospel of Luke: A Commentary on the Greek Text* (NIGTC; Grand Rapids: Eerdmans, 1978), p. 320.

56. Cf. Jean-Luc Nancy, *Listening* (trans. Charlotte Mandell; New York: Fordham University Press, 2007), p. 43. Cf. Julia Kristeva, '*"Nous Deux"* or a (Hi)Story of Intertextuality', *Romanic Review* 93 (2002), pp. 7-13 (7).

The fourth mode appears in this chapter in the interrupting descriptions of ancient papyrus manufacture and contemporary issues around the making of Bible paper. One way of reading these interruptions may be to understand the prevalence of Bibles over two millennia (and their seeming increase in this era of celebrated post-Christendom) as an exemplar of, or evidence for, the wide and imprecise dissemination of the seed/word, to whose ecological effects we need turn. In what ways can we understand the matter of the text to be at play in ecocritical biblical studies accountable for these effects?

### *The Matter of the Text and a Material Intertextuality*

When considering biblical texts, scholars usually refer to the interplay of author, text, and reader, aware of the different social and cultural contexts of all three. Taking shape in relation to specific readers/hearers, the text relies on, but is other than, the material artefact in which particular words, spaces, punctuation and structure present themselves to reading.[57] For a biblical passage, myriad such material artefacts, versions, translations and readings exist. The transferability of a passage to a variety of material media and reading contexts over many centuries gives priority to its words rather than the matter supporting them. Indeed, the priority of the word all but effaces the material medium that supports it.[58]

> The complexity of the paper issue means that firm conclusions are hard to draw. All paper manufacture causes harm to the environment and more often than not the determining factors in a paper mill's environmental performance are not the process, paper type or fibre source but the location, mill practice and mill operator.
>
> Friends of the Earth Briefing Sheet, 'The Environmental Consequences of Pulp and Paper Manufacture'

Although effectively invisible in most contemporary biblical studies, the material medium of a passage is not without effect. While a survey of ways different media affect readings is beyond the scope of this book, one may wonder what styles of interpretation seem most compatible, for example, with a parchment codex such as those produced at the order of Constantine as Christianity became the religion of the empire. In what ways were the lives and labours of animals and humans reflected in interpreters' effacement, or otherwise, of the agency of animal and slave characters in biblical narratives? How different were the readings of these characters when Bibles were produced with illuminations of plants and animals and human scribes twining through and around the pages? With the advent of printing and then,

57. I am grateful to Shane Mackinlay for our conversation concerning 'what is a text?'.

58. Kirk, review of *Oral and Manuscript Culture*; Aichele, 'Reading beyond Meaning'.

after the industrial revolution, the mass production of standardized Bibles in Hebrew, Greek and in translation, to what extent did the thin pages of modern Bibles influence interpretation of a scriptural world thinned of its material context?[59]

In the second and third century CE, the codex form of the book came to prominence in Christianity before it was popular in the ancient Mediterranean.[60] Larry Hurtado suggests that a Christian preference for the codex, in particular for reproducing its Scriptures, had a theological purpose reflected in the linking of texts—such as the letters attributed to Paul—in single volumes, rather than series of scrolls.[61] While not all texts so linked became canonical, the early linking of texts in codices moves in the direction of canon.[62] Further, the Christian preference for the codex in the second and third centuries CE and the adoption of Christianity by Constantine in the fourth are key moments in Western book production, leading to contemporary industrialized manufacture of Bibles and all that entails in terms of ecological cost.[63]

In the context of the history of Bible production, it is insufficient to describe the text as completely separate from the material artefact by which it presents itself to be read, because this then separates the text from its underlying material givenness.[64] Instead, a *text* can be defined as an interrelationship between the written, proclaimed, or remembered text, its readers/hearers/interpreters, and the medium/media in which the text presents itself. This text holds a complex relationship of dependence on, and embeddedness in, a more-than-human Earth community. Can we extend intertextuality to *a material intertextuality* in which the material givenness of the text irrupts in our reading?

For Kristeva, because the *chora* is ordered by the maternal body, the intertextual interruption of the semiotic returns us to our embodiment as living organisms, marked by biochemical processes of separation and con-

59. Adrian Johns, *The Nature of the Book: Print and Knowledge in the Making* (Chicago: University of Chicago Press, 1998), demonstrates the complexity of the move to the modern printed book and the accompanying concept of the fixity of the text.

60. Hurtado, *Earliest Christian Artifacts*, pp. 43-93. See also Harry Y. Gamble, 'Bible and Book', in *In the Beginning: Bibles before the Year 1000* (ed. Michelle Brown; Washington, DC: Freer Gallery of Art and Arthur M. Sackler Gallery Smithsonian Institution, 2006), pp. 15-35 (16).

61. Hurtado, *Earliest Christian Artifacts*, pp. 69-83.

62. Cf. Gamble, 'Bible and Book', pp. 31-35.

63. Note also the role of Christian monasteries; see Diringer, *Book before Printing*, pp. 275-82.

64. Cf. Jerome McGann's reflections on 'what is a text?', in Jerome J. McGann, *The Textual Condition* (Princeton, NJ: Princeton University Press, 1991), pp. 177-86. See also Aichele, *Sign, Text, Scripture*, pp. 12-13.

nection and biological limits and controls as well as social ones.[65] Biological operations have a relation of *différance* with respect to signifying operations and social codes; while subject to these, 'they infringe the code in the direction of allowing the subject to get pleasure from it, renew it, even endanger it'.[66] To describe the intertextual operation of the semiotic, Kristeva introduces two further terms: (i) the *genotext* is a process foundational to language, in broad terms the underlying and dynamic social, familial, biological, ecological environment of language, through which the semiotic functions; (ii) the *phenotext* is a structure of language, serving to communicate.[67] Because humans are embodied and embedded in a (more-than-human) sociality, the material given, through the genotext, is already intertextual with texts.

Nevertheless, no simple parallel exists connecting the relationship between child and mother that erupts in language and the relationship between texts and their more-than-human contexts. The intensity of the child/mother relation and the forgotten dramas of speculation and castration that produce the thetic phase are not replayed in the relationship between texts and the material given. However, that pregnant bodies, bodies and the social are each paradigmatic of the material given and that the maternal via the semiotic and the social via orality remain as traces in sign systems suggest that the rhythms of the semiotic *chora* may be evoked in modes of reading texts intertextually with their more-than-human contexts.[68]

Reading Mark's Gospel 'concretely' as a Derridean postcard, Stephen Moore offers an example:

> Writ(h)ing in pain on his cross, Jesus can at last be read: 'Truly this man was a son of God' (15:39). He is in the process of becoming book. Nailed, grafted onto the tree, Jesus' body is becoming one with the flesh of the wood. His flesh, torn and beaten to a pulp, joined by violence to the wood, is being transformed into processed wood-pulp, into paper, as the centurion looks on. As tree and budding book, Jesus is putting forth leaves, the leaves of a gospel book, whose opening sentence the centurion has just read: 'The beginning of the good news of Jesus Christ, son of God' (1:1).[69]

65. Julia Kristeva, 'The System and the Speaking Subject', in *The Kristeva Reader* (ed. Toril Moi; Oxford: Basil Blackwell, 1986), pp. 24-33 (29).

66. Kristeva, 'System', p. 30.

67. Kristeva, *Revolution*, pp. 87-88.

68. I am grateful to Julie Kelso for her emphasis on the mode of reading.

69. Stephen D. Moore, 'Illuminating the Gospels without the Benefit of Colour: A Plea for Concrete Criticism', *JAAR* 60 (1992), pp. 257-79 (262-63). Cf. Alan H. Cadwallader, *Beyond the Word of a Woman: Recovering the Bodies of the Syrophoenician Women* (Adelaide: AFT Press, 2008), p. xxxix. See also, on concrete theology, Aichele, *Sign, Text, Scripture*, p. 19.

In Moore's reading, the Bible as thing—both Earth product and object of consumption within global markets—speaks back to the text through the imaginative mode of his reading.

As books, Bibles have become objects of production and consumption. William Irwin writes, 'Intertextuality defies the capitalist paradigm by presenting the text not as a product ready for consumption, but as a growing, evolving, never-ending process.'[70] Rosalind Coward and John Ellis comment concerning Kristeva's work on 'the process of signification as the process of the subject itself', and suggest that especially her understanding of the way in which the intertextual ingress of the semiotic puts the subject on trial or in process can contribute to a material theory of language, in terms of Marx's dialectical materialism.[71] Nevertheless, Irwin objects, 'use of the term *intertextuality* ... implies that language and texts operate independently of human agency'.[72] But the interrelatedness of language and the maternal simultaneously affirms human agency and calls it into question as recoverable. While author and reader are agents, the text is more than their different agencies; the medium of the text, and its underlying relation to the material given, may also be agential.

Nevertheless, the physical medium of the text continues to occupy a relation of otherness to the meaning of the text, and the agency of the material givenness of a particular text cannot be articulated in a reading.[73] Yet reading remains an embodied process and bodies, embedded in a more-than-human sociality, are affected by reading.[74] Ecocriticism wagers that reading practices can shape relationships between readers and their more-than-human environments, so that reading both emerges from and prompts embodied practices of ethical engagement in an Earth sociality critically at risk.

Ecomimesis is one form of reading/writing practice that seems to parallel the mimesis Kristeva celebrates. Timothy Morton understands the genotext to be the 'environment' to the phenotext of ecomimesis.[75] This environment or ambience both separates and connects the material subject and

70. William Irwin, 'Against Intertextuality', *Philosophy and Literature* 28 (2004), pp. 227-42 (232).

71. Rosalind Coward and John Ellis, *Language and Materialism: Developments in Semiology and the Theory of the Subject* (London: Routledge & Kegan Paul, 1977), esp. p. 152.

72. Irwin, 'Against Intertextuality', p. 240.

73. Aichele, *Sign, Text, Scripture*, pp. 19-20.

74. Cf. Judith Butler, *Bodies That Matter: On the Discursive Limits of 'Sex'* (London: Routledge, 1993); David Bleich, 'The Materiality of Reading', *New Literary History* 37 (2006), pp. 607-29.

75. Timothy Morton, *Ecology without Nature: Rethinking Environmental Aesthetics* (Cambridge, MA: Harvard University Press, 2007), p. 77.

its representation in writing. While celebrating what cannot be said of the other, the ecomimetic performance of the uncertain relation 'between' the word and the thing can also serve to reinforce the distance it was meant to negotiate.[76] Instead, Morton argues, neither inside nor outside exists, nor nothingness between them. Despite this seeming apophasis, he eschews a negative poetics.[77] Morton suggests that, recognizing the extent of our responsibility for ecological destruction, ecocritics acknowledge and live with the distance between the word and the thing and engage with a 'dark ecology' of ecological lamentation.[78]

Accepting that the material givenness of a text is withdrawn from us as we read, we confront a loss that we can allow to resonate with the losses the text's production brings about. If the Bible is 'a text that thrusts its words into [our] losses', biblical readers attentive to the matter of the text can allow these losses to resonate in modes of 'reading Earth' intertextually with the text.[79] Norm Habel suggests that when we read biblical texts as matter we are reading Earth, an Earth Luke's parable of the sower characterizes (unfairly) as bad or good according to its receptivity to the seed.[80] As we move from seed to word to book (and screen), we engage with reading practices both colonizing of, and attentive to, an Earth community where parable becomes lament:

> *A seeder went out to seed the seed, and as he seeded some fell into papyrus swamp, some into goat herd, some into old-growth forest and some into recycling bin.... And the parable is this: the seed is the book, produced a billionfold.*

76. Morton, *Ecology without Nature*, pp. 29-78.

77. Morton, *Ecology without Nature*, esp. p. 46. Cf. Kate Rigby, 'Earth, World, Text: On the (Im)Possibility of Ecopoiesis', *New Literary History* 35 (2004), pp. 427-42.

78. Morton, *Ecology without Nature*, pp. 181-201. Cf. Rigby, 'Writing after Nature', where the focus is on response rather than mimesis.

79. Kristeva, 'Reading the Bible', p. 119. See also Wesley A. Kort, *'Take Read': Scripture, Textuality, and Cultural Practice* (University Park: Pennsylvania State University Press, 1996), esp. p. 117.

80. Norman C. Habel, review of *An Ecological Feminist Reading of the Gospel of Luke: A Gestational Paradigm* (Lewiston, NY: Edwin Mellen Press, 2005), by Anne Elvey, in *Australian Religion Studies Review* 21 (2008), p. 116. Also personal communication, e-mail 19 March 1999.

# 3

## 'I'm holding in my hand': A Material Reading

Michele Boisseau's poem 'Parchment', which forms an epigraph to this book, describes the speaker holding in her hand an illuminated prayer book (perhaps a Psalter) made from calf skin. In Lk. 4.16-20, which appears at the beginning of Chapter 1 in an English translation from the NRSV, the Lukan Jesus unrolls and rolls up a scroll of the prophet Isaiah made from animal skin or plant fibre. Between this textual touching of the material artefact and my readings of Luke in this book lie myriad reproductions of the text. These include those texts of the Gospel of Luke with which I am working: versions of the Greek New Testament published in 1983 as a modern book on cream Bible paper and an electronic reproduction on CD-ROM; a New Revised Standard Version on lighter weight fine white Bible paper and a reproduction on CD-ROM. I can look up electronic reproductions of the Great Isaiah Scroll and parts of Codex Sinaiticus on the Internet. I can look at pages of ancient codices and papyri under glass at the British Library and turn some of their pages virtually. The few verses I have cut and pasted in this book appear to me, as I scroll to them, as dark marks (which I have learned have the shape of words) against a background of white (light and shade) that is 'written' somewhere inside the machine as binary code. It will appear later to my reader as ink on paper, I hope from plants from sustainable plantations or already once or more recycled. But behind that reproduction are myriads of reproductions on animal skin, woven papyrus, and manufactured paper, myriads of scribes and printers labouring to produce and reproduce the text, which seems less and less a material thing, but nevertheless is. To varying degrees, the reader's engagement with the material artefact in which a writing presents itself is mediated by the senses. This chapter begins with explorations of the trace of the materiality of the text as it appears both in the scroll of Luke 4 and in Lukan references to 'the writings' or 'it is written'. Then I draw on Michel Serres and Jean-Luc Marion to suggest a mode of sensual reading open to the materiality of a text that can be seen, spoken, heard and touched.

*'He unrolled'... 'he rolled up'*

The programmatic proclamation of Lk. 4.18-19, bringing together two quotations from Isaiah (Isa. 58.6; 61.1-2), nestles between the actions of Jesus' unrolling and rolling up the scroll (4.17; 20a), themselves situated in a wider field of action:

> And he went into Nazareth (εἰς Ναζαρά)
>     where he was brought up (nourished) (οὗ ἦν τεθραμμένος)
> and, as was his custom on the Sabbath day, he entered the synagogue
>     and stood up (ἀνέστη) to read (ἀναγνῶναι).
> and the scroll (βιβλίον) of the prophet Isaiah was given (ἐπεδόθη) to him
>     and unrolling (ἀναπτύξας) the scroll (τὸ βιβλίον)
> he found the place (τὸν τόπον)
>     where it was written (οὗ ἦν γεγραμμένον):
> ...
>     and rolling up (πτύξας) the scroll (τὸ βιβλίον)
> giving it back (ἀποδούς) to the attendant
>     he sat down (ἐκάθισεν)
> and the eyes of all in the synagogue were fixed on him.

The field of action, in which Jesus handles the scroll, has several threads Luke weaves through the text and sets up as chains, parallels and contrasts. Nazareth provides the overall setting of place, the home town (4.22b, 23), which becomes both focus (4.23-24) and site of the conflict between Jesus and his hearers (4.28-29), a conflict which arguably he prompts (4.23). Within Nazareth, the synagogue (4.16) is the local site of the action and becomes linked to the response of the hometown people assembled there (4.20, 28). In this framework of place, Jesus acts and is acted on; with a series of aorist active indicative verbs, he comes to Nazareth, enters the synagogue and stands up (4.16).

Interrupting this action are descriptive clauses and phrases: Nazareth is the place *where he was brought up, nourished, or made to grow*; *according to his custom on the Sabbath day*, he enters the synagogue; he stands *to read*. Providing a contextual field for Jesus' action, these descriptions suggest familial, religious, and educational, as well as topographical, relations. When Jesus stands to read, the action shifts. The scroll is given to him. Then his action of unrolling the scroll is described in a participial phrase leading to the main action, designated by an aorist active indicative verb, followed by a further clause: he found *the place where it was written*. The construction οὗ ἦν γεγραμμένον echoes the construction οὗ ἦν τεθραμμένος. In this shared grammatical construction, Nazareth, *where he was nourished*, and the place, *where it was written*, mutually reflect each other.

Let me note a further element of the field of action in which Jesus handles the scroll. The passage the Lukan Jesus reads from Isaiah in 4.18-19 is framed by the phrases: (i) unrolling the scroll; rolling up the scroll; (ii) being given the scroll; giving back the scroll; and the decisive action: (iii) he stood up to read; he sat down. Neatly Luke holds the passage between these customary actions for a reader in a synagogue, such as those Luke knew. When Jesus sits, all in the synagogue initially respond with expectation: their eyes were gazing at him/fixed on him (4.20b). Their sense of sight is engaged. Jesus begins to speak to them, shifting the focus to the writing they have just heard him read: 'Today this writing/scripture (ἡ γραφὴ αὕτη) has been fulfilled in your ears' (4.21). We are returned to the place (ὁ τόπος) where it was written (οὗ ἦν γεγραμμένον) read in the place where Jesus was nourished (οὗ ἦν τεθραμμένος). At this juncture, where the question of what has been fulfilled rings in the ears of those gathered, the narrative continues to play with the interrelationship between Jesus, all in the synagogue, and the place that is his home town. The fulfilment is multi-dimensional: written in a place found in the scroll; recited in Jesus' voice and in their ears; a prompt for tension with the home place that is set up both in parallel and contrast to the written place. Does the scroll take over from the home town as where he is nourished? Is writing a form of nourishment? The appeals to Elijah and Elisha further the engagement with written and/or heard story and with the question of nourishment, and open up the question of who receives nourishment and healing (4.25-27). I will return to this point in my discussion of ἄφεσις below, but will first expand the context for understanding the agency of the scroll.

The most common word in the Hebrew Bible to be translated in the Septuagint by ἡ βίβλος or τὸ βιβλίον is ספר, occasionally מגלת־ספר (the latter at Jer. 36.2-32; Ezek. 2.9; 3.1-3; Zech. 5.1-2; Ps. 40.8; Ezra 6.2). Like ἡ βίβλος or τὸ βιβλίον, ספר refers to scrolls, letters, accounts or papers, but where the Greek words have a direct etymological connection with the underlying material medium, namely papyrus, the Hebrew ספר seems to be more likely connected with the content of the written text. According to Brown, Driver and Briggs, ספר probably comes from the Assyrian *šipru*, missive or message, and relates to notions of sending and commissioning, for example, prophets (BDB, 709). In a collection of cuneiform texts, however, a Babylonian letter from the king dated to between 710 and 704 BCE, concerning the language the Aramaic Sin-iddinam should use in writing to the king, refers to *šipru.* Here *šipru* relates to alphabetic script written on skin; it is unclear from the translation whether *šipru* refers simply to skin or to the inscribed skin.[1] In either case, this understanding of *šipru* leaves open the possibility that ספר, too, refers to the materiality of inscribed skin.

1. See 'Letters in Babylonian Script' from Jeannette C. Fincke, 'The Nineveh Tablet Collection', http://www.fincke.uni-hd.de/nineveh/babylonian/letter.htm.

The occasional addition of מגלת may refer more directly to the papyrus or parchment scroll.[2]

The biblical uses of ספר, however, do not focus on its animal or plant foundations. Rather, ספר appears as a thing that carries a memory to be recited (Exod. 17.14); as guarantor of the story, especially in the appeal to the annals of the kings variously of Israel, Judah or both (1 Kgs 14.19, 29; 15.7, 23, 31; 16.5, 14, 20, 27; 22.39, 45; 2 Kgs 1.18; 8.23; 10.34; 12.19; 13.8, 12; 14.6, 15, 18, 28; 15.5, 11, 15, 21, 26, 31, 36; 16.19; 20.20; 21.17, 25; 23.28; 24.5; 1 Chron. 9.1; 2 Chron. 16.11; 20.34; 24.27; 25.4, 26; 27.7; 28.26; 32.32; 34.21, 24, 31; 35.12, 27; 36.8); as record of the law and the covenant and importantly as witness (Deut. 28.58, 61; 30.10; 31.24; Josh. 1.8; 8.31, 34; 23.6; 24.26).[3] The king must have a copy of the Torah written for him *into a scroll* (Deut. 17.18-20). Moses, described as a scribe of the book of the Torah (Deut. 31.24), commands the Levites, 'Take this book (ספר) and place it beside the Ark of the Covenant of Yhwh your God; let it remain there as a witness against you' (Deut. 31.26). The materiality of the ספר makes possible both the aura it gains through its physical situation beside the Ark of the Covenant and its agency as witness against the people. In each case, this agency occurs within a network of relationships and action, which includes principally the Mosaic and prophetic scribes, the chroniclers, the people and their God.

In addition to the scroll of the law, the annals of kings, and the prophetic scrolls are other writings on stone, stone tablets, stones covered with plaster and wooden tablets (Job 19.24; Exod. 34.1; Deut. 27.2-3; Isa. 30.8; Hab. 2.2). In particular, Exodus 24 sets a narrative in which Moses writes the laws and the ordinances Yhwh told him in the Book of the Covenant, beside a narrative in which Yhwh gives Moses 'the tablets of stone with the law and commandment which [Yhwh has] written for their instruction' (Exod. 24.12; cf. Josh. 8.30-32). There may be both parallel and contrast here between the more fragile substance of the scroll and the more permanent substance of the stone tablet (generally hide wears more quickly than stone). But there may also be a conflation of traditions of receiving and writing the Torah that preserve both divine and human authorship. Notably, even the divine scribe requires a material medium.

ספר appears also as a material thing that can be burnt (Jer. 36.1-32) or found (2 Kgs 22.1-20; 2 Chron. 34.8-21), prompting further action. Its materiality allows for a self-referential quality in texts, when they refer to what is written and hence attested 'in this scroll' (בספר הזה Deut. 28.58; 29.19,

2. Ernst Würthwein, *The Text of the Old Testament: An Introduction to the Biblica Hebraica* (trans. Erroll F. Rhodes; Grand Rapids: Eerdmans, 2nd edn, 1995), p. 5.

3. See Ferdinand Deist, *The Material Culture of the Bible: An Introduction* (ed. Robert P. Carroll; Sheffield: Sheffield Academic Press, 2000), pp. 226-32.

26; Jer. 25.13). In having Jesus refer to 'this writing' (ἡ γραφὴ αὕτη, 4.21), Luke plays with textual self-reference; *this writing*, referring to a place in the scroll from which Jesus reads, also has a place in Luke's text when Luke reproduces texts from Isaiah there. This self-referential quality comes back in the later Johannine writings, at John 20.30 and 21.25, and notably in the book of Revelation with reference to τὸ βιβλίον τοῦτο (Rev. 22.7, 9, 10, 18, 19). A writing has a physical place in the material artefact that is scroll, codex or book. Although through reproductions of the text the material artefact changes, in the internal self-reference to 'this scroll' a trace remains of the materiality not only of the current artefact (in my hands or before my eyes) but of those from which this current artefact has been copied. So, the material place of a writing (even where this place is on-screen) is a nesting of many artefactual places where the writing has appeared and from which it has been copied.

As considered above, in Lk. 4.16-30 this place (τόπος) of a writing resonates with the geographic place in which the narrative is set. Moreover, the geography is also marked by a particular Lukan temporality: today (σήμερον) is for Luke the time of birth (2.11), fulfilment (4.21) and salvation (19.9), parallel to the season that marks the imminence and immanence of the βασιλεία of God. The interplay between the place of writing and the home place, as the place of hearing and responding, occurs in this heightened temporality, the season of divine visitation. The scroll as the material place of a writing, parallel to the geographic places of its setting, is not incidental to the central themes of Luke's Gospel. One difficulty for ecological readings of the Second Testament, however, centres on the question of relationship to place.

Where the First Testament, in the Hebrew Bible and Septuagint, carries strong traditions in which the relationship between the land, the people and God is critical, in the Second Testament relationship to the land seems to have receded. Under the influence of Roman imperialism, the early Jewish hearers of the Second Testament writings are displaced from, or dispossessed within, their homelands. The home town seems less part of a covenantal relationship between the people and their God. Moreover, while retaining its Jewish roots in the First Testament, early Christianity opens to a Gentile mission, which becomes in a different sense its cultural home territory. This interplay of Jewish and Gentile cultures already influencing Hellenistic Judaism informs Luke's Gospel, so that relations to geographic place need to be understood in this wider cultural milieu, not only of imperial dispossession from traditional lands but of human relations to imperial cities and the pathways between them (including the sea). In this context, we may suspect that the written text of Scripture replaces the land as locus of relationship between God and the people.[4] Is this what Luke is doing in 4.16-30, and if so, what does the Scripture he has Jesus read communicate about this re-place-ment?

### *A Place in the Skin/Bark/Scroll*

Within the frame of Jesus' unrolling and rolling up the scroll is a proclamation of liberation (Lk. 4.18-19). The key word ἄφεσις—which also occurs at several other places in Luke (1.77; 3.3; 4.18; 5.20-21, 23-24; 7.47-49; 11.4; 12.10; 17.3-4; 23.34; 24.47)—and its related verb ἀφίημι (4.39; 5.11; 6.42; 8.51; 9.60; 10.30; 12.39; 13.8; 13.35; 17.34-35; 18.16; 18.28-29; 19.44; 21.6) refers to liberation, and more generally allowing, letting be and letting go, even leaving (BAGD, 125-26). More particularly, ἀφίημι is one of the two verbs used for 'to forgive'. The other, ἀπολύω (2.29; 6.37; 8.38; 9.12; 13.12; 14.4; 16.18; 23.16, 18, 20, 22, 25), has a similar range of meaning (BAGD, 96). Etymologically, ἄφεσις is related to freedom from captivity and oppression.[5]

In the Septuagint, ἐνιαυτὸς ἀφέσεως σημασία αὕτη (Lev. 25.10), the cycle (year) or extended time of this signalling (or commanding) of liberty, designates what has come to be known as the Jubilee, described in Lev. 25.8-55 as occurring in the fiftieth cycle or year. Here ἄφεσις interrupts the usual social cycles with freedom upon the land/earth for all its inhabitants (ἐπὶ τῆς γῆς πᾶσιν τοῖς κατοικοῦσιν αὐτήν, Lev. 25.10 LXX). Agricultural labour is suspended (Lev. 25.11) and from the open country (ἀπὸ τῶν πεδίων) the people are to eat the land's products (τὰ γενήματα αὐτῆς, Lev. 25.12). Moreover, ἄφεσις extends to the way the people buy and sell the land and its produce; the Jubilee interrupts the capacity for anyone to own the land (Lev. 25.13-17). On the principle that the land belongs to Yhwh (Lev. 25.23), the people are tenants who must keep the land (Lev. 25.23-24) in such a way that they enable the divine blessing to be effective in the season of Jubilee (Lev. 25.18-22). They must provide for the redemption of the land (Lev. 25.24-28) so that all can return to their ancestral holdings as to a gift. In this dispensation of liberation (ἄφεσις), kin who fall into difficulty are not to be treated as slaves, but as paid workers who are

4. This parallels William Scott Green's claim concerning the relationship between the book and the building, specifically the Torah and the Temple in Judaism. See Green cited in S. Balentine, '"He Unrolled the Scroll ... and He Rolled up the Scroll and Gave It Back"', *Cross Currents* 59.2 (2009), pp. 154-55.

5. This paragraph and the three that follow first appeared substantially in Anne Elvey, 'Can There Be a Forgiveness That Makes a Difference Ecologically? An Eco-Materialist Account of Forgiveness as Freedom (Ἄφεσις) in the Gospel of Luke', *Pacifica* 22 (2009), pp. 148-70.

released from the authority of the house in the Jubilee, returning to their ancestral holdings (Lev. 25.40-41).[6]

In Luke this Jubilee obligation toward kin comes under the influence of the redefinition of neighbour in the parable of the Good Samaritan (10.25-37), where the neighbour is the other who enacts divine mercy.[7] The interruption of social cycles signalled by ἄφεσις plays out in the Lukan motif of reversal. Even as it assumes a hierarchy of master over slave, the Gospel of Luke undermines the master/slave relation through a series of reversals integral to the programme of the Gospel (1.46-55; 6.20-26; 16.19-31).[8] In the Magnificat, God appears as the primary agent of reversal (Mary celebrates God's doings in 1.51-53). But in the parable of the rich man and Lazarus, the reversal of fortunes occurs through the mediation of angels (16.22), a 'great chasm' reflecting the social chasm between the two men (16.25-26), and as an effect of the rich man's neglectful exercise of his agency (16.19-21). In the Lukan beatitudes and woes, the agent of reversal is hidden in the passive, usually taken as code for divine agency. Read between the Magnificat and the parable of the rich man and Lazarus, the reversal of fortunes in Lk. 6.20-26 may be understood in a wider framework of more-than-human agency, neither solely divine nor solely human, rather an interplay of divine, human and other-than-human agents of blessing and woe.

A further clue to Luke's unsettling of a master/slave dynamic appears when a master is depicted as serving his slaves:

> Be dressed for action and have your lamps lit; be like those who are waiting for their master to return from the wedding banquet, so that they may open the door for him as soon as he comes and knocks. Blessed are those slaves whom the master finds alert when he comes; truly I tell you, he will fasten his belt and have them sit down to eat, and he will come and serve them. If he comes during the middle of the night, or near dawn, and finds them so, blessed are those slaves (12.35-38 NRSV).

This unsettling of the master/slave dynamic reappears in the context of Jesus' final meal with his disciples before his arrest, trial and execution, where he describes himself as 'one who serves':

> A dispute also arose among them as to which one of them was to be regarded as the greatest. But he said to them, 'The kings of the Gentiles

6. The servant of God tradition underlies this principle (Lev. 25.42, 55). Nevertheless, it is problematic that other peoples may be kept as slaves (Lev. 25.44-46).

7. See Brendan Byrne, *The Hospitality of God: A Reading of Luke's Gospel* (Strathfield, NSW: St Pauls, 2000), p. 101; Elvey, *Ecological Feminist Reading*, p. 242.

8. While at times these reversals seem to reinstate the master/slave, self/other, dynamic they are intended to replace, this is not the whole story. On the dual effect of these reversals, see Mark Coleridge, 'In Defence of the Other: Deconstruction and the Bible. [Applied to Luke's Infancy Narrative]', *Pacifica* 5 (1992), pp. 123-44.

> lord it over them; and those in authority over them are called benefactors. But not so with you; rather the greatest among you must become like the youngest, and the leader like one who serves. For who is greater, the one who is at the table or the one who serves? Is it not the one at the table? But I am among you as one who serves' (22.24-27 NRSV).

An implicit assumption of the 'naturalness' of the relation between slave and master becomes the background for a radical displacement of that relation, so that when in the narrative the disciple responds to the divine purpose in the character of a slave, she or he responds as the divine agent, Jesus, does himself.[9] Luke's appeal to Isaiah in Jesus' preaching in the synagogue in Nazareth (4.16-30) situates this theme of reversal at the heart of Jesus' message and mission, where the interruption of social relations signalled by ἄφεσις marks a divine visitation (1.77-78).

The proclamation of this divine advent of liberation, characterized by nourishment, healing and forgiveness and linked with the Levitical Jubilee proclamation of freedom upon the land, is *placed* in multiple intersecting τόποι. First, described as where Jesus was brought up or nourished (τεθραμμένος, 4.16), the geographic place Nazareth has links with the maternal, and hence the material givenness, which forms the understory of Jesus' life. From the verb τρέφω, meaning 'to nourish', τεθραμμένος recalls both the divine nourishment of birds (12.24) and a mother's breastfeeding her child (23.29).[10]

Second, the socio-religious place of the synagogue, a place of assembly, 'represents both an institutional linkage to the Temple and a modification of its function in society'.[11] Like the move from oral tradition to written text in the wake of the destruction of the Temple in 586 BCE and the exile, the rise of the synagogue responds to changing religious needs especially in the wake of the destruction of the Second Temple in 70 CE. In contrast to the Temple as site of divine presence in the Holy of Holies, a presence that is arguably an absence or distance approachable by a priestly elite, the synagogue offers a different place, where through reading and interpretation of written texts the divine is approached or encountered in the assembly.[12] In this context, the synagogue provides a physical place in which the written text

9. This assumption and unsettling of the master/slave relation may be part of a strategy of covert resistance to the imperial Roman social framework in which Luke and his community find themselves. See Gary Gilbert, 'Luke–Acts and the Negotiation of Authority and Identity in the Roman World', in *The Multivalence of Biblical Texts and Theological Meanings* (ed. Christine Helmer, Charlene T. Higbe and Brenna Moore; Atlanta: Society of Biblical Literature, 2006), esp. pp. 100, 104; Kahl, 'Reading Luke against Luke', esp. p. 75.

10. Elvey, *Ecological Feminist Reading*, p. 156; Marshall, *Gospel of Luke*, p. 181.

11. Balentine, 'He Unrolled the Scroll', p. 159.

12. Balentine, 'He Unrolled the Scroll', p. 159.

can be read and interpreted. As such, the reading is place-specific, situated in the socio-political networks associated with its particular geography: the Roman Empire, Galilee, a type of religious freedom for Jews within, and under, an imperial religious context. Samuel Balentine comments that 'even in the synagogues, according to the archaeological evidence from the Galilee area, the visible symbols of Judaism had likely been amalgamated with images from a status-quo culture that diminished their claims on a people formed by distinctive memories'.[13] The reading of Scripture in this place and the authority attributed to it are shaped by the authority of the Roman Empire and its particular exercise in a Jewish village in the Lower Galilee.[14] Together Nazareth and the synagogue form a fractured place where the Lukan Jesus encounters, and prompts, resistance and hostility. They stand for and open into two Lukan threads: a displacement of the maternal (see esp. 8.19-21; 11.27-28) and a failure to recognize the divine visitation (see esp. 7.29-30; 19.41-44).[15] Notably, the theme of failure to recognize the divine visitation connects the synagogue in Nazareth with the Temple and the city of Jerusalem, in particular their destruction.

Third, the Lukan Jesus finds a place in the scroll, a place where ink inscribes animal skin or plant fibre, from which he reads a divine visitation marked by ἄφεσις. Fourth, between the unrolling and the rolling up of the scroll, the place of writing has become the place of hearing, which Jesus then proclaims: 'Today this writing/scripture (ἡ γραφὴ αὕτη) has been fulfilled (πεπλήρωται) in your ears (ἐν τοῖς ὠσὶν ὑμῶν).' (4.21) For Michel Serres each of the sensory organs of sight, hearing, taste and smell is a folding in of the primary organ of sense, the skin.[16] In Lk. 4.16-21, the sensory place of reception of the word, the *ears* of those gathered, represents a station in the movement from skin to skin, from the skin of the scroll, through the eyes and mouth of Jesus to the ears of the assembled. In the enfolded skin of the ears that are always open to sound, the writing is subject to a fullness. In 4.21, the verb used, πεπλήρωται, is a third singular perfect passive of πληρόω, 'to fill, fulfil, or bring to completion'. The perfect tense suggests that what is filling their ears is both complete and in the process of completion. This becoming full is signalled by the filling up of, and from, the organs of sense (eyes 4.20; ears 4.21; mouth 4.22).

In Lk. 4.16-30, the response of the assembled to Jesus' reading from the place in the scroll is first remarked in the eyes fixed on him (4.20). But the Lukan Jesus then moves the focus to the ears in which the writing is being

13. Balentine, 'He Unrolled the Scroll', p. 157.

14. Balentine, 'He Unrolled the Scroll', pp. 156-57.

15. See Elvey, *Ecological Feminist Reading*, esp. Chapters 4–6.

16. Michel Serres, *The Five Senses: A Philosophy of Mingled Bodies*, I (trans. Margaret Sankey and Peter Cowley; London: Continuum, 2008), p. 53.

fulfilled (4.21). The assembled comment on what comes from his mouth (4.22). At this point, their receptivity falters. The earlier reference to Nazareth placed Jesus in relation to the maternal and more generally the material given (4.16); now the assembled comment on his lineage as Joseph's son (4.22). There is a turn in relation to the place. While Joseph must be included among the more-than-human community who contributed to the nourishment/upbringing of the Lukan Jesus, Luke has already unsettled the identity of Jesus in relation to Joseph (3.23). The question of the assembled prompts a provocative response from Jesus, which turns on the question of the receptivity of the home town, namely Nazareth (4.23-24). This place enters a chain of places that fail to receive the divine visitation.

The stories of Elijah and Elisha to which Jesus refers come as recollected writings with their own nested places in series of scrolls (4.25-27). These nested sites of writing form the fifth place within the multiple intersecting τόποι among which Luke places the proclamation of the divine advent in 4.18-19. The failure of receptivity to this advent is signalled by a movement from the specific sense organs—eyes and ears and mouth (4.20-22)—to the more general 'when they heard this' (4.28). A fracture in receptivity to the divine visitation in Jesus is matched by a fracture between skin and skin. This fracture is characterized by the threat of violent touch (4.29) which, at this stage of the narrative, Jesus avoids (4.30). The threatened body of the Lukan Jesus is the sixth and final site, the implied place of the fulfilment of this writing of ἄφεσις that Jesus has found in a synagogue in his home town Nazareth in a place in the scroll of the prophet Isaiah.

Geographic and socio-religious locations, the place of a writing in a scroll, the corporeal sensory sites of reading and receptivity, the nested material places of remembered narratives, and the threatened place of the speaker/reader, namely the body of Jesus, are intersecting τόποι in Lk. 4.16-20. Their complex interplay suggests that rather than re-place-ing the relationship to the land, the τόπος of a writing is in a complex network of relationships to the material given. Land and bodies, and the exercise of political power over bodies and land, are part of a material givenness that includes the complexities of human sociality within a wider more-than-human sociality in a particular here and now. The writing of a divine visitation as ἄφεσις received through the senses speaks to the relations of political power to land and bodies, and by extension the material given more generally.

### *'It Was Written'*

When Luke places a writing on the skin of a scroll, this place is marked by the multiple intersecting τόποι of bodies, senses, skin, political power, geographic and socio-religious locations. In Luke, then, the refrain 'it is/

was written' can be read as evoking the materiality of an artefact in which a writing has a place that is itself already multiple. The word γέγραπται evokes both the materiality of the medium and the labour of the scribe. The most common constructions used in Luke for an appeal to Jewish Scriptures are the third person singular perfect passive form γέγραπται, it is/was written; the phrase πάντα τὰ γεγραμμένα, all that is/was written, where the neuter plural γεγραμμένα is a form of the perfect passive participle; and the related τοῦτο τὸ γεγραμμένον (3.4; 4.4, 8, 10-11, 12; 7.27; 10.26; 18.31; 19.46; 21.22; 22.37; 24.27, 32, 44, 45, 46). The perfect captures the character of writing as both a past activity and a continuing material presence. Moreover, these constructions invite us to recall the agency of the medium on the type of writing. For example, the properties of clay lent themselves to cuneiform script.[17] The scroll lent itself to longer continuous works; the codex to collections of works. Was it the intense human labour of scribes to inscribe a scroll or codex, the orality of reading in the ancient world and the persistence of oral tradition that allowed a running together of words? Did a certain distance from origins and oral memory prompt the introduction of vowels in some Hebrew, and punctuation in many later Christian reproductions of the Greek and Hebrew, texts? What relations of skin to skin—inscribed animal skin and plant fibre to human memory and imagination—influenced the particular material embeddedness of writing?

Luke sets out to write (γράψαι) in an orderly way for his addressee, Theophilos (1.3). At the beginning, there is a self-referential quality to Luke's account, a self-consciousness of Luke as writer that is far less evident in the Gospels of Matthew and Mark. While, as Nancy argues, every book is an address to a reader, Luke's Gospel is self-consciously so.[18] Luke situates his work in a tradition of existing accounts as an orderly writing, intended to communicate assurance to his addressee, Theophilos (1.1-4). I use the masculine pronoun advisedly, under the influence of Luke's self-designation with the masculine singular dative of the perfect active participle παρηκολουθηκότι, from παρακολουθέω, 'to follow closely'. The introduction signals a carefulness, both in the writer's claimed attention to the emerging traditions about Jesus, and in his intention to provide a reliable and safe account for a reader constructed as God-loving, of higher social class, and Gentile. This careful introduction to a writing precedes Luke's evocation of the imaginary of a thoroughly Jewish temple-based religion, governed by what is written in the law/Torah of Yhwh (καθὼς γέγραπται ἐν νόμῳ κυρίου, 2.23; cf. Deut. 28.58, 61; 29.19, 20, 21, 26, 27; 31.9, 24, 26). For Luke this writing in/of the law/Torah is an address, a writing to (and for) others, as the Lukan Jesus declares to the Sadducees: Μωϋσῆς

17. Diringer, *Book before Printing*, p. 54.
18. Nancy, *Commerce of Thinking*, p. 10.

ἔγραψεν ἡμῖν, 'Moses wrote to/for us' (20.28). It is also an invitation to read; the Lukan Jesus addresses the lawyer who has approached him: 'In the law what is written (γέγραπται)? How do you read (ἀναγινώσκεις)?' (10.26).

Only in 4.16-21 does Luke refer explicitly to the place (τόπος) of the writing in the material artefact that is a scroll. However, this reference can inform Luke's other references with an underlying materiality that intersects with the corporeality (which is also a materiality) of the memory of the one who recites or alludes to the recollected verse/s, who is at once the writer of the Lukan text and the Lukan character who makes reference to what is/was written. Usually Luke has Jesus or the narrator refer to what is/was written or to the writings (Jesus: 4.4, 8, 17; 7.27; 10.26; 18.31; 19.46; 20.17, 28; 21.22; 22.37; 22.44, 46; narrator: 2.23; 3.4; 24.27, 45). Exceptions occur twice. In the Lukan interchange between the devil (ὁ διάβολος) and Jesus, the devil mimics Jesus by referring to what is written (4.10-11); after Jesus has disappeared from them, the two who encounter him on the Emmaus road echo the narrator (24.27) when they reflect on the effect of Jesus' interpreting/opening the writings for them (24.32). In the Acts of the Apostles, key figures such as Peter, Stephen, James and Paul refer to what is/was written or to the writings (1.20; 7.42; 13.29, 33; 15.15; 17.2, 11; 23.5; 24.14). As in Lk. 4.16-30, the synagogue is a focal site for the reading and interpretation of Jewish Scriptures (see esp. Acts 13.15; 17.2). But it is not the exclusive site for such interpretative activity. Jesus interprets the writings on the road to Emmaus (Lk. 24.13-27); Philip interprets the writings to an Ethiopian eunuch on a wilderness road from Jerusalem to Gaza (Acts 8.26-35). Each act of interpretation is followed by what will become an early Christian ritual, the breaking of bread (Lk. 24.28-31) and baptism (Acts 8.36-39), requiring respectively the life-sustaining material elements of bread and water.

Reading and interpreting what is written become in Luke–Acts part of early Christian practice. This early Christian engagement with Jewish writings has a particular focus in Luke and Acts. Acts 17.1-3 is paradigmatic in this regard:

> After Paul and Silas had passed through Amphipolis and Apollonia, they came to Thessalonica, where there was a synagogue of the Jews. And Paul went in, as was his custom, and on three sabbath days argued with them from the scriptures (ἀπὸ τῶν γραφῶν), explaining (διανοίγων) and proving that it was necessary (ἔδει) for the Messiah to suffer and to rise from the dead, and saying, 'This is the Messiah, Jesus whom I am proclaiming to you.'

The clause 'as was his custom' links the activity of Paul in Acts with that of Jesus in Lk. 4.16, both in attending the synagogue on the Sabbath and interpreting the writings there. The act of interpreting is a form of opening (διανοίγων).

In Lk. 24.32, the two who have encountered Jesus on the Emmaus road exclaim to one another, 'Were not our hearts burning (in us) as he spoke to us on the way, as he opened (διήνοιγεν) the writings (τὰς γραφάς) to us?' The materiality and material embeddedness of the scroll echo in this reference to opening the writings. In the previous verse, the narrator reports that following the breaking of the bread (24.30), their eyes were opened (διηνοίχθησαν) and they knew or recognized Jesus (24.31). The opening of the eyes is a metaphor for knowledge or recognition of something previously hidden (see also Gen. 3.5, 7; Prov. 20.13 LXX). The metaphor has its ground in the senses as ways of knowing through experience and experiment. In 24.45, Luke makes explicit this link with knowledge in relation to opening the writings: τότε διήνοιξεν αὐτῶν τὸν νοῦν τοῦ συνιέναι τὰς γραφάς, 'then he opened their minds to understand the writings'. Similarly, one's heart can be opened to listen (Acts 16.14; cf. 2 Macc. 1.4). διανοίγω is also used in relation to opening the womb, particularly the opening that occurs in the birth of the first offspring, for both humans and other animals (Lk. 2.23; Exod. 13.2, 12, 13, 15; 34.19; Num. 3.12; 8.16; 18.15). Thus, opening the writings to understanding has resonances of the maternal and the sensual, the creativity of birth and the embodied knowing of the senses that informs, and is informed by, the mind, heart, imagination and memory.

In Acts 17.1-3 Paul's opening of the writings focuses on the passion, death and resurrection of Jesus as elements of a divine necessity. The Gospel of Luke refers five times to this divine necessity:

> The Human One must (δεῖ) undergo great suffering, and be rejected by the elders, chief priests, and scribes, and be killed, and on the third day be raised (9.22; NRSV modified).
>
> For as the lightning flashes and lights up the sky from one side to the other, so will the Human One be in his day. But first he must (δεῖ) endure much suffering and be rejected by this generation (17.24-25; NRSV modified).
>
> For I tell you, this scripture must be fulfilled in me (τοῦτο τὸ γεγραμμένον δεῖ τελεσθῆναι ἐν ἐμοί), 'And he was counted among the lawless'; and indeed what is written about me is being fulfilled (22.37; NRSV modified).
>
> Remember how he told you, while he was still in Galilee, that the Human One must (δεῖ) be betrayed into the hands of sinners, and be crucified, and on the third day rise again (24.7; NRSV modified).
>
> Then he said to them, 'Oh, how foolish you are, and how slow of heart to believe all that the prophets have declared! Was it not necessary (ἔδει) that the Messiah should suffer these things and then enter into his glory?'

> Then beginning with Moses and all the prophets, he interpreted to them the things about himself in all the scriptures (24.25-27; NRSV).

The Lukan divine necessity relates to a particular interpretation of the Jewish Scriptures, as applied to the life of Jesus of Nazareth, and a particular interpretation of his life in relation to these writings. The interpretation, or opening, has its parallel in an awakening of the senses, and particularly the inner sense (of heart or mind), to the lived experience of Jesus of Nazareth as a fullness and end (*telos*) of the writings.[19]

When we focus on the materiality evoked by 'the writings', 'it is written' and 'what is written', the opening of the writings onto the body of Jesus at once displaces and continues the engagement with the materiality of the text. The appeal to what is written, as simultaneously a past event of writing and a material presence open to reading and interpretation, connects with the divine necessity that is expressed in the suffering, death and resurrection of the Lukan Jesus. This writing on, and of, the body occurs through the violent laying on of human hands (see also Lk. 18.31).

Written of (and on) the body of Jesus is a fulfilment or end of a divine purpose. For Luke this purpose expressed in Jewish writings on animal skin or plant fibre becomes a divine necessity, an effect of divine providence, neither fully identifiable with Greek notions of fate (that is, of events as wholly determined without the effect of human will or action) nor with Jewish scriptural notions of divine election.[20] For Charles Cosgrove the divine δεῖ points to God's plan or purpose in history, calling forth a response.[21] Although understood to be free, human responsiveness to (and cooperation with) the divine purpose is likened to that of a slave (for example, Lk. 1.38; 17.10).[22] Nonetheless, often a coincidence exists between divine call and human response. Ensuring the divine plan, the divine necessity signals a co-agency between God and humans in the freedom of human response to

19. As Regina Schwartz (*Curse of Cain*, esp. p. 174) argues, a mode of Christian interpretation of Jewish Scriptures that focuses on fulfilment is problematic, in that it tends to freeze the meaning of the text, obscuring both the specificity and the multiplicity of the text it sets out to interpret. See also Robbins, *Prodigal Son/Elder Brother*, esp. pp. 2, 9.

20. Charles H. Cosgrove, 'The Divine Δεῖ in Luke–Acts', *NovT* 26 (1984), pp. 168-90; see also Mark Reasoner, 'The Theme of Acts: Institutional History or Divine Necessity in History?', *JBL* 118 (1999), pp. 635-59; Elvey, *Ecological Feminist Reading*, p. 97.

21. Cosgrove, 'Divine Δεῖ'.

22. Cf. John T. Squires, *The Plan of God in Luke–Acts* (Cambridge: Cambridge University Press, 1993), pp. 177-78.

the divine purpose, even where this response is a refusal.[23] The divine δεῖ continually returns 'to surprise or interrupt history'.[24]

Moreover, Luke links this divine necessity with the fate of Jerusalem and the Second Temple. As I will consider in Chapter 6, the stones of the Temple and the body of Jesus stand in parallel and contrast (see, for example, 20.17). Signifying the destruction of Jerusalem and the Temple, these stones are also the subject of an interpretation of what is written (19.41-46; 21.20-22). What is written, in a place in a scroll, is central to Luke's writing. What is written can be opened to the eyes and ears, hearts and minds of its hearers. An inscription on animal skin or plant fibre in turn inscribes a divine purpose on the body of the Lukan Jesus and the place of Jerusalem. This writing on body and place is the result of human response (signified by voice and hand, ear and heart) to a divine visitation marked by ἄφεσις. As I will consider more closely in Chapter 7, the materiality of the writing remains for Luke a witness, in particular a witness that comes into play through readings that, in opening up a writing, open the senses to meaning. Appeals to, or inscriptions of, particular authorized or canonical readings can circumscribe meaning. However, such appeals do not wholly contain the activity of reading that is an engagement with the senses, a movement from skin to skin.

## *Skin to Skin: Sensual Reading as Saturated Communion*

### *Skin to Skin*

To explore the activity of reading as a movement from skin to skin, I turn to Michel Serres's work on the five senses, where he appeals to six fifteenth-century CE tapestries, *The Lady and the Unicorn*, in the Cluny Museum. Each of five tapestries depicts one of the five senses with a final tapestry relating 'to the sensorium in general'.[25] The tapestries depict one or two women on a blue island against a reddish background; a lion and a unicorn also appear as key characters in each tapestry. The scenes are full

23. This is particularly evident in the passion predictions (esp. 9.22; 17.25) where the rejection by the religious authorities that leads to Jesus' death (and for Luke also the destruction of Jerusalem, 19.41-44) is co-agential with the divine necessity. The point is a subtle one: while there is for Luke an inevitability to the divine purpose, nonetheless this does not render human acceptance or rejection of that purpose, and hence human response, irrelevant. But it does suggest that the divine necessity has a resilience that is not destroyed by human intransigence or refusal.

24. Robert Brawley, *Centering on God: Method and Message in Luke–Acts* (Louisville: Westminster John Knox, 1990), pp. 123-24, argues that this capacity to surprise adds complexity to a Lukan characterization of divine superiority with respect to changing circumstances.

25. Serres, *Five Senses*, p. 55.

with animal and plant life, including fruit trees; and one or more characters in relation to an object depict each of the external senses. For sight, the unicorn sees its reflection in a mirror held by the woman. For hearing, the woman and another woman, perhaps an attendant, finger a musical instrument, a positive organ. For taste, the attendant offers a dish from which the woman takes candy; as an interpretative key, the monkey is also eating. For smell, the attendant presents a basket of flowers to the woman; the monkey holds a flower to its nose. For touch, there is no separate object; instead, the woman touches the horn of the unicorn.[26] As Serres notes in relation to the materiality of the woven tapestry, and elsewhere in relation to writing, the depiction of the senses as engagements on skin already occurs on skin.[27]

Likewise, in Lk. 4.17-20 the Lukan Jesus is depicted on skin (the surface of the Lukan text) proclaiming from skin (the scroll of Isaiah), the sensory engagement of skin (the enfolded skin of eye, mouth and ears) with a writing. Moreover, as noted in Chapter 2, for Luke the ear, the heart and the earth are related metaphorically and metonymically as sites of receptivity to the divine word/seed. The ear, heart and earth both parallel and supplant the receptivity characterized by the maternal body. The external senses, in particular hearing, suggest what Serres calls an internal sense, in which the heart becomes a site of divine writing (cf. Jer. 31.33).

In the sixth Cluny tapestry, the woman stands on the island before an open tent, with her attendant holding open a casket into which the woman places a necklace; the lion stands to one side of the two women, the unicorn to the other. Serres draws on this tapestry as indicating an internal sense: 'Indeed a sixth sense is necessary, in which the subject turns in on itself and the body on the body: a common or internal sense, indeed a sixth island was necessary, a doubly enclosed island for the body itself.'[28] For Serres, touch as a 'factor common to four external senses, an open and closed sense in itself, ... protects the internal sense and begins to construct it'.[29] The organ of touch, the skin, on which 'the world is printed' is 'a wax garment that surrounds and clothes us, that now offers us an intimate habitat'.[30] Luke's linking of ear and heart resonate with Serres's 'internal sense', in which the sensual tattoo on the skin becomes an internal writing. For Luke, this sensual writing on the heart echoes both in the sowing of the earth (8.4-15) and the interpretation of the Scriptures (24.32), and

26. Serres, *Five Senses*, p. 53.
27. Serres, *Five Senses*, p. 53.
28. Serres, *Five Senses*, p. 54. See also Aristotle, *De an.* 2.11.
29. Serres, *Five Senses*, p. 55.
30. Serres, *Five Senses*, p. 55.

has resonance in the later association of the Books of Nature and Scripture.

Jane Walling describes a tradition and mode of reading the Book of Nature 'where sensual reading of phenomena is combined with penetration beyond them'.[31] The senses are traditionally the means and mode of knowing a more-than-human world. Writers such as Goethe have drawn on this sensory mode of knowing to express a deeper knowing about the more-than-human Earth community.[32] While a metaphor of penetration, such as that used by Walling, may recall problematic symbols of knowing as undressing, mining and mastering the Earth, the relation between sensory knowing and a beyond can echo Serres's understanding of a relation between the senses and the inner sense.[33] Moreover, this sensory engagement with the phenomenon implies that 'the knower is not just an onlooker or reader but a participant in nature's processes and the state of being known [and I would add, more particularly the state of knowing through the senses] can be seen as an evolutionary development of nature itself'.[34] Here, Walling claims, 'the phenomenon itself ... appears in consciousness when it is known', and this knowing 'is not a subjective human activity' but part of 'the development of the phenomenon'.[35] Below I will appeal to Jean-Luc Marion's understanding of saturated phenomena to offer a different nuance to this relationship between the human subject and the more-than-human phenomenon with which he or she is engaged in an interpretative act. For now, I want to expand the question of the relation of the senses to the Book of Nature.

In Chapter 1, I made reference to a long tradition of two books, the Book of Nature and the Book of Scripture, which come together in an approach to the Bible as a material artefact, in Eastern tradition 'a verbal icon'. My reading of Luke's attention to what is written as evoking the place in the material artefact as a nested set of places, with which the reader, interpreter and hearers engage through the senses, is coherent with this intersection of the two books. Moreover, the appeal to the senses as modes of knowing the Book of Nature cannot be limited to that book but offers a mode of engage-

31. Jane Walling, 'Reading (in) Proust: With the Senses, beyond the Senses', in *Sensual Reading: New Approaches to Reading in its Relation to the Senses* (ed. Michael Syrotinski and Ian Maclachlan; London: Associated Universities Presses, 2001), pp. 271-91 (272).

32. Walling, 'Reading (in) Proust', pp. 272-74.

33. See, in particular, Carolyn Merchant's critique of Bacon in Carolyn Merchant, *The Death of Nature: Women, Ecology and the Scientific Revolution* (originally published 1980; republished with new preface; San Francisco: Harper & Row, 1990), esp. pp. 164-91.

34. Walling, 'Reading (in) Proust', p. 275.

35. Walling, 'Reading (in) Proust', p. 275.

ment with the Book of Scripture, more particularly, 'the writings' to which Luke alludes and the writing that is the Gospel of Luke. Even where we have forgotten them, our senses are engaged with the material text in the act of reading. In this act of reading, the text as inscribed skin meets the enfolded skin of the human senses.

*A Saturated Communion*

These senses are modes of perception linking the one who senses with the thing sensed. This connection between the one sensing and the thing sensed is twofold. First, the thing sensed is afforded a priority, since without the sense-object the faculty of sensation remains potential rather than actual (Aristotle, *De an.* 2.5); this implies that in Lk. 4.17-20 the material scroll precedes the engagement of the hands, eyes, ears and mouth of the Lukan Jesus. Second, a hermeneutic relationship is established between the one who senses and the thing sensed. The thing sensed is perceived within the interpretative framework of the prior experience of the one sensing; before he proclaims (and interprets) the writing in the scroll, the Lukan Jesus has already received this material artefact as an inscribed skin that may be read, rather than as a garment to be worn around his shoulders.[36]

Further, sense experience becomes 'a form of communion' with the other, in which the body surrenders itself to the sensible.[37] In Lk. 4.17-22 both the interplay of senses signalled and the tenor of expectation conveyed suggest that the body of the Lukan Jesus is engaged with the scroll and its writing, through eyes, voice, breath and hearing, even to the extent that he embodies that to which he corporeally surrenders his senses (4.21). For Maurice Merleau-Ponty, this corporeal surrender signals a shift from an 'expectation of a sensation' to which one has given eye or ear to being overtaken by the sensible which 'takes possession' of one's ear or one's gaze.[38] The sensible is 'a certain way of being in the world' precisely insofar as it is 'seized and acted upon by [a] body ... capable of doing so'.[39] The capacity to sense and the act of sensing, which actuates this capacity in relation to another thing, become a different *thing* that is the communion formed through sensation. In the case of the Lukan Jesus in 4.17-22, this communion is a fully embodied proclamation of a material text.

To explore this sensual communion further, I turn to Jean-Luc Marion's 'saturated phenomenon' to describe material or sensual reading as a

36. Maurice Merleau-Ponty, *Phenomenology of Perception* (trans. Colin Smith; London: Routledge Classics, 2002), p. 60.

37. Merleau-Ponty, *Phenomenology of Perception*, p. 246.

38. Merleau-Ponty, *Phenomenology of Perception*, p. 246.

39. Merleau-Ponty, *Phenomenology of Perception*, p. 246.

saturated communion.[40] 'Saturation' is a term Marion applies to particular phenomena that present themselves to experience in a heightened manner.[41] Luke's depiction of the programmatic scene in 4.17-22 could be understood as depicting this quality of saturation in the way it portrays Jesus' act of reading from a place in the scroll, his interpretation and the people's reception of his action and interpretation as exceeding expectation.

Important for an understanding of Marion's saturated phenomena, and the excess it denotes, is a distinction between intuition and concept received from Immanuel Kant. Intuition refers to 'an immediate and singular representation' of a thing, that is, what is apprehended empirically through sensation or purely as the particular spatial and temporal form of things.[42] Concept refers to 'a general representation of an attribute or mark of a class of objects', that is, what is thought about a thing, its comprehension within a certain frame of thinking, as an abstraction from the thing intuited.[43] As Shane Mackinlay explains, 'Sensibility "gives" objects to us in intuition, while the understanding "thinks" these objects by means of a concept'.[44] For Marion, intuition and concept can be related in three ways.

First, the concept and the intuition correspond, so that there is a relation of adequation or sufficiency between them, with the intuition filling the concept precisely. Second, the concept may exceed the intuition, for example, in the case where the abstract idea conveyed by the concept of a cube includes rear and bottom surfaces I do not see when viewing it from a certain angle, and an interior volume I do not touch when I hold it in my hands. To these Marion brings a third relation, where the intuition exceeds the concept. For example, in a work of art, the concepts of colour, line, shape, and texture—and the concepts named in titles, such as 'Blue Poles' or 'The Gleaners' or 'David'—neither constitute the painting or sculpture nor make it comprehensible as an object. In a canonical text, such as the Gospel of Luke, the meaning of the text as sacred Scripture exceeds both the concept of a writing that presents itself in a place in a material artefact

40. Jean-Luc Marion, 'The Saturated Phenomenon', *Philosophy Today* 40 (1996), pp. 103-24.

41. Already to use the adjective 'heightened' is to be imprecise concerning the relationship between experience and the phenomena that Marion describes as 'saturated'.

42. Paul Guyer, *Kant* (London: Routledge, 2006), pp. 53-55, 375.

43. Guyer, *Kant*, p. 374.

44. Shane Mackinlay, *Interpreting Excess: Jean-Luc Marion, Saturated Phenomena, and Hermeneutics* (Perspectives in Continental Philosophy; New York: Fordham University Press, 2009), p. 64.

and the concepts, such as ἄφεσις, to which the writing itself pertains.[45] In such cases, one is confronted by a saturated phenomenon.[46]

As Marion writes of the work of art, the phenomenon presents itself to intuition as itself, and as itself 'comes upon me' in excess of my expectation of it.[47] Such a phenomenon saturates experience, unsettling my egocentric subjectivity. 'My horizons are overwhelmed and submerged by it [a saturated phenomenon]. I am more the subject constituted by its givenness than it is the object constituted by my subjectivity.'[48] The unsettling of subjectivities described in Chapter 1 in relation to both the icon and the Bible as verbal icon resonates with this experience of the saturated phenomenon.

The priority Marion accords the phenomenon in his account of saturation is both attractive and problematic. From an ecological perspective, the notion of phenomena appearing prior to the hermeneutic activity of a human subject is attractive. However, Shane Mackinlay finds a tension between Marion's theoretical description of saturated phenomena as appearing prior to any interpretation and accosting the subject who becomes their passive recipient, and Marion's examples of saturated phenomena, which give the subject a more active role in their reception and interpretation.[49] Moreover, if considered in relation to the senses discussed above, the intuition of phenomena through sensation implies a hermeneutic communion between the thing presenting itself and its interpreter. Mackinlay poses Marion the following question: 'Is not all phenomenology necessarily hermeneutic, because interpretation is part of the very structure of the appearing of phenomena?'[50]

From an ecological perspective, Marion's concept of saturation is important for its critique of a phenomenology that reduces phenomena 'to projections of the subject'.[51] A saturated phenomenon arrests one at the point where self-projection passes into transcendence of the self (but not simply as self-transcendence). Here one becomes *l'adonné*, 'the one "given over", gifted, or devoted to the self-giving phenomenon, the one who receives

45. Jean-Luc Marion, 'They Recognized Him; and He Became Invisible to Them', *Modern Theology* 18.2 (2002 ), pp. 145-52 (147); Kevin Hart, 'Poetry and Revelation: Hopkins, Counter-Experience and *Reductio*', *Pacifica* 18 (2005), pp. 259-80 (276).

46. Jean-Luc Marion, 'The Banality of Saturation', in *Counter-Experiences: Reading Jean-Luc Marion* (ed. Kevin Hart; Notre Dame, IN: University of Notre Dame Press, 2007), pp. 383-418 (391-93).

47. Marion, 'Banality of Saturation', p. 393.

48. Merold Westphal, 'Transfiguration as Saturated Phenomenon', *Journal of Philosophy and Scripture* 1 (2003), pp. 26-34 (26).

49. Mackinlay, *Interpreting Excess*, pp. 54-56.

50. Mackinlay, *Interpreting Excess*, p. 36.

51. Mackinlay, *Interpreting Excess*, p. 47.

itself from what it receives'.[52] Applying this to Lk. 4.16-20, I could say that Luke depicts Jesus not simply as actively reading from a place in a scroll, but as corporeally and sensorially 'given over' to the writing he reads. Moreover, in the preceding narrative of Lk. 1.1–4.15, even before he has unrolled the scroll to read, Jesus is already given over to the writing (ἡ γραφή) that presents itself materially. This giving over, exemplified in the Lukan usage of the divine necessity as a fulfilment of the writings, can be understood not only by way of Jesus receiving himself in receiving the saturated phenomenon of divine appointment, but also as a self-reception that arrives from the Earth community, in the materially mediated writing from which he proclaims his appointment.

The encounter with a materially mediated writing is an encounter with an Earth that gives itself to a human person who is thereby gifted (*adonné*). Moreover, the one gifted is also part of the Earth community that is given. However, 'For Marion, there is no sense of an *encounter* between an *adonné* and that which is given, but simply a *transmission* of an already-determinate package'.[53] If this is the case, the interrelatedness that characterizes a more-than-human Earth community is elided. If, however, as Mackinlay suggests, saturated phenomena need to be understood in terms of a mutuality between the thing that gives itself and the one it gifts (*adonné*),[54] and if this mutuality is characterized by hermeneutics of openness and response to the thing so given, then an understanding of saturated phenomena may enhance a consideration of a more-than-human interrelatedness. In this latter sense, and diverging somewhat from Marion, a saturated phenomenon appears not so much in the thing that gives itself as in the communion occurring between the given and the gifted (*adonné*) in a hermeneutic space opened between them.[55]

This hermeneutic space is opened uniquely by the given and by the gifted, so that the thing gives itself to interpretation and the one to whom it is given interprets, and has their interpretation interrupted by, the thing. When the thing that gives itself is a biblical text, the hermeneutic space opened between text and interpreter is no guarantee that a critical interpretative response will be forthcoming. Rather, the hermeneutic space opens as a summons to interpret the text as a thing, saturated both in its material givenness and in its play of words, images, structure and flow. Reading becomes a saturated communion with the text.

52. Robyn Horner, 'Translator's Introduction', in *In Excess: Studies of Saturated Phenomena,* by Jean-Luc Marion (New York: Fordham University Press, 2002), pp. ix-xx (xv).

53. Mackinlay, *Interpreting Excess*, p. 49.

54. Mackinlay, *Interpreting Excess*, p. 14.

55. Cf. Mackinlay, *Interpreting Excess*, p. 177.

### *Reading with and through the Senses*

As a saturated phenomenon, which may engage a reader in a saturated communion, a text is indeterminate. 'It is not an object that can be put away on a shelf or placed on a table, but neither is it this printed text found on its pages. Instead, it shifts from one to the other, or else resides in the tension between the two.'[56] There is an oscillation between the both/and and the either/or that characterizes the undecidability concerning the text as material thing and its saturation.[57] The text is always in excess of its materiality, and this materiality remains in excess of the text it mediates. The text is both the material artefact, in which it presents itself to reading, and the writing that can be found in a *place* in the artefact; at the same time the text is neither wholly one nor the other: neither artefact nor writing.

The text is also part of a commerce of ideas and interpretation not fully contained in the economics of its production and trade. This commerce informs, and is informed by, the being in common, the common life, of human community.[58] Central to this common life is the notion of communication, including the interrelatedness, commonality and complex communicability of thought.[59] Communication requires transformation, translation and interpretation.[60] Communication entails, moreover, a saturated communion that holds a text before the eyes, in the ears or in the hands; that touches a writing in a place in a skin; that translates from skin to skin through the senses.

This sensory communication requires a common sense, in the mode of Hans-Georg Gadamer's common sense as 'the sense that founds community'.[61] For my eco-materialist approach this common sense has two interrelated aspects: First, it resonates with Serres's understanding of

56. Nancy, *Commerce of Thinking*, p. 2.

57. Compare with the use of this oscillation in Jacques Derrida, *On the Name* (trans. John P. Leavey, David Wood, Jr, and Ian McLeod; Stanford, CA: Stanford University Press, 1995), p. 91; John D. Caputo, *The Prayers and Tears of Jacques Derrida: Religion without Religion* (Indiana Series in the Philosophy of Religion; Bloomington: Indiana University Press, 1997), p. 35. On the 'constructive ambivalence' of both/and; either/or, see also Catherine Keller, *Apocalypse Now and Then: A Feminist Guide to the End of the World* (Boston: Beacon Press, 1996), p. 24, and Elvey, *Ecological Feminist Reading*, p. 105.

58. David Wills, 'Translator's Foreword: Thinking Singular Plural', in *On the Commerce of Thinking: Of Books and Bookstores,* by Jean-Luc Nancy (New York: Fordham University Press, 2009), pp. xiii-xx (xvi-xviii).

59. Wills, 'Translator's Foreword', pp. xviii-xix.

60. Wills, 'Translator's Foreword', p. xix.

61. Hans-Georg Gadamer, *Truth and Method* (trans. Joel Weinsheimer and Donald G. Marshall; London: Continuum, 2nd rev. edn, 2004), p. 19.

the internal sense that 'makes sense' of the senses; second, in its making sense of the senses it provides a basis for being with a more-than-human community, as a mode of attentive knowing. In reading the relation between the senses and the common sense from the Lady and the Unicorn tapestries, Serres already situates the common sense in a more-than-human context, the more-than-human community of the island. Resonating with the characterization of the internal sense of the heart/mind, which Luke links with the ear and the earth, the common sense opens to *reading with the senses* the multiple intersecting *topoi* of a writing. Moreover, a text itself mirrors the relation between the senses and the common sense. Nancy comments, 'The book lays out its end in itself and comports itself as the envelope of an interiority.'[62] The crossing in the writing between the opened book or the unrolled scroll and its meaning parallels the crossing in reading between text skin, human skin and the internal sense.

The following five chapters each focus on one of the senses as a mode of attentiveness to the text of Luke's Gospel. In each chapter, I engage with a particular sense, drawing on critical theory to describe a phenomenology of the sense and bringing this into creative conversation with a reading of the sense as it is characterized in the text and as it informs an engagement with the text as material artefact. In a recent article Dorothy Lee explores the interrelated symbolic, theological and christological import of the five senses in the Gospel of John, with brief reference to the materiality of the text in a footnote.[63] While there are some parallels, my focus on the senses is somewhat different; my emphasis is on an engagement with the senses as a mode of exploring a material intertextuality.

Michael Syrotinski comments, 'language seems to interfere with the immediacy one normally associates with sense experience', indicating 'a senselessness at the heart of language'.[64] He suggests that sensual readings play with this tension between sense experience and language. Addressing the text as both/and, neither/nor material artefact and writing, my readings engage the senses across this tension, affirming that every reading involves sense experience, whether we acknowledge it or otherwise. Moreover, every reading from a place in an artefact is an engagement with multiple intersecting places. As Lorraine Code indicates, ecological thinking expands the situation of the question—'whose knowledge are we talking about?'—to

62. Nancy, *Commerce of Thinking*, p. 15.

63. Dorothy Lee, 'The Gospel of John and the Five Senses', *JBL* 129 (2010), pp. 115-27, esp. p. 26 n. 40.

64. Michael Syrotinski, 'Introduction: *Hors d'oeuvre*', in *Sensual Reading: New Approaches to Reading in its Relation to the Senses* (ed. Michael Syrotinski and Ian Maclachlan; London: Associated Universities Presses, 2001), pp. 7-12 (9).

such multiple intersecting places, of power, privilege, authority, and I would add a more-than-human materiality.[65] A sensual reading affirms the situatedness of interpretation, not only in the embodiment and material embeddedness of the interpreter but also in the nested places of the materiality of a text.

65. Lorraine Code, *Ecological Thinking: The Politics of Epistemic Location* (Oxford: Oxford University Press, 2006), p. 21.

# 4

## Touching (on) Death: On 'Being toward' the Other

He took him in his arms and praised God ...

Lk. 2.28 (NRSV modified)

Mankulla gaiya bon noa gikoug kin turrug ka, gatun pitalma now bon Eloinug, gatun wiyelliela ...

Lk. 2.28 in *The Gospel by St Luke Translated into the Language of the Awabakal,* by L.E. Threkeld (Sydney: Charles Potter, Government Printer, 1891)

On one page of the thirteenth-century CE Parisian *Bible moralisée*, an infant nestles in a partly open Bible. The scene recalls the presentation. A woman appears with the child and two men are present. The men stand together. The gaze of one rests on the woman; the gaze of the other is directed toward the child. In the image to the left, ties or clasps secure the book holding the child. The book is close/d around him. Above left, a child appears swaddled; and directly above, he lies in a basket afloat on a river among the rushes. A woman inclines toward the child at a similar angle to that with which the woman bends toward the child in the book. The eyes of the former woman are closed while the latter's focus on the child. The words to the side of the images suggest that these narratives are about Moses and his sister Miriam (Marie). But the images link Jesus and Moses and suggest at this level that the book represents the Torah, the law of Moses, referred to in Luke's account of the presentation (2.22-24). There is a crossing between basket/manger/cradle/book. A white scroll falls from the draped hand/arm of Miriam/Marie, and could also hint at the prophet Anna. The Lukan story unfolds in relation to a woman called Mary/Marie/Miriam. One tradition has Luke as the painter of the icon of Mary; another has Mary as Luke's informant. For Luke, she is the keeper of all these things: the story, the Torah, the word (2.19, 51). In the moment represented in the *Bible moralisée* illumination, the Bible (as manger/basket) is the intermediary between

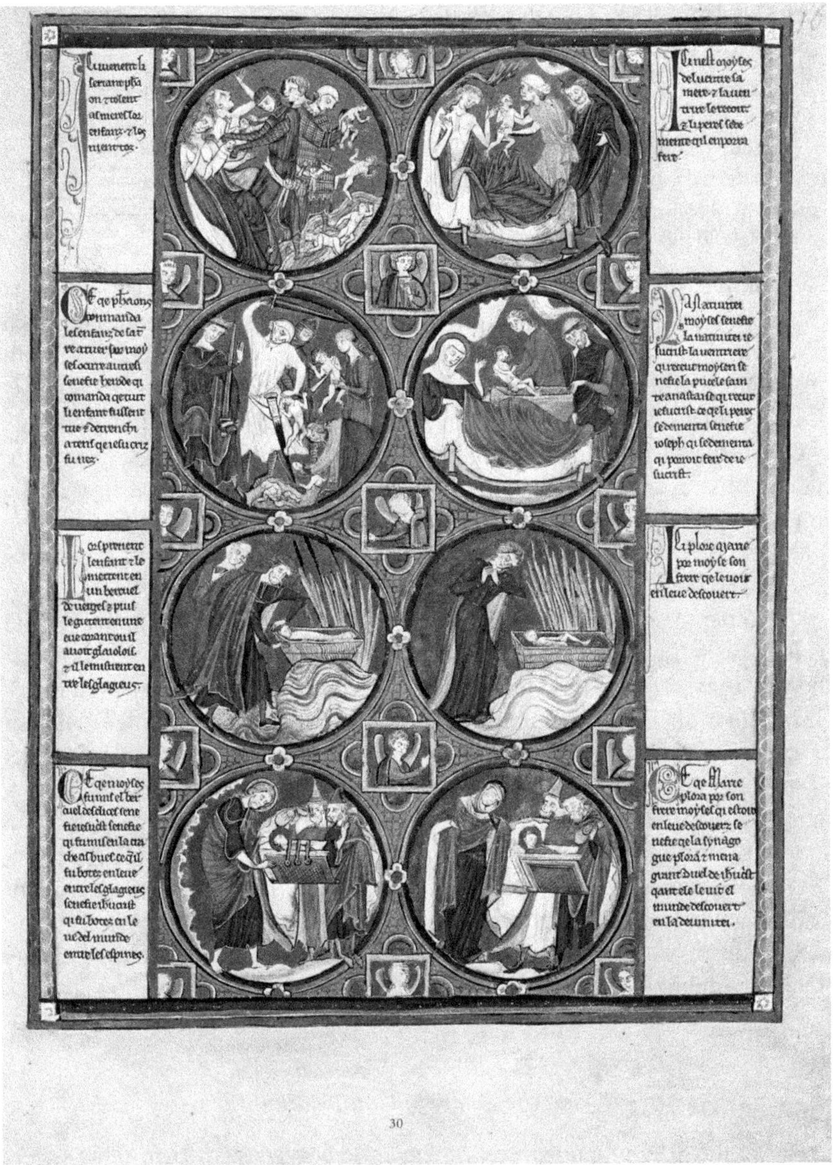

Fig. 1. *Bible moralisée.* Cod. 2554, fol. 16r. Copyright Austrian National Library Vienna, Picture Archiv+Signature.

the touch of the sister/mother and the touch of the elders. Here the materiality of the text touches the materiality of the body.[1]

Jean-Luc Nancy writes of texts and bodies:

> Bodies, for good or ill, are touching each other upon this page, or more precisely, the page itself is a touching (of my hand while it writes, and your hands while they hold the book). This touch is infinitely indirect, deferred—machines, vehicles, photocopies, eyes, still other hands are all interposed—but it continues as a slight, resistant, fine texture, the infinitesimal dust of a contact, everywhere interrupted and pursued.[2]

The complexity of the touch of the text as a material artefact comes to the reader by way of a network of writing and reading contexts, material media and their situations of embeddedness in a more-than-human sociality. With this more-than-human sociality in view, I would argue that the touch is finitely, rather than infinitely, indirect and deferred. The multiple deferrals and material mediations of the touch of the text in front of the reader are indeterminate, but finite, existing within, and touching on, the limits of a finite Earth. Nevertheless, Nancy's point that the material text touches the material body is central to this chapter, which brings the sense of touch represented in the text and the touch of the text into conversation.

This chapter explores the touch of the biblical text and touch in the Gospel of Luke as a touching on life and death. Beginning with a consideration of the way in which the Bible touches bodies, communities and land as a material artefact of European colonization of Australia, I then consider a pattern of compassionate touch in the Gospel of Luke that may unsettle patterns of violent relatedness. Reading this compassionate touch as marked by a touching (on) death, I take up Nancy's notion of a consent to the body (and so to mortality) as the taking place of being. In this corporeal taking place, skin answers to skin—with violence, compassion, indifference, salve-ation/healing, love. Here, death is part of the life process, and the body, in its being toward death and life, is a focus of the material embeddedness of things (including human bodies and Bibles) in their more-than-human socialities.

## *Contact: The Bible as Material Artefact and the Touch of Colonization*

Showing the Torah/manger holding the child Moses/Jesus before his sister/mother and two elders, the mediaeval *Bible moralisée* image references the

1. I am grateful to art historian Dr Claire Renkin for alerting me to this *Bible moralisée* page and for her helpful discussion of the images.

2. Jean-Luc Nancy, *Corpus* (trans. Richard A. Rand; Perspectives in Continental Philosophy; New York: Fordham University Press, 2008), p. 51.

Lukan presentation narrative (2.22-35).[3] In Luke's narrative, the Torah is the prompt for the presentation of the mother and child. The days of purification are numbered 'according to the law of Moses' (κατὰ τὸν νόμον Μωϋσέως) (2.22); the firstborn is presented 'as it is written in the law of the lord' (καθὼς γέγραπται ἐν νόμῳ κυρίου) (2.23-24); the parents bring 'the child Jesus, to do for him what was customary under the law' (κατὰ τὸ εἰθισμένον τοῦ νόμου) (2.27). Simeon is a righteous representative of Israel, expecting the Christ and inspired by the Holy Spirit (2.25-27). When Simeon takes Jesus in his arms (2.28), he speaks first of peace, salvation, revelation and glory; the primary sense evoked is sight (2.29-32). Following the parents' amazement, he turns to Mary and speaks of the conflict the child will occasion and the violent touch she herself will suffer: 'a sword will pierce your own soul, too' (2.33-35). As the aged Simeon nears his own death, the materiality of the text touches the materiality of the vulnerable body of the child; Simeon's words of expectation fulfilled are traced with the touch of Jesus' violent death and the maternal suffering to come.

In the *Bible moralisée* page, the right-hand images from top to bottom show the birth of a child, the lying in the cradle/manger, the discovery of Moses among the rushes, and the presentation of the child in the book. There is a crossing between the hands of the midwife, the manger, the reed basket and the book as the place that touches and holds the child and keeps him safe. The left-hand column provides a contrast. From top to bottom are images of children taken from their mothers and slaughtered with the sword; of Moses left on the river because of Pharaoh's cruelty; of the book closed around the child. The mediaeval images of violence against children are uncanny in their resonance with the Indigenous Australian experience of colonization, of forced removal of children and massacres. For many the Bible has become part of this ongoing story of dispossession, resistance, survival and cultural negotiation.

Signifying touch, 'contact' is a word used for the colonizing meeting of invader or settler with Aboriginal and Torres Strait Islander peoples. Australian scholars such as Roland Boer, Mark Brett and Deborah Rose have considered aspects of the use and impact of the Bible in a period of contact that continues. For example, the Bible has informed explorer and settler perceptions of their enterprises and relationships to land, has authorized the suppression and destruction of indigenous cultural practices, and has prompted critique of the violence and dispossession accompanying colonization.[4] Jeremy Beckett argues that once colonization has occurred, mate-

3. The symbolism of such mediaeval images was multivalent, drawing on figurative interpretation that linked Miriam and Mary, Moses and Jesus.

4. See Roland Boer, *Last Stop before Antarctica: The Bible and Postcolonialism in Australia* (Sheffield: Sheffield Academic Press, 2001); Mark G. Brett, *Decolonizing*

rial artefacts such as Bibles become resources for ongoing meaning making within indigenous cultures.[5] At the same time, traditional material symbols, such as message sticks and coolamon, become part of Aboriginal and Torres Strait Islander inculturation of Christianity.

Some indigenous Christians in Australia, for example, are recovering the coolamon as a way of representing the infancy story liturgically. Throughout the season of Advent, the coolamon, a curved, open receptacle of bark or wood for carrying infants and also food, lays face downward. At Christmas, the coolamon is turned over, and the doll representing the child Jesus placed in it.[6] If I were to attempt to translate the *Bible moralisée* image in this context, I might suggest that the Bible stands in the place of the coolamon, as receptacle for the child. The child is presented to the elders of the people in the Bible/coolamon. I do not know if Aboriginal and Torres Strait Islander children are routinely presented to their elders in anything like a ritual sense, nor, if they are so presented, whether the coolamon features as part of such a ritual. To a non-indigenous person such as me, the evocation of the coolamon reinforces the Lukan symbol of the manger as the feedbox that becomes the receptacle for the child, which suggests that the child is in some sense nourishing for the community. The manger and the coolamon and, in the *Bible moralisée* image, the Bible itself—as both Torah and Christian Bible—also mediate the touch of the semiotic, as a separation from the maternal body.[7] The adoption of the coolamon as an Aboriginal Christian symbol, and my appeal to it here, also touches on the agency of the Bible as material artefact in the history of colonization, the way the Bible touches on the bodies, communities and cultures of colonized and colonizer.

In the wake of colonial dispossession and displacement which is not past, one negotiation of meaning for Aboriginal Christians in this (post-)colonial context is an appeal to two laws, that parallels but differs from traditional Christian appeals to an old law, represented by the Torah, and a new, represented by Jesus of Nazareth as the Christ. Diane J. Austin-Broos relates a story in which an Aranda elder refers to two laws, Aranda law and God's/Bible law, seeing both as resources for survival, but differently in that while

*God: The Bible in the Tides of Empire* (Sheffield: Sheffield Phoenix Press, 2008), pp. 7-31; Deborah Bird Rose, *Reports from a Wild Country: Ethics for Decolonisation* (Sydney: University of New South Wales Press, 2004).

5. Jeremy Beckett, 'Aboriginal Histories, Aboriginal Myths: An Introduction', *Oceania* 65.2 (1994), pp. 97-115 (99).

6. Aboriginal Catholic Ministry Victoria has gifted this symbol of the coolamon to the wider Australian church for the liturgical celebration of Advent and Christmas. See Elizabeth Pike, 'The Power in the Story: Advent Leads Us to Christmas', *Madonna* (Nov.–Dec. 2001), pp. 27-28.

7. On the semiotic, language and the maternal, see the discussion in Chapter 2 above.

biblical religion has taught that Aranda law is not 'proper', God's law is lacking as it 'doesn't say anything about country'.[8] Warramirri elder David Burramurra also poses the question of the relationship between the God of the Bible and the land. Without the lens of biblical religion, 'would he [God] look like the natural world?'[9] Burramurra describes a sacred Yolngu word that is 'our word for God', encompassing 'ceremonial beliefs and cultural traditions' and having manifestations like 'the Bible, Cross, flying fox, or cuttlefish'.[10] This suggests to me that the Bible, as material artefact, interpretative story and interpreter of story, is assimilated to country, as one among many sources of life.

Ian McIntosh describes further some ways in which the Aboriginal community of Elcho Island negotiates meaning and survival in relation to their traditional beliefs and Christianity. He relates a story told by Buthimang, a senior member of the Wangurri clan at Elcho Island, that 'there were two types of Balanda [non-Aboriginal people]. One had a gun and the other a book (i.e. the Bible), and only the latter could be trusted'.[11] Nevertheless, he notes, 'The local view [is] that there is little respect among Balanda for Yolngu understandings or ways of doing things and yet Aborigines have needed to make substantial changes in their own ways to accommodate Balanda ideas and structures'.[12] As regards the Bible, one aspect of this accommodation has been in relation to language. In many cases, Aboriginal and Torres Strait Islander people have been introduced to the Bible in English, the language of the colonizer, as part of the process of cultural damage that accompanied colonial education.[13] Some attempts were made to translate the Bible into local languages. The translation of the Bible into Aranda language has impacted the language, shifting the meaning of some concepts, notably, for example, 'the moralization of various terms concerned

8. Diane J. Austin-Broos, '"Two Laws" Ontologies, Histories: Ways of Being Aranda (Aboriginal People) Today', *Australian Journal of Anthropology* 7 (1996), pp. 1-20 (11).

9. David Burramurra and Ian McIntosh, '*Motj* and the Nature of the Sacred', *Cultural Survival Quarterly* 26.2 (Summer) (2002), http://www.culturalsurvival.org/our-publications/csq/article/motj-and-nature-sacred. See also Rose, *Reports from a Wild Country*, p. 178.

10. Burramurra and McIntosh, '*Motj*'.

11. Ian McIntosh, 'Anthropology, Self Determination and Aboriginal Belief in the Christian God', *Oceania* 67 (1997), pp. 273-88 (276).

12. McIntosh, 'Anthropology, Self Determination', p. 286.

13. In 2007, the Kriol Bible was published in Australia. 'Kriol, an Australian Creole language developed out of contact between European settlers and the indigenous people in the northern regions of Australia is presently spoken by 30,000 people across the Top End'; see http://www.kriol.info/about_kriol_bible.php.

with physical well-being'.[14] In the nineteenth century with his Aboriginal mentor and friend Birabahn (Johnny Magill), Reverend Lancelot Threlkeld attempted to translate the Bible into the Awabakal language.[15] His translation of Lk. 2.28 appears in the epigraph to this chapter.[16] Where Threlkeld could not find words in the Awabakal language for concepts in the biblical text, he introduced Greek or Hebrew words.[17] Among his published research is an incomplete Awakabal–English lexicon.[18] While his project set out to respect the language and culture of the Awakabal, it did little to ensure the survival of the people whose language it celebrated.[19]

Indigenous writer Oodgeroo Noonuccal situates her writing as a material alternative to the Bible for her people, a translation of an oral Aboriginal voice in writing.[20] Anne Brewster relates:

> The decision to work with the written word was a conscious political decision for Noonuccal. She describes in an interview how old Aboriginal men would express themselves at public meetings through the Bible, and that the sight of this prompted her to write them 'a book they could call their own' ('Recording the Cries' 18). She describes seeing, after the publication of *We Are Going*, the same old man who used to quote the Bible, reciting her poetry at a meeting, despite the fact that he could 'neither read nor write; he had got his white friends to read it to him and had memorised it' (23). ... Noonuccal concluded her anecdote about the old man and how *We Are Going* replaced the Bible, with an explanation for the popularity of the book: 'for the first time the Aboriginals had a voice, a written voice' ('Recording the Cries' 19).[21]

Writing in response to an issue of the Friends of the Earth magazine *Chain Reaction*, which focused on the positive role faith traditions could play in

14. Austin-Broos, '"Two Laws"', p. 7. See also Brett, *Decolonizing God*, pp. 60-61. Concerning the way in which the call of a dove has been reinterpreted by Yolngu Bible translator Maratja Dhamarrandji, see Fiona Magowan, 'The Joy of Mourning: Resacralising "the Sacred" in the Music of Yolngu Christianity and an Aboriginal Theology', *Anthropological Forum* 9 (1999), p. 32.

15. David Andrew Roberts, '"Language to Save the Innocent": Reverend L. Threlkeld's Linguistic Mission', *Journal of the Royal Australian Historical Society* 94.2 (2008), pp. 107-25. See also Boer, *Last Stop*, pp. 160, 169-70.

16. L.E. Threkeld, *The Gospel by St Luke Translated into the Language of the Awabakal* (Sydney: Charles Potter, Government Printer, 1891).

17. L.E. Threkeld, *An Awabakal–English Lexicon to the Gospel by St Luke* (Sydney: Charles Potter, Government Printer, 1892).

18. Threkeld, *Awabakal–English Lexicon.*

19. Roberts, '"Language to Save the Innocent"', pp. 120-21. See also Boer, *Last Stop*, pp. 94-95.

20. Anne Brewster, 'Oodgeroo: Orator, Poet, Storyteller', *Australian Literary Studies* 16.4 (1994), pp. 92-104 (101).

21. Brewster, 'Oodgeroo', p. 101.

response to ecological crisis, Yorta Yorta elder Monica Morgan points out that religions such as Judaism, Christianity, Islam, and Buddhism are introduced to Australia.[22] They are 'man-made' insofar as they are not of the land.[23] She is strongly critical of Christianity:

> Christianity is especially divisive and dangerous. At its core is the need to control resources—it promotes wealth, elitism, the benefits of a few at the expense of the many; it is almost like a feudal system. It benefits a few and captures the rest—in effect becoming like slaves. Then the bounty of the earth becomes the property of those in charge.
>
> The Catholic church has been one of the worst. They have stolen the most from our peoples. They have store houses of sacred objects: Churingas, sacred stones, human remains and other objects, carefully taken and catalogued, our culture and history taken and archived; it's like stealing DNA because these objects are the very core of our being. And once they stole our objects, and controlled our symbols, they replaced them with their own—the cross, the Bible.[24]

Of the relationship of 'white fellas' to the land, she continues:

> They have brought their religion to this place and just rolled it over the top of what was here before, just like their gardens of plants and lawn are rolled over the top of the real plants. None of the introduced religions have evolved to the point where they understand where they are and what that means.[25]

Palawa womanist theologian Lee Miena Skye is similarly critical of the failure of white Australians to understand the spiritual being (which she calls 'spiritualness') of indigenous people, especially as regards their connection to country, a 'spiritualness' she regards as inherited through genetic memory in spite of colonial dispossession.[26]

This 'spiritualness', for Skye, is counter to a Western and colonialist dualistic framing of spirit in opposition to matter.[27] Skye describes the Christianity inculturated by indigenous women as different from the Christianity of the colonizer, 'presenting an image of Christ that is One-with-Creation'.[28] For Skye, the problem with the Bible is in its destructive misinterpretation by those who brought it to Australia.[29] She comments that for the Austral-

22. Monica Morgan, 'Colonising Religion', *Chain Reaction* Summer (2005/2006), pp. 36-37.

23. Morgan, 'Colonising Religion', pp. 36-37.

24. Morgan, 'Colonising Religion', p. 37.

25. Morgan, 'Colonising Religion', p. 37.

26. Lee Miena Skye, *Kerygmatics of the New Millennium: A Study of Australian Aboriginal Women's Christology* (Delhi: ISPCK, 2007), pp. 48-76 (66).

27. Skye, *Kerygmatics*, esp. p. 97.

28. Skye, *Kerygmatics*, pp. 48-76 (66).

29. Skye, *Kerygmatics*, esp. pp. 15, 82-83.

ian Aboriginal Christian women she interviewed and for herself, 'the Bible validated their "experience" of Christ; in other words, the Bible was not their "first" introduction to and experience of Christ'.[30] Their experience of Christ is embedded in the sacredness of the land and reflects the experience of their own suffering, which cannot be separated from the suffering of the land. Properly inculturated into country, biblical story is reshaped by these indigenous women and becomes part of an ongoing narrative of relationship to country and kin, which, Skye argues, can form the basis for an ecological Christology.[31]

Wiradjuri and Kamilaroi artist Michael Riley's images of the Bible pick up something of the tension that inheres in the touch of the Bible as a material artefact accompanying colonization. In his *flyblown* series, a Bible lies/floats open face down on a shallow puddle on red-brown earth. Another image in this series shows a dead galah on baked red-brown earth. In his *cloud* series, a Bible floats open face down against blue sky and luminous cloud. Other images in the series show a crow's left wing, split and open; a cow; a locust with wings open wide as if pinned to a board; a boomerang; and a feather, floating or positioned against a similar blue sky with white sometimes luminous cloud.[32] The audio commentary that accompanies *untitled* [*bible*] from the *cloud* series says:

> The Church had a seminal impact on Michael Riley's childhood through the weekly visits of the Aboriginal Inland Mission. Michael's mother, Dorothy, recalled how Michael loved to attend Sunday School. However, in his later years, Riley referred to his Christian experience as 'creepy'. The floating Bible appears in other photographic series, often associated with images of the cross set against a brooding sky. In this series of photographs, the Bible, identified by the cross on the cover, floats alone. The book is open. Its pages are invisible behind the cover and the cross is aimed downwards like an arrow, like a weapon.[33]

In Riley's *flyblown* and the *cloud* series, the Bible appears as a material artefact in parallel and contrast with images of sky, earth, colonization, death, drought, rain and spirit. This multiple imagery echoes the multiplicity of the touch of the Bible on people and country.

Aboriginal and Torres Strait Islander people have never ceded sovereignty to their colonizers. In my limited understanding, such indigenous sovereignty

30. Skye, *Kerygmatics*, p. 69.

31. Skye, *Kerygmatics*, esp. pp. 77-98.

32. For a retrospective of Riley's work, including the images cited, see Brenda L. Croft, *Michael Riley, Sights Unseen* (Canberra: National Gallery of Australia, 2006).

33. Transcribed from audio commentary on Michael Riley's *untitled* [*bible*] from the series *cloud*, National Gallery of Australia, Canberra, 'Michael Riley, Sights Unseen', www.nga.gov.au/Exhibition/RILEY.

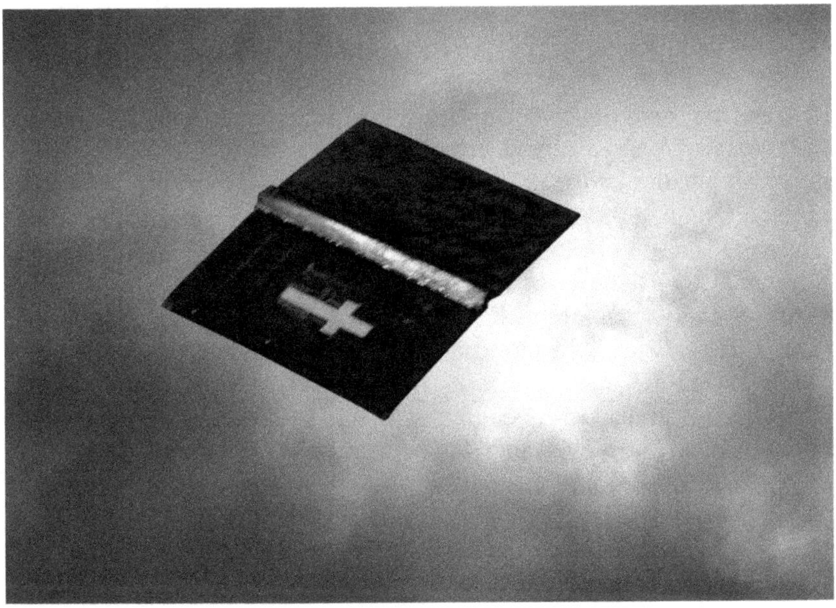

Fig. 2. Michael Riley, *untitled [bible]* from the *cloud* series, National Gallery of Australia, Canberra.


in Australia inheres in a deep, experiential relationship of embeddedness in, and responsibility for, country, to which the colonizers (and I include myself) were and are almost universally blind. Because this sovereignty is about indigenous being-in-place, it cannot be ceded. As Skye points out, white Australia routinely and effectively denies such indigenous being-in-place; this denial is a violent touch on Aboriginal and Torres Strait Islander bodies and communities.[34] Because of the relationship between people and country, this denial also touches violently on the land.[35] The Bible as a material artefact of colonization is implicated in this contact.

### *Contact: Bodies and Communities, Writing and Land*

That this impact of the Bible as a material artefact of the colonizer can fall under the term 'contact' occurs because the term itself is in debt to the more general sense of contact as the touch of one person or thing on another. In this section, I explore the notion of touch with particular reference to rep-

34. Skye, *Kerygmatics*, esp. pp. 1-24.
35. Skye, *Kerygmatics*, esp. pp. 1-24.

resentations of touch in the Gospel of Luke (a Gospel that, in being translated into Awakabal, is part of a history of colonial contact). Touch is the primary sense insofar as all the senses depend on touch (Aristotle, *De an.* 3.13) and are forms of contact, of being touched by, and touching, another.[36] Such contact is inescapable: the contact of my feet with my socks; of my eyes with photons of light, indeterminate as they may be; of air on skin, molecules surging into nostrils; of sound waves pressing against the drum of an ear; the always being-in-contact of matter with other matter; the touch of one human on another, of one culture on another.[37]

As a primary agent of touch, the hand (ἡ χείρ) appears several times in Luke. Jesus extends his hand to touch as part of healing (5.13); he takes a child's hand as part of her resuscitation (8.54); Jesus, and in Acts the disciples, lays on hands in healing (4.40; 13.13; Acts 6.6; 8.17, 19; 9.12, 17; 13.3; 19.6; 28.8). The hands can be instruments of violent touch (9.44; 20.19; 21.12; 22.53; 24.7); the hand of the betrayer rests on the table at the Last Supper (22.21). As election and blessing, the hand of God is on the infant John the Baptist (1.66). The hand of Jesus can denote his role as eschatological harvester and judge (3.17). Angelic hands may be protective (4.11). The disciples use their hands to pick and prepare grain to eat on a Sabbath day (6.1); in juxtaposition, on another Sabbath Jesus heals a man's withered hand (6.6-11). The dying Jesus commends himself into the hands of God (23.46); the risen Jesus offers his hands and feet to be touched (24.39, 40); he raises his hands in blessing (24.50).

In his own touching on Jean-Luc Nancy, Jacques Derrida comments on Jesus as the Toucher who is touched.[38] For Derrida, 'the Gospels present the Christic body not only as a body of light and revelation but, in a hardly less essential way, as a body touching as much as touched, as flesh that is touched-touching. Between life and death.'[39] A middle verb, the Greek ἅπτομαι means to touch or take hold of and can refer to touch as 'a means of conveying a blessing', but also as bringing harm or injury (BAGD, 102-103). In Luke ἅπτομαι is used of Jesus touching: a leper (5.13); a bier (7.14); children (18.15); the ear of the high priest's slave (22.50). There is little sense in any of these cases that the touch is violent, unless it is the violence of transformation (even when transformation is healing or restorative). Other more precise words refer to violent touch: to whip (μαστιγόω,

36. Jean-Luc Nancy, *The Sense of the World* (trans. Jeffrey S. Librett; Minneapolis: University of Minnesota Press, 1997), pp. 15, 63.

37. Jean-Luc Nancy, 'Corpus', in *The Birth to Presence* (trans. Brian Holmes *et al.*; Meridian; Crossing Aesthetics; Stanford, CA: Stanford University Press, 1993), p. 203.

38. Jacques Derrida, *On Touching—Jean-Luc Nancy* (trans. Christine Irizarry; Meridian; Crossing Aesthetics; Stanford, CA: Stanford University Press, 2005), p. 100.

39. Derrida, *On Touching*, pp. 99-100.

18.33), to beat (δέρω, 22.63), to strike (παίω, 22.64), to discipline or scourge (παιδεύω, 23.16, 22). These words describe the power the agents of the Roman Empire wield against the body of Jesus.

The verb ἅπτομαι is also used of people touching Jesus, for example, the crowd (6.19), the woman who washes and anoints his feet (7.39) and the woman with the flow of blood (8.44-47). In these instances when he is touched, Jesus responds. In response to the desire of the crowds to touch him, Jesus speaks the beatitudes and woes of 6.20-26. In Luke 8 when a bleeding woman who is probably close to death touches him seeking healing, Jesus feels her touch as an outpouring of power from him (8.46).[40] Jesus' response to the woman's touch suggests the ambiguity of a touch that is at once mutual and unequal. A little earlier in the narrative, the Lukan Jesus is challenged by the unspoken question of why he allowed a woman considered to be a sinner to touch him. In response he speaks of a creditor and two debtors, of forgiveness and love (7.40-47), of his receipt of the woman's touch as an act of loving hospitality prompted by the divine hospitality of forgiveness (7.44-47).[41] While underscored with difference, the reciprocity of their touch brings their bodies into being in a particular time and place as 'absolutely separated and shared'.[42]

Derrida takes up a phrase from Nancy, *se toucher toi*, 'to self-touch you', to describe the way in which in touching the other I am already touching myself, but also the way in which I cannot touch myself without touching or being in touch with an other, even if that other is my own skin. 'To touch', writes Derrida, 'so one believes, amounts therefore to letting oneself be touched by what one touches....'[43] Moreover, through touching I experience myself as tangible (as a being touched by another). When in Luke 8 a woman touches Jesus, he feels his power expended (8.46). Despite her apparent timidity, the touch initiated by the woman is an act of power that draws forth his power to heal. She consents to the risky intersubjectivity of touch, of self-touching another. Not only is she touched by her touching him, but the Lukan Jesus is given to himself by the touch of the woman.[44]

40. Annette Weissenrieder, 'The Plague of Uncleanness? The Ancient Illness Construct "Issue of Blood" in Luke 8:43-48', in *The Social Setting of Jesus and the Gospels* (ed. Wolfgang Stegemann, Bruce J. Malina and Gerd Theissen; Minneapolis: Fortress Press, 2002), pp. 207-22.

41. Byrne, *Hospitality of God*, pp. 73-76.

42. Nancy, 'Corpus', p. 204; Nancy, *Sense of the World*, p. 60.

43. Jacques Derrida, '*Le toucher*', *Paragraph* 16.2 (1993), pp. 122-57 (136); Nancy, *Corpus*, p. 45.

44. Cf. Jean-Louis Chrétien, *The Call and the Response* (trans. Anne A. Davenport; New York: Fordham University Press, 2004), pp. 85-86, 120.

Nancy extends this mutuality of touching/being touched by the human other. The inescapability of the simplest touch or contact between things and the pervasiveness of the phenomenon of touch arise from and express 'the being-toward of one thing toward the other' that constitutes the sense of the world.[45] This 'being-toward' echoes the quality of interconnectedness expressed in the Earth Bible ecojustice principle: 'Earth is a community of interconnected living things that are mutually dependent on each other for life and survival.'[46] As Nancy notes, 'There is no *intact* matter; if there were, there would be nothing'.[47]

The interconnectedness expressed in the language of touch refers not only to physical contact—flesh to flesh, flesh to stone, even stone to soil—but also to the effects of writing. Being touched, gently, violently, or passionately (even tactlessly) by an action, conversation or writing *is* a physical touching, felt in the viscera of the human body. Luke makes this connection in the Emmaus story, where the two whom Jesus encounters on the road say to each other, 'Were not our hearts burning within us while he was talking to us on the road, while he was opening the scriptures to us?' (24.32). The writings that carry the touch of myriad material artefacts and embodied memories touch the bodies of Jesus and his companions on the road.

The pattern of call and response, focused in the divine visitation in Jesus, is mediated by a touch in which 'the flesh listens'.[48] The words of the risen Jesus are felt as a 'burning' in the heart (ἡ καρδία ἡμῶν καιομένη, 24.32). The verb καίω means to burn or burn up. Another word not used here but closely related to touch means to ignite, namely ἅπτω, from which the middle ἅπτομαι comes. The burning of the heart suggests a touch that is transformative, as fire transforms. Derrida writes of the heart as always the heart of the other, the other heart.[49] The two on the road to Emmaus say to each other 'our heart'; the heart that burns here in response to a word is a singular shared heart; for each it is the heart of the other.[50] Touching/being touched by the other is the basis of shared life, that is, community.

For Rosalyn Diprose, the uniqueness and difference of bodies is the 'life-blood' of community: 'Community lives on difference, on the touch of

45. Nancy, *Sense of the World*, p. 15.

46. Habel (ed.), *Readings from the Perspective of Earth*, p. 24. See also Sallie McFague, *Super, Natural Christians: How We Should Love Nature* (London: SCM Press, 1997), pp. 93-95.

47. Nancy, 'Corpus', p. 203, emphasis added.

48. Chrétien, *Call and the Response*, p. 130.

49. Derrida, *On Touching*, p. 283.

50. As noted in Chapter 2, for Luke the ear/heart/earth intersect as places of response to the word/seed.

difference of other bodies that cannot be assimilated to mine.'[51] She explains, 'The difference community lives from is the other's difference that I cannot grasp but that initiates my movement towards the other and towards the world.'[52] Diprose describes the touch of bodies on bodies as 'a cut that opens bodies to each other in community'.[53] Much as ancient writing on a tablet or skin was an inscription (a cut), the cut that occurs in the touching and being touched at the limit that is the skin is a writing in one's blood.[54] By referring to touch as a cut, Diprose echoes Derrida's assertion of the violence pertaining in even the most tactful touch.[55] Considering the treatment of asylum seekers in Australia, Diprose distinguishes between the trace of violence in the tactful touch that is necessary for the corporeal sociality of community, and *a touch that violates* the other in the name of community, for example, through hate speech or laws enacted to excise from the community a particular group identified as alien.[56] As Skye argues, this latter touch is destructive of bodies and communities, country and land.[57]

Writing in relation to the contemporary plight of refugees throughout the world, Nancy describes compassion as a kind of *contact* that counters violence:

> What I am talking about is compassion, but not a compassion as a pity that feels sorry for itself and feeds on itself. Com-passion is the contagion, the contact of being with one another in this turmoil. Compassion is not altruism, nor is it identification; it is the disturbance of violent relatedness.[58]

The violent relatedness of colonization, the ongoing violence of contact it occasions and the treatment of more-than-human others as expendable adjuncts to our existence form a contemporary context for the question of touch in, and of, Luke and the extent to which the Lukan text can reinforce and disturb such patterns of violent relatedness.

51. Rosalyn Diprose, 'The Hand That Writes Community in Blood', *Cultural Studies Review* (*Affective Community,* ed. Chris Healy, Stephen Muecke and Linnell Secomb) 9 (2003), pp. 35-50 (39).

52. Diprose, 'Hand That Writes', p. 40.

53. Diprose, 'Hand That Writes', p. 36.

54. Diprose, 'Hand That Writes', pp. 36, 45.

55. Derrida, '*Le toucher*', pp. 122-57; Jacques Derrida, *Le toucher, Jean-Luc Nancy* (Paris: Galilée, 2000); Derrida, *On Touching*. See also Kevin Hart, 'Horizons and Folds: Elizabeth Presa', *Contretemps* 2 (2001), pp. 171-75.

56. Diprose is referring particularly to the policies of the Howard Coalition government, especially between 2001 and 2007, but her remarks could be applied to more recent Labor government policies concerning asylum seekers arriving by boat.

57. Skye, *Kerygmatics*, pp. 5-23.

58. Jean-Luc Nancy, *Being Singular Plural* (trans. Robert D. Richardson and Anne E. O'Byrne; Meridian; Crossing Aesthetics; Stanford: Stanford University Press, 2000), p. xiii.

### *Patterns of Touch in the Gospel of Luke*

For Luke, the theme of divine hospitality forms a pattern in which compassion, divine and human, is mediated by touch felt in the gut. Early in the Gospel of Luke, Zechariah proclaims a divine visitation that brings liberation (1.68), an arrival that delivers from violent touch: the hand (ἐκ χειρός) of enemies, those who hate (1.71, 74). Imaged as the daily visitation of the sun, this visitation heralds the gut-felt mercies (σπλάγχνα ἐλέους) of the divine (1.78). Gut-felt mercies find an echo in the verb σπλαγχνίζομαι, 'to have compassion' or 'feel sympathy', literally 'to be moved in the guts'. The stem of the Greek verb σπλαγχνίζομαι, 'to have compassion' or 'feel sympathy for' is related to the noun σπλάγχνον, meaning 'inward parts' or 'entrails', sometimes also 'womb', and refers figuratively to the seat of the emotions, and thus echoes with the crossing between κοιλία (womb) and καρδία (heart) that Luke entertains (BAGD, 762-63).[59]

Σπλαγχνίζομαι occurs three times in the Lukan narrative (7.13; 10.33; 15.20). The first occurrence is in the story of the restoration of the widow's son outside the town gate of Nain (7.11-17); the second in the parable of the Good Samaritan (10.25-37); the third in the parable of the Prodigal Son (15.11-31). In each case, there is a moment, which is also a movement, of compassion. Luke describes a situation in which someone is an extremity: a widow whose only son has just died (7.12); a person who has been robbed and beaten and left half-dead by the roadside, whom passers-by see but ignore (10.30-32); a younger son who has squandered his share of the family estate only to return destitute and ashamed (15.11-19).[60] Each time someone sees: Jesus sees the widow (7.13); a Samaritan sees the half-dead stranger (10.33); the father sees in the distance his son (15.20). Each is physically moved by compassion (7.13; 10.33; 15.20) toward the other (7.14; 10.34; 15.20).

Prompted by an inner touch, the movement is directed toward an outward touch: Jesus touches the bier (ἥψατο τῆς σοροῦ, 7.14); the Samaritan bandages the person's wounds (κατέδησεν τὰ τραύματα, 10.34); the father falls on the son's neck and kisses him (ἐπέπεσεν ἐπὶ τὸν τράχηλον αὐτοῦ καὶ κατεφίλησεν αὐτόν, 15.20). A restoration follows this compassionate contact. In 7.16 the crowd recognizes this movement of compassion as a divine

59. In Hebrew, the connection between compassion (רחמים) and womb (רחם) is even more pronounced. See Thomas Staubli and Silvia Schroer, *Body Symbolism in the Bible* (trans. Linda M. Maloney; Collegeville, MN: Liturgical Press, 2001), pp. 71-73. On the crossing between κοιλία (womb) and καρδία (heart) (BAGD, 437); see also Elvey, *Ecological Feminist Reading*, p. 182.

60. Derrida also notes the first of these three gut-felt movements, to touch; Derrida, *On Touching*, p. 101.

visitation. When read in conjunction with the Benedictus, where the gut-felt mercies of God signify and accompany a divine visitation, this pattern of compassionate responsiveness in 7.11-17; 10.30-37; and 15.11-24 is also a pattern of divine visitation expressed in a touched-touching, a contact.[61]

In the Lukan narrative the compassion that touches the other, that makes compassionate contact with the other, is predicated on a certain kind of seeing. The seeing that prompts compassion stands in contrast to other kinds of seeing. From an ecotheological perspective, Sallie McFague distinguishes between the arrogant and the loving eye.[62] '[T]he ecological model of the self' which gives rise to the 'loving or attentive eye' is grounded in touch as the primary sense.[63] In this model attentiveness to the other—both human and other-than-human—has characteristics of 'intimacy and distance, with affection and respect for difference'.[64] In the story world of the parable, the seeing of the Samaritan (10.33) stands in contrast to the seeing of the priest (10.31) and the Levite (10.32). For these latter two, seeing prompts not compassion but neglect of the other. In 7.36-50, where the Lukan Jesus receives the loving hospitality of the woman's touch, seeing is also at issue. The seeing of a Pharisee named Simon prompts a misjudgment of the woman and a misinterpretation of her touch (7.39). In the question 'Do you see this woman?' (7.44), Simon is challenged to see as the Lukan Jesus sees and to recognize the visitation of God in the hospitality both of the woman's touch and of divine forgiveness.[65] Elsewhere in Luke, seeing and knowing stand in parallel (19.42); seeing prompts knowing (21.30-31). What is needful is to know the time of the visitation (of God) (19.44). Not knowing this moment of divine hospitality (19.44), not knowing and seeing 'the things that make for peace' (19.42), is to be implicated in a pattern of violent relatedness manifest historically in the destruction of Jerusalem (19.43-44). Jesus' seeing the city prompts his compassionate grief (19.41).[66]

61. Concerning this pattern of compassionate responsiveness, see further Anne Elvey, 'To Bear the Other: Toward a Passionate Compassion (an Ecological Feminist Reading of Luke 10:25-37)', in *Sea Changes: Journal of Women Scholars of Religion and Theology* 1 (2001), http://www.wsrt.com.au/seachanges/volume1/elveyframes.html.

62. McFague, *Super, Natural Christians*, pp. 67-117.

63. McFague, *Super, Natural Christians*, p. 116.

64. McFague, *Super, Natural Christians*, p. 116.

65. Barbara E. Reid, '"Do You See This Woman?" A Liberative Look at Luke 7.36-50 and Strategies for Reading Other Lukan Stories against the Grain', in *A Feminist Companion to Luke* (ed. Amy-Jill Levine with Marianne Blickenstaff; London: Sheffield Academic Press, 2002), pp. 106-20 (110).

66. In the context, too, of the destruction of the Temple, there is in *3 Enoch* 48A a wonderful apocalyptic image of the relationship between touch and the divine visitation of compassionate grief: the weeping hand of God (*3 Enoch* 48A.4). But here the

In this representation of the gaze, the one *seeing* is touched or better grasped in the guts by compassion for the other. Such a gaze disrupts the violent relatedness that sees the other within the ambit of the same, appropriating the other to the same or denying the claim of the other: the violent relatedness of a master-slave imaginary and practice, of the colonizer over the colonized. Within the Lukan narrative, approved characters such as Jesus, the Good Samaritan and the father of the Prodigal Son respond to the claim of the other in a pattern of touch. Through the contact of sight, the person seeing is moved to compassion—a touch felt in the guts—and this internal touch prompts the person to touch the other (7.13-14; 10.33-34; 15.20; see also 13.12-13).

There are several aspects to the touch of the other within these narratives. First, according to Jewish custom there is a question of ritual uncleanness, which is as I understand it a question of bodily integrity and sometimes also (metaphorically at least) of moral integrity. Scholars are divided on the question of the role first-century CE systems of purity (both in Jewish and Greek contexts) play in Luke, and it is likely that this is not a key focus of these and other Lukan narratives.[67] A more important aspect of this touch is its excess.[68] For example, in the parable of the Good Samaritan, the Samaritan's actions surpass what would be expected even in regard to one's neighbour. They surprise 'not by unfulfillment but by overfulfillment'.[69] Most importantly for my argument, in each narrative, the protagonist touches (on) death.

Jesus touches a bier, a litter bearing a corpse (7.14); the Samaritan touches a person who is 'half-dead', who might very soon die (10.30, 34); the father embraces a son who has been living dissolutely, working with pigs and eating their food, who has in the father's words been dead (νεκρός, 15.24). What is touched is *the other's death.* To touch with compassion,

tears that fall from the divine hand bring destruction upon earth before a merciful Messianic advent (*3 Enoch* 48A.4-10). See James H. Charlesworth (ed.), *The Old Testament Pseudepigrapha.*I. *Apocalyptic Literature and Testaments* (Garden City, NY: Doubleday, 1983), pp. 300-302; Staubli and Schroer, *Body Symbolism*, pp. 179-80.

67. For discussion of the issue of purity in the first-century CE world of the Gospel of Luke, see Bruce J. Malina, *The New Testament World: Insights from Cultural Anthropology* (Louisville, KY: Westminster John Knox, 3rd, rev. and exp. edn, 2001), pp. 161-97; Jerome H. Neyrey, 'Clean/Unclean, Pure/Polluted and Holy/Profane: The Idea and System of Purity', in *The Social Sciences and New Testament Interpretation* (ed. Richard Rohrbaugh; Peabody, MA: Hendrickson, 1996), pp. 80-104; Weissenrieder, 'Plague of Uncleanness?'

68. Sally B. Purvis, 'Mothers, Neighbours and Strangers: Another Look at Agape', *JFSR* 7 (1991), pp. 19-34; Byrne, *Hospitality of God*, pp. 129-30; Elvey, 'To Bear the Other'.

69. Purvis, 'Mothers, Neighbours', p. 30.

and so to touch the death of the other, is marked by an excess in which the self is never solely singular, but in Nancy's terms 'singular plural'.[70] In this context, to touch compassionately is to be open, to offer oneself in a particular way to the in-breaking (*effraction*) of the other.[71] In such touching, I am drawn in the direction of 'consenting to the body'.[72] To so consent is to be open precisely to the otherness of the corporeal and hence also to death.[73] Compassion signals an openness to the in-breaking of the other whereby in touching the other I touch myself, but this touch is an exposure to death—to finitude—both the other's and my own. In touching the death of the other, I touch my own mortality.[74]

The proximity of touch masks the material interval (air or water) between toucher and touched.[75] Contact requires but ignores this interval.[76] The representation of touch in a pattern of compassionate responsiveness in Luke as touching the death of the other suggests that this material interval is marked by mortality, both as the finitude of the toucher and the touched and what is at stake in touching any other. With Levinas in mind, I would suggest that touching another always resonates with the imperative 'thou shalt not murder'. For Luce Irigaray reading Levinas critically, the death of the other, and especially woman as other or the other as woman, inheres in a caress that assimilates the other to the same, the woman to the man.[77] In the frame of (post-) colonial contact, the touch of the other is inhabited by the other's death: assimilation, damage to culture, loss of traditional languages, appropriation of country, and genocide. In an ecological frame, touching–being touched by the other is resonant with the death of species and the destruction of habitats, both for other species and future generations of our own.

The power of touch to harm or to heal, to destroy or to further life, is embedded in the mutuality of a sense that is intrinsically relational. Within the pattern of compassionate responsiveness outlined above, when Jesus touches the bier, immediately the bearers stand still (7.14). In the parable of the Good Samaritan, we do not hear any response from the other to the touch of the Samaritan (10.34), but his actions undo the violent touch of

70. Nancy, *Being Singular Plural,* pp, 1-99.

71. Derrida, '*Le toucher*', p. 137.

72. Derrida, '*Le toucher*', p. 137; Nancy, *Corpus*, p. 47.

73. Derrida, '*Le toucher*', p. 139.

74. Cf. John Donne, 'Meditation XVII *Nunc lento sonitu dicunt, morieris*', *Devotions upon Emergent Occasions* (1624), www.luminarium.org/sevenlit/donne/meditation17.php.

75. Chrétien, *Call and the Response*, pp. 88-89.

76. Chrétien, *Call and the Response*, pp. 88-89.

77. Luce Irigaray, *An Ethics of Sexual Difference* (trans. Carolyn Burke and Gillian C. Gill; Ithaca, NY: Cornell University Press, 1993), pp. 185-217 (210-14).

the robbers (10.30). In the parable of the Prodigal Son, the son responds to the father's embrace with his prepared speech concerning his unworthiness (15.21).

To touch the other, to touch the other's death and so my own, is also not to touch. In the Lukan narrative three figures, moved by compassion, touch the other, and in touching the other who is dead, near-death, or socially or morally dead touch (on) the death of the other. But what is touched is also not death: Jesus touches a bier not a dead body; the Samaritan touches someone near-death but alive; the father embraces a living son. In each case the protagonist both touches and does not touch the death of the other. This Lukan patterning of touch describes a particular mode of sociality or interconnectedness between self and other; touched by the sight of the other, I feel the internal grasp of compassion and am prompted to touch the other. So touching the other, I touch (and do not touch) the other's death and am touched (impossibly) in turn by my own mortality, that reality of human embodiment and embeddedness in the Earth community before which we tremble and toward which we tend whether we wish it or not. Moreover, the text touches me as reader through a representation of touch as touching (and not touching) death, as putting the one who touches in touch with her or his own mortality—a being-in-touch with human embodiment and embeddedness in the Earth community made possible by the other who calls forth compassion.

## *Touching (on) Death in the Gospel of Luke*

The text touches its readers through the way it touches not only *on* touch and compassion but also *on* death. In the Lukan narrative, the representation of death is problematic in at least two ways. First, the narrative construction of its other in relation to the death of Jesus can be taken up in anti-Jewish polemic and violence. Second, the notion of resurrection can valorize an otherworldly life beyond death, which devalues Earth. With these problems in mind, I turn now to consider some ways in which the Lukan narrative touches on death.

### *Death as Divine Necessity*

There are many places in which the Lukan narrative touches on death (for example, 1.79; 2.26; 7.11-17, 22; 8.42, 52-53; 9.7, 27, 60; 15.24, 32; 16.22, 30-31; 20.28-29, 31-32, 35-38; 21.16; 22.33; 23.15, 22), but a particular death underwrites the text. The suffering, rejection, death and raising of the Lukan Jesus are characterized as a divine necessity, indicated by the Greek δεῖ (9.22; 17.25; 22.37; 24.7, 26).[78] Within the Gospel of Luke, there is a concatenation between themes of divine necessity, purpose, visitation and hospitality. Compassion is a mark or trace of divine visitation. God arrives in the person of a guest to whom hospitality is due. In the narratives I have addressed, compassion is a form of hospitality. Moreover, in the course of the Lukan narrative, in welcoming this divine visitation one receives the hospitality of God.[79]

As Derrida and Dufourmantelle suggest, however, within the dynamic of hospitality there is a crossing between host and *hostis*, host and enemy.[80] In the characterization of the Pharisees in Luke and Acts this crossing between host and enemy also occurs.[81] The ambiguous character of visitation is evident in the Lukan characterization of Jerusalem. Doubly the site of death, the death of Jesus and the later destruction of the city itself by the Romans in 70 CE (21.20-27), Jerusalem becomes the spatial focus of the Lukan divine necessity (18.31-33; see also 13.22, 33; 17.11; 19.11, 28; cf. 9.57). More particularly for Luke, Jerusalem is the site of failure of hospitality toward Jesus.

From the Lukan perspective, whereby every occurrence from the death of individuals to the destruction of cities is governed by the divine purpose, this failure is the reason for the later destruction of the city (19.41-44; cf. 21.20-27). This Lukan interpretation of the fall of Jerusalem as consequent on a refusal of divine hospitality gives rise to violent relatedness exemplified in the othering of the Pharisees and lawyers (7.30) and tends to elide Roman responsibility for Jesus' execution and the destruction of the city.[82] But in 10.25, a figure of these others, a lawyer, poses a question that allows for the telling of the parable of the Good Samaritan and a redefinition of the other. As suggested above, here the violent relatedness of othering is called into question by compassionate responsiveness. While the writing that is the Gospel of Luke might be thought to touch violently on the other, to touch the other with violence, to touch (on) the death of the other through violence, this writing also calls into question such violent contact and offers

78. On the force of the divine δεῖ in the Gospel of Luke, see Cosgrove, 'Divine Δεῖ', pp. 168-90.

79. Byrne, *Hospitality of God.*

80. Jacques Derrida and Anne Dufourmantelle, *Of Hospitality* (trans. Rachel Bowlby; Cultural Memory in the Present; Stanford, CA: Stanford University Press, 2000).

81. Note particularly Gowler's *Host, Guest, Enemy and Friend.*

82. Anne Elvey, 'Legacies of Violence toward the Other: Toward a Consideration of the Outsider within the Lukan Narrative', *Colloquium: The Australian and New Zealand Theological Review* 34 (2002), pp. 21-34. For an alternative view of Luke's representation of Jerusalem, see Merrill Kitchen, 'The Good News of Restoration: Reading Luke–Acts Then and Now', *Pacifica* 23 (2010), pp. 157-72.

a pattern of compassionate responsiveness: a gut-felt impetus toward the mortal other. This mortality is already a human necessity, part of the material givenness of the Earth-being of humankind.

*The Materiality of Death*

As Val Plumwood points out, however, from an ecological perspective representations of death in Western and Christian thought are at best ambiguous:

> For both Platonic and Christian systems, the meaning of death is that the meaning of human life is elsewhere, not to be found in the earth or in human life as part of nature, but in a separate realm accessible only to humans (and only to certain chosen of these), the world of the Forms and the world of heaven. The salvation awaiting them beyond and above the world of nature, a fate marked out for humans alone, confirms their difference and separation from the world of nature, and their destiny as one apart from that of other species.[83]

In what ways then are we to understand the human necessity of death in the Gospel of Luke? Within the Lukan narrative, the human necessity of death is multifaceted. There are frequent references to violent death or the threat of violent death at the hands of others (for example, 9.22), by way of accident (for example, 13.4), or through natural disaster such as a storm (for example, 8.24). In Luke's use of the verb ἀπόλλυμι there is a correlation between death (6.9; 11.51; 13.33; 19.47), material destruction (5.37) and loss (15.4, 6, 9, 17, 24, 32; 19.10). These themes of death, destruction and loss come together in the sayings concerning eschatological expectation in 17.22-37. The Lukan narrative distinguishes between death as destruction of the body (12.4) and a metaphorical death or loss of one's self (ψυχή) occasioned by personal action and divine judgment (9.12; 12.5; 13.3, 5; 17.33). Underlying this distinction is a first-century CE apocalyptic imaginary in which death is not the end of the human story, but where divine judgment figures not only in an end-time scenario but also for individuals in a life after death (16.19-31). Within this imaginary, death is also a metaphor for the imprisonment of sin (1.79; cf. Ps. 107.10).[84] For the Lukan Jesus life after death is continuous with, but qualitatively different from, everyday human life (20.27-40).

Nonetheless, in Luke the language surrounding death is sensually material. A person sees and tastes death (2.26; 9.27). The reader is mortal (9.27; 21.16). Tragic deaths are not themselves the result of divine judgment or punishment (13.1-5). Just as the Lukan God has power to open the womb (1.25; cf. Gen. 29.31; 30.22), this God has authority over death. Within

83. Plumwood, *Feminism and the Mastery of Nature*, p. 100.

84. Joseph A. Fitzmyer, *The Gospel according to Luke I–IX: Introduction, Translation, and Notes* (AB; New York: Doubleday, 1981), p. 388.

the Lukan narrative, the raising of the dead is one of the signs Jesus offers John's disciples concerning his advent (7.22); it is a sign of divine visitation (7.16). In the tragedy of deaths that occur through patterns of violent relatedness between humans, a divine purpose is also at work (11.49; 13.31-35). This is particularly the case in the death of Jesus, which (as already noted) Luke interprets as a divine necessity (9.22; 17.25; 22.37; 24.7, 26).

### *The Death of Jesus*

Looking at the Lukan passion narrative with an eye to the materiality of Jesus' death (22.1–23.56), I am struck first by the way in which this movement toward death—situated for Luke in the space and time of a Passover meal—is already in debt to another death, the ritual slaughter of the Passover lamb. That this death is embedded within the logic of the text, the logic of a divine necessity, is seen in 22.7:

> He sent Peter and John saying, 'It is necessary (ἔδει) to sacrifice/slaughter the Passover lamb.'

Here θύεσθαι from θύω refers to the ritual slaughter of τὸ πάσχα, the Passover lamb. The word πάσχα is repeated six times until the slaughter of the lamb, the eating of its meat, and the imminent suffering (22.15) of Jesus form a well-know metonymy, such that Jesus becomes the paschal sacrifice, the body given and the blood shed are his (22.19-20). Through the motif of divine necessity and the metonymy of human and other-than-human animal bodies, the narrative connects the 'destiny' of the human representative, Jesus, and other species, represented in the lamb.[85]

There is a change, too, in that instead of the body of the animal, what Jesus shares are cups and bread.[86] There is also question of whether the Lukan Jesus joins in eating and drinking (22.15).[87] Jesus *will* eat in the appearance narrative of 24.36-43, but there the emphasis on the physicality of the body in v. 43 is overtaken by a focus on the word (24.44-47). But as the narrative of Luke 22 continues, in the hand of the betrayer (22.21) and the necessity of swords (22.36-38) there are intimations of a violent touch. The cup returns as a symbol of divine purpose (22.42). In what is probably an addition to the text, the body and an interrelationship with earth are once more foregrounded when in agony Jesus' sweat falls as blood on the earth (22.44).

85. Cf. Carol J. Adams and Marjorie Procter-Smith, 'Taking Life or "Taking on Life"?', in *Ecofeminism and the Sacred* (ed. Carol J. Adams; New York: Continuum, 1994), pp. 295-310 (306).

86. See also John Berkman, 'The Consumption of Animals and the Catholic Tradition', in *Food for Thought: The Debate over Eating Meat* (ed. Steve F. Sapontzis; New York: Prometheus Books, 2004), pp. 198-208 (203).

87. Ringe, *Luke*, p. 261.

In the passion narrative proper, however, the body is all but absent. Gregory Sterling and others argue that the text presents the death of Jesus as a noble death, in the tradition of the deaths of Socrates and of Jewish martyrs.[88] The everyday human necessity of death is overshadowed not only by a divine necessity but also by the apparent 'calmness' with which the innocent man undergoes his execution.[89] Nevertheless, within the passion narrative, there are repeated indications of violent touch (22.21; 22.36-38, 53, 54, 63). The violence of the hands is matched by the violence of the tongue (22.63-64) and of words that authorize a violent touch (23.16, 22, 23-25).

In the Gospel of Luke, the interplay between body and word is intimate and complex. From the multiple intimacies of the meal where the words of the Lukan Jesus bring together body and bread (22.19), cup and blood (22.20), and the touch of betrayal (22.21), the narrative moves to the words of the Lukan Pilate and the crowds that bring violence and death to the body of Jesus (23.13-25). But both in between and after, the words of the Luke's narrative serve to efface the suffering body. A movement from body to word has already occurred in 8.21 and more particularly in 11.27-28 in relation to the maternal body. There is one moment in the passion narrative, however, when the bodies of women come to the fore as markers of the suffering to come (23.27-31). But as the Lukan Jesus is crucified there is no description of the body, of the physical process of execution, no crying out 'I thirst' (23.32-43; cf. Jn 19.28).

As death approaches, however, there is resonance in the Earth community: darkness comes over the land; the sun that dawned in Luke 1 with the visitation of divine compassion is eclipsed (23.44-45). Then the body, which has been largely absent in the passion narrative, becomes focal in death. Joseph of Arimathea goes to Pilate to ask for the body (23.52). Like the Lukan Mary at the birth of Jesus, he takes it, wraps it and lays it (23.53; cf. 2.7). Some women take note of the position of the body in the tomb (23.55). Their return to the empty tomb after the Sabbath prompts the question, 'Where is the body?' (24.3, 23).

### *The Body in Death*

In coming to minister to the dead body of Jesus, the women arrive seeking to touch an absence. In the face of the empty tomb, this absence takes on a different character. The absence of the living Jesus becomes the absence of the

88. Gregory E Sterling, '*Mors Philosophi*: The Death of Jesus in Luke', *HTR* 94 (2001), pp. 383-402. See also Peter J. Scaer, *The Lukan Passion and the Praiseworthy Death* (NTM, 10; Sheffield: Sheffield Phoenix Press, 2005).

89. Cf. Judith Lieu, *The Gospel of Luke* (Epworth Commentaries; Peterborough: Epworth Press, 1997), p. 195.

corpse. But what does their desire to touch this absence signify? Whether we see death as transition to another world, as part of a natural cycle of birth, growth, death and birth, as return to the land, or as part of embeddedness in place, there is an alterity to death. This otherness is characterized by Derrida in his *Adieu to Emmanuel Levinas* as the 'non-response' of the corpse.[90] But there is also a hiatus between the breathing body and the corpse, both of which can be touched. The moment of death is other, a space between the breathing body and the corpse; in our contemporary setting, it is a space between the heartbeat measured on a screen and a flat-line, between activity in the brain and the absence of such activity.

In Luke, the otherness of death is uncannily captured in the appearance narrative of 24.36-43, where the body is foregrounded. Jesus appears to the eleven and their companions gathered in Jerusalem (24.33-36). They respond to the apparition with fear, believing it to be a spirit (ghost; breath), πνεῦμα (24.37). This is the first time the term πνεῦμα occurs since Jesus' death, where he gives up his spirit (breath) (πνεῦμα), signifying his whole person, into the hands of the divine and takes his final breath (ἐξέπνευσεν): 'Then Jesus, crying with a loud voice, said, "Father, into your hands I commend my spirit." Having said this, he breathed his last' (23.46).[91] The dying Jesus invokes the divine touch as the end of his death. Now appearing post-death he offers an invitation, 'Look at my hands and my feet; see that it is I myself. Touch me and see; for a ghost (πνεῦμα) does not have flesh and bones as you see that I have' (24.39). The invitation draws attention to the body, to hands and feet, flesh and bones. Where John's Gospel makes explicit the relation of Jesus' risen body to the suffering body of the dying Jesus (Jn 20.27), Luke's reference to Jesus' hands and feet makes a similar connection implicitly. There is a turn: the eleven and their companions are joyful but still disbelieving (24.41a). Jesus asks for something to eat, is offered fish and eats (24.41b-43; cf. 8.55). The focus on the materiality of the body, hands and feet, flesh and bones, is intensified by the physicality of eating which marks human dependence on, and continuity with, the wider Earth community. As Sjef van Tilborg and Patrick Chatelion Counet note, in this section there is an answer to the question raised in the two preceding narrative sections: Where is the body? (24.3, 23).[92] The body that, touched by a divine necessity, has suffered violent touch at the hands of Roman executioners returns (albeit transformed) as palpably material.

90. Jacques Derrida, *Adieu to Emmanuel Levinas* (trans. Pascale-Anne Brault and Michael Naas; Meridian; Crossing Aesthetics; Stanford, CA: Stanford University Press, 1999), p. 6.

91. Green, *Gospel of Luke*, p. 826 n. 57.

92. Sjef van Tilborg and Patrick Chatelion Counet, *Jesus' Appearances and Disappearances in Luke 24* (Leiden: E.J. Brill, 2000), p. 96.

*Consenting to the Body*

As noted above, Nancy writes of 'consenting to the body'. This consent is a 'yes' to the interconnectedness mediated by the touch of self and other, the self-touching that occurs in touching the other; a 'yes' to a compassionate touch that undoes the touch of violent relatedness; a 'yes' to mortality, when in touching the other's death, I touch my own. It is also a 'yes' to the alterity of death and more particularly to the alterity of the other.[93] For Luke, it is also consent to the body of the risen Jesus that is in continuity with the suffering body.

In the Gospel of Luke, the body (σῶμα) is subject to death (12.4). But the body is more than human anxieties about survival (12.22-23). In 11.33-36 the Lukan Jesus speaks of the eye as the lamp of the body. The eye and the body are related metonymically so that the whole or healthy eye signifies the whole or healthy body. Read in conjunction with the pattern of compassionate responsiveness outlined above, the Lukan narrative suggests that the healthy eye sees compassionately; the healthy body gives itself to the touch of the other's (and hence one's own) death. This understanding of embodied wholeness returns in the Lukan account of the Last Supper:

> Then he (Jesus) took a loaf of bread, and when he had given thanks, he broke it and gave it to them, saying, 'This is my body, which is given for you' (22.19 NRSV).

Unlike some twenty-first-century discourses around health, this is not a bodily wholeness that protects one from, or postpones, one's death. For Luke, in ways that remain problematic from a contemporary ecological perspective, the body subject to death also transcends death. Consenting to the body implies not only a consent to death, but also to the materiality of this transcendence of death. From an ecotheological perspective Rosemary Radford Ruether writes of a problematic 'cultural avoidance of death', asking what kinds of human relationships with more-than-human nature might be imagined if we understood our bodies in death as compost for life?[94] Luke's Jesus says, Τοῦτό ἐστιν τὸ σῶμά μου τὸ ὑπὲρ ὑμῶν διδόμενον (This is my body that for you/on your behalf/for your sake is being given). The body is being given for others; similarly, the blood is being poured out.

In the appearance narratives, Luke emphasizes not the raising of Jesus' ψυχή nor the return of his πνεῦμα, but the physicality of a risen body that can be seen and touched, that eats and speaks, that is being given and poured out for others. The emphasis on the body is matched by a (re)turn of

93. Cf. Jacques Derrida, *The Gift of Death* (trans. David Wills; Religion and Postmodernism; Chicago: University of Chicago Press, 1995), p. 82.

94. Rosemary Radford Ruether, *Gaia and God: An Ecofeminist Theology of Earth Healing* (San Francisco: HarperCollins, 1992), p. 53.

focus toward earth. At the beginning of Acts, the apostles stand gazing up toward the skies. They are challenged by two men in white robes: 'Why are you looking up toward heaven (the skies)?' (Acts 1.10-11). The disciples' gaze is redirected earthward.[95] In two other episodes, namely the transfiguration (9.28-36) and the empty tomb (24.1-12) narratives, the appearance of two men is announced in the same words: ἰδοὺ ἄνδρες δύο (9.30; 24.4; Acts 1.10). In the transfiguration account where the two men are identified as Moses and Elijah, the εἶδος, the form or outward appearance of Jesus' face, becomes other (ἕτερον); his clothes become 'dazzling white' (9.29). This moment of otherness and δόξα (9.31-32) occurs on a mountain, an earthly space, and refers directly to the ἔξοδος to be accomplished through Jesus' passion and death in Jerusalem (9.31). After Jesus' death, the women arrive at the tomb, but they find no body (24.1-3). Two men in dazzling robes appear, asking, 'Why do you look for the living (τὸν ζῶντα) among (or with) the dead (μετὰ τῶν νεκρῶν)?' (24.5). When the eleven and their companions encounter the risen Jesus (24.36-43), it becomes clear that the materiality of the body is an essential characteristic of the living (τὸν ζῶντα). In the heightened moments of transfiguration, resurrection and ascension when earth and skies (heaven) meet, heaven is turned toward earth; ψυχή and πνεῦμα are interconnected with σῶμα. The body subject to death is no longer with the dead.

*Summary*

Coming from outside the text, two deaths are central to the Lukan narrative: the death of Jesus and the death/destruction of Jerusalem. Writing from and toward these deaths, Luke gives an account of divine visitation, expressed as necessity, hospitality, forgiveness and compassion. While this account has its own violent legacies, it also presents a patterning of touch in which the touch of the other through sight provokes a compassionate contact that puts the protagonist in touch (impossibly) with her or his own death. In turn, this pattern of touching (death) suggests a focus on the way Luke touches *on* death. The focus on death, the alterity of which inheres in its everydayness, makes space in Luke for a kind of seeing that is toward the body. Not only does this seeing call forth compassion, but for Luke it also invites contact with the materiality and material dependence of the body that in the risen Jesus is with the living.

95. I am indebted to Melbourne priest Michael Casey of St Ambrose's Church in Brunswick for this insight concerning the ascension narrative.

### *Touching the Text*

Nancy introduces a term 'exscription' to describe the way in which any writing is engaged already with the materiality and material dependence of the body. 'Exscription' is a writing from and toward its outside; a writing 'from a place outside itself and other'.[96] For Nancy, the body of Jesus is the paradigm for the body that is both outside and the subject of writing. He writes:

> There is only exscription through writing, but what's exscribed *remains* this other *edge* that inscription, though signifying on an edge, obstinately continues to indicate as its own-other edge. Thus, for every writing, a body is the own-other edge: a body (or more than one body, or a mass, or more than one mass) is therefore also the traced, the tracing, and the trace (*here*, see, read, take, *hoc est enim corpus meum* ...).[97]

Nancy begins his dense reflection on the body and bodies with reference to the Latin phrase *hoc est enim corpus meum*, 'this is my body'. He returns to this phrase repeatedly.[98] The body is the taking-place of being, the being-in-place first of human beings, but also of a writing as a body, the material being-in-place (as scroll, page, screen) of a writing. The materiality of a writing touches on the materiality of an already-given body. The body is nonetheless shaped, and reshaped, in and by writing. Moreover, writing is a response to the body.

The complexity of Nancy's *Corpus* replays the complexity of this contact between bodies and writing, between writings, things and places. In the ravelled and unravelled skein of connection between writing, bodies and places, bodies are violated en masse every day.[99] Exscription describes an opening to the other, a *being-toward* the other, for which Luke's pattern of compassionate responsiveness suggests an ideal mode. The responsive orientation to the other is a space or spaciousness from, and within which, writing takes place in matter, where writing engages with, and opens to, the sense of the world: 'to go up and touch the concretion of the world'.[100] This mutual touch of writing and 'the concretion of the world' takes place both in the material artefact of a text and in the material reciprocity in which the world shapes writing and a writing shapes a world, a world where violent relatedness can

96. Peggy Kamuf, 'Introduction', *Paragraph* 16.2 (1993), pp. 103-107 (106).

97. Nancy, *Corpus*, p. 87, emphasis in original.

98. Nancy, *Corpus*, pp. 2-7, 12-13, 26-29, 32-33, 38-39, 52-53, 72-73, 76-79, 110-11, 118-19.

99. Nancy, *Being Singular Plural,* p. xiii.

100. Nancy, *Sense of the World*, p. 14.

be countered with compassion. The touch of matter and writing in the material artefact is necessary to the world-shaping writing of compassion.

Nevertheless, the material artefact as the taking place of a writing is itself dead insofar as the writing that touches, and touches on, the body is transferable to a variety of media. This obscuring of the particular instance of a writing as it presents itself in this book, on this screen or in this photocopy parallels the transferability of bodies and places as labour and sites of production in our contemporary context of global consumerist capitalism. William Cavanaugh describes the way in which consumerism works through our detachment from production, producers and products.[101] We make very little of what we consume; the lives and working conditions of those who make what we consume are largely hidden from us; the desire for the new encourages us not to become too attached to the things we already own and use; and in-built redundancy consolidates this detachment from the things we own as we feel forced to participate in a 'throw-away' society.[102] Similarly, in our reading of a biblical text we are largely detached from the particular material artefact, its condition of production, and the chain of material artefacts and their material dependence that form the being-in-place of the writing before us.

Michael Riley's images of floating Bibles, especially the cloud Bible, where the pages are hidden, suggest something of the complexity of this detachment. In a colonial context, the Bible as a material artefact is both more and less than its writings and their interpretation. It is a potent image that as David Burramurra and Monica Morgan point out stands with the cross as one of two central symbols of Christian culture and belief, which can be understood in parallel and tension with key indigenous cultural symbols. In Riley's work, the Bible and cross stand in parallel in separate images with the cross also inscribed on the book of the Bible itself. The Bible is inscribed with the death by imperial Roman execution that its Gospel writings narrate. Moreover, the Bible as material artefact and symbol of Christian culture accrues meaning both by and in excess of certain readings of its writings that situate Christian culture in competition with, and superior to, other cultures.

The pattern of compassionate responsiveness I have read in Luke with an ear to some contemporary theory of touch, especially that of Jean-Luc Nancy, offers a counter to the violent relatedness of the colonial expansion that brought the narrative of Luke's Gospel to Australia. Such a reading of touch in Luke cannot undo the damage of colonization, nor is it an apologetic for the cultural touch of the material artefact that has become

101. William T. Cavanaugh, *Being Consumed: Economics and Christian Desire* (Grand Rapids: Eerdmans, 2008), pp. 35-47.

102. Cavanaugh, *Being Consumed*, pp. 35-47.

in Riley's cloud Bible image a book with its pages hidden. Mine is not a *true* reading of a misinterpreted text, but a possible reading of ourselves as readers of Luke. Luke touches (on) death through a pattern of compassionate responsiveness and through the being-given of the body of the Lukan Jesus, and in so doing is in touch with the concretion of a world in which certain writings can be interpreted to give meaning to religious and political violence. This particular meaning-making in turn shapes a world. Insofar as Luke writes to account for the tragedy of Jesus' death and the destruction of Jerusalem, his touching (on) death touches on the tragedy of bodies (and concomitantly lands) violated en masse every day.

Does my focus on death rather than birth, however, reinforce the violent relatedness of colonization of lands, people, communities and bodies?[103] The focus on death as part of a pattern of compassionate relatedness is consonant with a focus on the maternal and birth, not only because of the linguistic link between compassion and womb. When in Luke Simeon holds the child in his arms he also holds death, both his own, before which he has hoped for this moment of contact, and the child's. The living body of the infant will become the dying body of the man, executed by the imperial occupiers. The holding is part of a pattern of holding that passes from the maternal body, through the manger to Simeon and to a Gospel inscribed in a book.

The material artefact that holds the story of the child, like the book holding the child Moses in the *Bible moraliseé* image, is part of a complex history of biblical production, reproduction and interpretation that touches, and touches on, bodies, communities and lands, where mortality and finitude are proper to their life and being. The violence remains; the potential for further violence remains. But the deconstruction of Christianity Nancy brings to the body and my reconstructive reading of touch in Luke suggest the possibility of rethinking the touch of the writing that is the Gospel of Luke as disturbing the violent relatedness of colonization. This interpretation of the touch of a writing cannot, however, account for the complex touch on the reader and on the Earth community of the material artefact in which the writing presents itself to reading.

## *Conclusion*

Every reading occurs within a more-than-human community of touching/being touched that includes not only the touch of the material artefact in which a writing presents itself to a reader but also the touching/being touched of bodies, communities, Earth and text. In reading and writing, we

103. Cf. Grace M Jantzen, *Becoming Divine: Towards a Feminist Philosophy of Religion* (Bloomington: Indiana University Press, 1999).

touch on the body and we touch bodies. Writing touches on bodies and land, for example, through the use of 'women', 'bodies' and 'land' as metaphors; through representations of human embodiment, relationships between men and women and between humans and land; and through the ways in which women, bodies and land are interconnected in the internal logic of a writing. Questions remain concerning elements of the Lukan narrative that eschew the body and the material text, and about a certain ambiguity regarding the maternal body in particular. Nonetheless, a kind of reading that consents to the body and to the reality of human mortality has wider implications. Perhaps the ex-scription of death—of the reality of human mortality as Earth beings, in our philosophical, economic and cultural thinking—can make space for a kind of seeing that invokes relations to the other, which are toward the body and toward Earth. Such a seeing in Luke not only prompts a compassionate touch but also touches the materiality of the body of the risen Jesus who is with the living. Can such seeing-touching disturb the violent relatedness of species extinctions, colonialist assimilation and ecological destruction?

A kind of connectedness is at work between the writing's touching *on* a subject, such as land, and the touch of the text as it affects land through the subsequent uses of the text to authorize particular relationships to land. But the temporal separation between the composition of a writing and its reading creates a disjunction between the material effects of a text (for example, on certain colonized lands and peoples) and any resonances in a writing of its underlying material embeddedness, its multiple touches on the places that support its being as matter. Through the material artefact in which a writing presents itself and the only partially traceable lineage of its artefactual production and reproduction, the touch between country/land/bodies and a writing bears complex and multiple relations to bodies and places. The process of reading a writing with land, bodies, women, Earth, death or the sense of touch itself 'in mind' may begin to connect the 'touching *on*' of the writing and its touch as a material thing that we encounter in reading. In the *Bible moralisée* image with which I began this chapter, the juxtaposition of a violent touching and the touch of safekeeping is mediated by the images of the material artefact as closed and open text.

# 5

## Incense and Ointment:
## Smell and the Absent Body/Text

> The women who had come with him from Galilee followed, and they saw the tomb and how his body was laid. Then they returned, and prepared spices and ointments. On the sabbath they rested according to the commandment. But on the first day of the week, at early dawn, they came to the tomb, taking the spices that they had prepared. They found the stone rolled away from the tomb, but when they went in, they did not find the body.
>
> Lk. 23.55–24.3 NRSV

A sixteenth-century icon from Novgorod housed in the State Tretyakov Gallery, Moscow, is entitled *Myrrh Bearers*. The icon presents three women toward the centre of the image. Before them in the lower centre of the icon is an open coffin. Inside the coffin are grave cloths but no body. Closest to the centre, a woman in red or deep orange is turned toward another in yellow/ochre. A third is behind them in a slightly deeper shade of red. The one in yellow carries a stoppered flask of myrrh. The Synoptic Gospels each tell the story of a group of women coming after the Sabbath to tend to the dead body of Jesus and finding the tomb empty (Mt. 28.1-8; Mk 16.1-8; Lk. 24.1-12). Luke gives more emphasis to the preparation and bringing of aromatic spices (ἀρώματα) and ointments (μύρα) than do Matthew and Mark (Lk. 23.56–24.1; cf. Mt. 27.61; 28.1; Mk 15.47–16.1). Where Matthew does not mention the spices and ointment directly, and Mark mentions spices for anointing, Luke writes of both the women's preparation of spices and ointments prior to the Sabbath and their bringing spices after the Sabbath. In the Gospel of John, Nicodemus brings the spices for Jesus' burial, and Jesus' corpse is anointed with the spices before burial (Jn 19.39-40). The *Myrrh Bearers* icon echoes the Lukan and Markan traditions, which juxtapose the bearing of the spices (and ointments) with the discovery of the empty tomb. The former signifies the expectation overturned by the latter. In the icon, the flask of myrrh remains closed in the face of an empty burial casket.

The scent that would emanate from the flask, the aroma of spice and ointment, is muted by this closure; the odour that would signify a decaying body is absent from the description of the empty tomb (cf. Jn 11.39; 12.3). Apart from the allusion to the preparation and bringing of spices and ointments, scent does not feature strongly in the scene. Indeed, descriptions of aromas and odours do not figure strongly in the Second Testament. The following few passages refer directly to ὀσμή (fragrance or odour) and εὐωδία (pleasant smell) and ὄζω (to smell sweet or to stink): 2 Corinthians 2.14-16; Ephesians 5.2; Philippians 4.18; John 11.39; 12.3. In one word for spice (ἄρωμα)—appearing at Mk 16.1; Lk. 23.56-24.1; Jn 19.40—we can hear the English word aroma. There are in Luke references to things the reader may expect to evoke certain scents, particularly the offering of incense (θυμιάω; θυμίαμα, 1.9-11) and anointing with ointment (μύρον, 7.37-38, 46). But Luke does not proffer appeals to fragrance such as those associated with divine wisdom in Ben Sira 24.15 and the divine realm, for example, in *1 En.* 24.4; 25.4-6; 32.3-6 and the *LAE* 29.1-6.[1] Nevertheless, smell was ubiquitous in the ancient world.

Constance Classen, David Howes and Anthony Synnott reconstruct the first-century CE Roman world of smell as follows:

> Walking through the streets of Nero's Rome in the first century AD, one would encounter the stench of refuse rotting by the wayside, the piercing fragrance of burning myrrh emanating from temples, the heavy aroma of food being cooked by street vendors, the sweet, seductive scents of flowering gardens, the malodour of rotting fish at a fishstand, the sharp smell of urine from a public latrine and perhaps the incense trail of a passing procession honouring a god or hero.[2]

What are we to make of the apparent absence of smelling in the Gospel of Luke, written as it was in a world of odours and aromas? Lyall Watson writes, 'Smell is the forgotten sense'.[3] He continues,

> There are no agreed measures of its nature, no societies dedicated to its appreciation, no descriptions of it except those borrowed from our overbearing sense of sight.... Smell is our most seductive and provocative sense, invading every domain of our lives, providing the single most pow-

1. See Susan Ashbrook Harvey, *Scenting Salvation: Ancient Christianity and the Olfactory Imagination* (Transformation of the Classical Heritage, 42; Berkeley: University of California Press, 2006), pp. 46-56.

2. Constance Classen, David Howes and Anthony Synnott, *Aroma: The Cultural History of Smell* (London: Routledge, 1994), p. 17.

3. Lyall Watson, *Jacobson's Organ and the Remarkable Nature of Smell* (New York: Norton, 2000), p. 3.

> erful link to our distant origins. But it is also mute, almost unspeakable, defying description and collection, challenging the imagination.[4]

In this chapter, I consider the sense of smell in the Second Testament, with particular reference to Paul's evocation of fragrance in 2 Cor. 2.14-16, and then give attention to the apparent absence of this sense in the Gospel of Luke. I suggest that the character of this Lukan absence has parallels with the apparent absence of the material artefact in our readings of biblical texts.

## *Artefacts and Absences*

As I read Lk. 23.55–24.3 onscreen at the head of this chapter, there is no scent that I can detect, neither of paper nor machine. My paper NRSV bears only a faint scent. My Greek New Testament a little more. Following a minority of ancient manuscripts, the NRSV ends Lk. 24.3 with, 'they did not find the body'. A small number also have the qualifier 'of Jesus' describing 'the body'. A majority of ancient manuscripts have 'the body of the lord Jesus'. Behind the discussion of the textual variant are ancient material artefacts, one might expect with their own scents conveying something of their materiality: from $P^{75}$ (Papyrus Bodmer XIV and XV), dated to the early third century CE, through the major codices, Sinaiticus, Alexandrinus and Vaticanus, to much later uncials, such as 0124, which each includes the phrase τοῦ κυρίου Ἰησοῦ. These artefacts, physically absent from the textual apparatus making reference to them, attest to a strange moment in these Lukan writings concerning the absence of the body. The women come expecting to find a dead body, but do not. By describing this body as 'the body of *the lord* Jesus', the writings anticipate the appearance of the risen body. There is no 'odour of the resurrection' in these accounts, except in the aromatic spices that remain closed in their flasks (as the icon *Myrrh Bearers* suggests), in the hands of the women who have no body to anoint.[5]

## *Smell*

In a first-century CE Mediterranean world saturated with scent, the absence of the dead body is also an absence of the odour of death. Do the aromas of spice and ointment linger in the narrative of Luke 24, even in their effective absence and the absence of the body (24.3) at this intersection of death and life? Michel Serres describes smell as 'the sense ... of the confusion

4. Watson, *Jacobson's Organ*, p. 3.

5. The 'odour of the resurrection' is a phrase used by Ambrose to describe scenting God as 'the smell of life as it would be fulfilled in immortality'; Harvey, *Scenting Salvation*, p. 132.

of encounters; the rare sense of singularities'.[6] The absence of the body in Lk. 24.3, provoking the question 'where is the body?', opens to a series of encounters with the risen Jesus, which emphasize the materiality and material embeddedness of the risen body. These material encounters would be saturated with scent: a road from Jerusalem to Emmaus (24.13), bread (24.30), fish (24.42), human bodies, but this world of smell receives little mention in Luke.

### *Smell as a Saturated Communion*

For Lyall Watson, the sense of smell 'almost slips entirely through the net of language'.[7] But Robert Burton describes a 'language of smell' whereby animals, human and other-than-human, communicate with one another, particularly with others within their own species.[8] As sense, smell puts subjects in material relationship with others, when they take in another's scent. This relationship is mediated by smell as both emission (or message) and sense (that receives and initiates a response). As emission, smell 'consists of molecules of a volatile substance that are carried in the air or, for aquatic animals, are soluble and carried in water'.[9] The sense of smell involves taking in the substance emitted by the other. As Fiona Borthwick argues, 'Olfaction opens the possibility, through the actual embodiment of the other, of another kind of sociality that acknowledges the interconnection with, not the complete separation of, the subject and the other.'[10] Thus, smell offers an alternative phenomenology to a Western metaphysical focus on the epistemologies of hearing and sight.

Moreover, 'not simply a biological and psychological phenomenon', smell 'is *cultural*, hence a social and historical phenomenon'.[11] In the ancient Mediterranean world, odours distinguished between rich and poor, various trades, city and country, freeborn and slave, war and peace, loss and victory, disease and health, death and life. Often a mark of wealth, use of perfume was also a sign of wastefulness; losing potency and effect quickly through evaporation, scents could not be passed on to the next generation (Pliny the Elder, *Nat.* 13.20; cf. Mark 14.4-5). Diffuse in nature, an odour's source is difficult to locate (Lucretius, *De rerum natura,* 4). Yet, for Lucretius, the embodied sense of smell and the associated scent of things give

6. Serres, *Five Senses*, p. 170.

7. Watson, *Jacobson's Organ*, p. 3.

8. Robert Burton, *The Language of Smell* (London: Routledge & Kegan Paul, 1976).

9. Burton, *Language of Smell*, p. 9.

10. Fiona Borthwick, 'Olfaction and Taste: Invasive Odours and Disappearing Objects', *The Australian Journal of Anthropology* 11.2 (2000), p. 135.

11. Classen, Howes and Synnott, *Aroma*, p. 3, emphasis in original.

evidence of the atomic nature of matter.[12] Fragrance becomes a metaphor for the soul; the parallel between scent and soul indicates the connectedness and interdependence of soul and body, as of the nature of human being (and well-being) (*De rerum natura,* 3). Moreover, this relationship between soul and body echoes in the olfactory sensuality of relationships between divine and human realms.[13] Inescapable and elusive, immediate and diffuse, material and ungraspable, sense and sensed—smell suggests something of the problematic of the interrelationship and interdependence between immanence and transcendence.

In Chapter 3, I drew on Jean-Luc Marion's notion of a saturated phenomenon to describe a saturated communion. A phenomenon can be described as saturated when my experience (my empirical apprehension) of the phenomenon exceeds my expectation of it, as a concept or category of thinking. Drawing on Shane Mackinlay's reading of Marion, I argued that the saturated phenomenon appears not so much in the thing that gives itself as in the communion occurring between the given and the gifted (*adonné*), in a hermeneutic space opened between them. The experience of smell as a material saturation that unsettles the distinctions between self and other can be understood as a saturated communion. The saturated communion expressed in the saturation of smell, which is both hermeneutic encounter and its interruption, is a counter experience.

Kevin Hart explains:

> 'counter-experience' ... contradicts the conditions of possibility for experiencing an object. The subject's intentional gaze is rebuked by the intuitions to which it is exposed, not necessarily because he or she is bedazzled but perhaps because of being disappointed by unfulfilled or displaced expectations, and in any case by the sheer resistance of the phenomenon to objectification.[14]

As a phenomenon characterized by a certain physical saturation, the sense of smell becomes a symbolic indicator of the counter-experiential interrelationship between matter and spirit, body and soul, the human and the divine. For Constance Classen and her colleagues, moreover, the interiorization of the other through the sense of smell contributes to 'the intimate and emotionally charged nature of the olfactory experience', ensuring that the cultural meanings of smell (as matter and sense) become 'deeply personal'.[15]

12. Lucretius, *Sensation and Sex* (trans. R.E. Latham; London: Penguin, 2005), p. 8.
13. Classen, Howes and Synnott, *Aroma*, pp. 18-48.
14. Hart, 'Poetry and Revelation', p. 276.
15. Classen, Howes and Synnott, *Aroma*, p. 3.

*The Evocation of Smell in 2 Corinthians 2.14-16*
Susan Ashbrook Harvey argues that the early Christians displayed ambivalence with respect to the sense of smell. While smells were ubiquitous in the ancient Mediterranean world, particular scents were associated with the Roman Empire, in particular those fragrances that accompanied incense offerings to the Roman gods. Although fragrance appeared in Jewish Scriptures, the Old Testament pseudepigrapha and the Greek and Roman worlds as imagery relating to the divine realm, the early Christians mostly eschewed the ritual use of fragrance. At a practical level, the business of trade in fragrance, its buying and selling, became problematic as such could implicate Christians in the imperial worship they sought to avoid. But aromatics also had a role in health and hygiene. Early Christians negotiated this difficult area by (i) cautiously affirming the practical use of ointments and fragrances, while avoiding their cultic uses; (ii) developing an ascetic approach to the sensing body; (iii) developing an imagery of fragrance that reflected spiritual realities rather than material ones, for example, the stench of a martyr's burning flesh could be reimagined, and even literally sensed, as a holy perfume and prayer became incense. From the time of Constantine this shifted, and the use of fragrance in liturgy became commonplace.[16]

Against this background, a small section in Paul's second letter to the Corinthians, 2 Cor. 2.14-16, stands out as the most developed appeal to the sense of smell in the Second Testament. Drawing on a variety of cultural meanings of smell to express a deeply personal understanding of his vocation, Paul uses two words for scent: ὀσμή and εὐωδία. While several commentators relate his use of ὀσμή to the fragrance arising from incense burnt during a triumphal procession,[17] the wider biblical usage of ὀσμή and εὐωδία suggests three points of connection to the relationship between the human and the divine—(i) sacrifice; (ii) wisdom; (iii) healing—each of which recalls a nexus between death and life.

In 2 Cor. 2.14, the manifestation of the fragrance of the knowledge of Christ (τὴν ὀσμὴν τῆς γνώσεως αὐτοῦ) occurs in parallel with an image of triumphal procession:

16. Harvey, *Scenting Salvation*, pp. 11-57.

17. See, for example, Charles H. Talbert, *Reading Corinthians: A Literary and Theological Commentary on 1 and 2 Corinthians* (New York: Crossroad, 1987), p. 141.

[God] ...
πάντοτε (at all times)
θριαμβεύοντι ἡμας (leads us in triumphal procession)
ἐν τῷ Χριστῷ (in Christ)
καὶ (and)
τὴν ὀσμὴν τῆς γνώσεως αὐτοῦ (the fragrance of the knowledge of him)
φανεροῦντι δι᾽ ἡμῶν (brings to light through us)
ἐν παντὶ τόπῳ (in every place)

φανεροῦντι δι᾽ ἡμῶν corresponds with θριαμβεύοντι ἡμᾶς and ἐν παντὶ τόπῳ matches the earlier πάντοτε so that the universality of God's action in Christ spans time and place in an encompassing excess. In a saturation of imagery matching the saturation of smell, the emotional urgency of the first part of the letter—arising both from Paul's confrontation with his own mortality and a painful sense of longing for reconciliation with the community (2 Cor. 1.8–2.11)[18]—erupts in the sensual imagery of scent in 2.14-16. Revelation is conveyed by a synaesthesia of sight and smell, when Paul writes of God bringing to light the fragrance of the knowledge of Christ (2.14).[19]

The parallel image of triumphal procession has vexed commentators. Paul writes of God at all times θριαμβεύοντι ἡμᾶς, leading us in triumphal procession in Christ (2.14). In Paul's time, the socio-political as well as the usual literary context for the expression refers to a triumphal procession of victorious generals who lead (θριαμβεύω) their captives, some toward death, the remainder into slavery.[20]

> Entering Rome through the triumphal arch, the general and his entourage would lead their captives through the city to the Capitoline hill. There,

18. Murray J. Harris, *Second Epistle to the Corinthians* (NIGTC; Grand Rapids: Eerdmans, 2005), pp. 164-82. Cf. Jerome Murphy-O'Connor, 'The Second Letter to the Corinthians', in *The New Jerome Biblical Commentary* (ed. Joseph A. Fitzmyer, Raymond E. Brown and Roland E. Murphy; London: Geoffrey Chapman, 1991), pp. 816-29 (817-18).

19. That ἐν τῷ Χριστῷ and τὴν ὀσμὴν τῆς γνώσεως αὐτοῦ stand in parallel suggests that the latter should be translated 'the fragrance of the knowledge of Christ'. For Marion, Revelation is the saturated phenomenon par excellence; see Jean-Luc Marion, *In Excess: Studies of Saturated Phenomena* (trans. Robyn Horner and Vincent Berraud; Perspectives in Continental Philosophy, 27; New York: Fordham University Press, 2002), pp. 158-62.

20. Harris, *Second Epistle to the Corinthians*, pp. 242-48; Talbert, *Reading Corinthians*, pp. 140-41; Margaret E. Thrall, *The Second Epistle to the Corinthians*, I (ICC; London: T. & T. Clark, 2004), pp. 194-95; Nigel Watson, *The Second Epistle to the Corinthians* (London: Epworth Press, 1993), p. 21. Note also the letter's recipients reside in Corinth, which having been destroyed in 146 BCE was rebuilt as a Roman colony in 44 BCE.

> they would offer a sacrifice of praise to Jupiter, the god who gave victory. After this, the prisoners of war would be executed. For the celebrants, the odor of burning sacrifice was the aroma of triumph; for the doomed captives, it was the smell of death.[21]

Many commentators, however, want to redeem the image, for example, by making Paul and his co-workers (or perhaps readers) soldierly partners in the divine triumph in Christ.[22] But the imagery resonates with Paul's self-designation as δοῦλος Χριστοῦ, slave of Christ (Rom. 1.1; Gal. 1.10; Phil. 1.1), and his comment to the Corinthians that in Christ freedom and slavery are reversed (1 Cor. 7.22). As Frank Matera explains:

> If *thriambeuō* normally means to lead someone in a triumphal procession as a captive, then Paul is presenting himself as God's captive, whom God conquered in order to be his apostle and ambassador.... God placed this 'obligation' on Paul when he 'captured' the former persecutor and made him his apostle and slave. Because he understands his ministry in this way, Paul preaches the gospel free of charge as an expression of the inner freedom he enjoys as Christ's slave (1 Cor. 9.15-18).[23]

In presenting himself as Christ's slave, Paul undermines any Corinthian expectation that he might belong to them.[24] But the language of slavery both reinforces and calls into question an underlying logic of mastery that, among other things, is problematic from an ecological perspective. This dual effect, at once unsettling and reinscribing the language of slavery, occurs quite explicitly in the post-Pauline letter to the Ephesians, where both master and slave come under the mastery of Christ (Eph. 6.5-9; see

21. Kevin Quast, *Reading the Corinthian Correspondence: An Introduction* (New York: Paulist Press, 1994), p. 119.

22. C.K. Barrett, *The Second Epistle to the Corinthians* (BNTC; London: A. & C. Black, 1973), p. 98; Colin Kruse, *2 Corinthians* (TNTC; Leicester: Inter-Varsity Press, 1987), pp. 85-86; Watson, *Second Epistle to the Corinthians*, p. 22. Cf. Harris, *Second Epistle to the Corinthians*, pp. 242-48; Thrall, *Second Epistle to the Corinthians*, pp. 194-95. The use of the first person plural pronoun (ἡμᾶς) allows an address of the reader and Paul's co-workers with Paul (and his ministry) in the Pauline self-reference of the text.

23. Frank J. Matera, *II Corinthians: A Commentary* (NTL; Louisville, KY: Westminster John Knox Press, 2003), pp. 72-73. See also Rudolf Bultmann, *The Second Letter to the Corinthians* (trans. Roy A. Harrisville; Minneapolis: Augsburg Publishing House, 1985), pp. 62-63; Jerry W. McCant, *2 Corinthians* (Readings: A New Biblical Commentary; Sheffield: Sheffield Academic Press, 1999), pp. 34-35.

24. McCant, *2 Corinthians*, pp. 34-35. Timothy Savage, *Power through Weakness: Paul's Understanding of the Christian Ministry in 2 Corinthians* (SNTSMS; Cambridge: Cambridge University Press, 1996), pp. 35-40, argues that the people belonged primarily to the 'upwardly mobile' class of 'freedman', a group often with weak ties to family or social inheritance.

also Col. 4.12). In 2 Cor. 2.14, a logic of mastery is unsettled when Paul invokes the shameful imagery of the humiliation of captives not at the point where he is describing the degradations he has suffered in the course of his ministry but paradoxically when he is evoking its efficacy, manifest as the fragrance of the knowledge of Christ (τὴν ὀσμὴν τῆς γνώσεως αὐτοῦ).[25]

Within the Second Testament, ὀσμή, fragrance, appears three times outside of 2 Cor. 2.14-16 (Eph. 5.2; Phil. 4.18; Jn 12.3). Ephesians 5.2 refers to Christ giving himself up (for us) as 'a fragrant offering (εἰς ὀσμὴν εὐωδίας) and sacrifice (θυσίαν) to God'. Philippians 4.18 describes the gifts from the community to sustain Paul's work as a fragrant offering (ὀσμὴν εὐωδίας) and a fitting sacrifice (θυσίαν δεκτήν). In the Septuagint, ὀσμή εὐωδίας describes the pleasing aroma arising toward God from sacrifices, in particular, the whole burnt offering, ὁλοκαύτωμα, of an animal (for example, Exod. 29.18; Lev. 3.5; 17.4; 23.18; Num. 15.3). Philo describes the whole burnt offering, on an altar anointed with very fragrant ointment (χρίσματος εὐωδεστάτου), in terms of its interrelationship with the four primary elements: earth, water, air and fire (Philo, *Vit. Mos.* 2.146-48).[26] Here, the offering of the animal body is both thanksgiving for, and reminder of, the sustenance of earth: the animal body, its carcass, flesh and blood recall food, clothing, shelter and life-giving water; the fragrance of the offering evokes the materiality of the air; the fire of the offering summons the necessities of heat and light (Philo, *Vit. Mos.* 2.146-48). With its explicit violence toward the other animal, the offering itself not only recalls for Philo's Moses (and Philo himself) dependence on, and interdependence with, the Earth community but also reminds readers of the sacrificial cost of human spending of Earth others. This cost has an eerie resonance in Paul's own self-understanding as slave, given up to death for the sake of the gospel (1 Cor. 9.19-23; 2 Cor. 4.11). This is especially so, because Paul's use of ὀσμή and εὐωδία in 2 Cor. 2.14-16 evokes both the Roman triumphal celebration of the sacrifice of the other in war and slavery and the ancient Hebrew sacrifice of other animals.

The imagery of fragrance, and the knowledge to which it is attached in 2 Cor. 2.14, also recalls the teaching of wisdom, whose fragrance is 'a sign of the divine presence'.[27] In the Septuagint Lady Sophia describes herself:

25. Cf. Jan Lambrecht, *Second Corinthians* (Sacra Pagina; Collegeville, MN: Liturgical Press, 1999), p. 38.

26. See also Mary L. Coloe, 'Anointing the Temple of God: John 12:1-8', in *Transcending Boundaries: Contemporary Readings of the New Testament* (Festschrift Francis J. Moloney; ed. Mary L. Coloe and Rekha Chennatu; *Biblioteca di scienze religiose;* Rome: Libreria Ateneo Salesiano, 2005), pp. 105-18.

27. Bultmann, *Second Letter to the Corinthians*, p. 64; Lambrecht, *Second Corinthians*, p. 39.

> Like cinnamon and aromatic aspalathos I gave fragrance (ὀσμήν),
> and like choice myrrh I spread my aroma (εὐωδίαν),
> like galbanum and onyx and stacte,
> and like the mist of frankincense in the tent (Sir. 24.15).

The reference to the tent recalls the cultic imagery of incense offering and sacrifice. Later when the scribe urges his faithful pupils to send out pleasing aroma, to blossom and to scatter fragrance, scent parallels and stands for singing praise to God (Sir. 39.14). Not only wisdom but also the scribe and the faithful pupils become themselves an incense offering. Paralleling Lady Sophia, the High Priest, entering the Holy of Holies, pours out 'a drink offering of the blood of the grape ... at the foot of the altar/a pleasing odour (ὀσμὴν εὐωδίας) to the Most High' (Sir. 50.15).[28] The pouring out echoes in Paul's and more particularly the Gospel accounts of the Last Supper where in the shadow of his death, Jesus pours out the drink offering which is his own life (1 Cor. 11.23-26; Mk 14.23-24; see also Mt. 26.27-28; Lk. 22.20).

The only other occurrence of ὀσμή in the Second Testament occurs in the Gospel of John immediately following Jesus' restoration of Lazarus from death to life (John 11). When Mary of Bethany, a sister of Lazarus, anoints the feet of Jesus, the fragrance of the myrrh completely fills the house (ἐκ τῆς ὀσμῆς τοῦ μύρου, 12.3). Mary's anointing of the feet parallels Jesus' washing of the feet in John 13, an act of loving service that in the context of Jesus' impending death subverts the usual relationship between master and slave.[29] The aroma of the pure nard Mary spills (12.3) contrasts with the stench of her brother's corpse (11.39). The fragrant ointment is medicinal, an agent of healing. The woman and the matter of the ointment are co-agents in the life-affirming action at the 'nexus' of life and death: 'the life given to Lazarus, the death faced by Jesus'.[30]

Underlying Mary's actions in John 12 may be the imagery of a single-use vessel, of which the neck is broken to release the ointment.[31] The breaking open of the vial, the spilling of its expensive contents and the filling of the whole house indicate a spending of not only fragrance but also the self of the giver. Paul expresses a parallel sense of spending himself for the Cor-

28. My thanks to Pamela Foulkes for alerting me to this reference.

29. Cf. Mary L. Coloe, 'Welcome into the Household of God: The Foot Washing in John 13', *CBQ* 66 (2004), pp. 400-15.

30. Dorothy Lee, *Flesh and Glory: Symbolism, Gender and Theology in the Gospel of John* (New York: Crossroad, 2002), pp. 202-203; Elaine Wainwright, *Women Healing/Healing Women: The Genderization of Healing in Early Christianity* (London: Equinox, 2006), p. 157. Two scenes later, Jesus enters Jerusalem in 'triumphal' procession (Jn 12.12-19).

31. I am grateful to Bernadette Kiley for this suggestion.

inthian community without asking for the sustaining donations that Philippians suggests he willingly accepted there as a fragrant offering (2 Cor. 11.7-11; Phil. 4.18). In the context of a meal between friends in whose presence Jesus abides (Jn 12.1-8; cf. 15.4), the universal dispersion of fragrance through Mary's loving act also echoes the symbolism of scent in the Song of Songs, where both the human lovers and the other-than-human habitat for their love exude perfume (Song 1.3, 12; 2.13; 4.10-16; 5.13; 7.8, 13).[32] Here love saturates the nexus of life and death (Song 8.5b-7). Fragrance also recalls for Paul this life/death nexus (2 Cor. 2.15-16). In being given over to the gospel as apostle and ambassador of Christ, Paul finds himself impelled by the love of Christ and his own affection for the community: 'you are in our hearts, to die together and to live together' (2 Cor. 7.3; see also 1.1; 5.14, 20; 6.12).[33]

Smell evokes a saturation at the nexus of life and death. When incense is burnt, an animal sacrificed or perfume spilt, the particles of scent carry in the air spreading and dissipating. Something is consumed; something is spent. But this consumption is also a consummation realized variously as a whole burnt offering, the wholeness of healing, the unbounded spread of the wisdom of the gospel, or the cost of loving. The uncanny face of this consummation shows itself in Paul's metaphor of the triumphal procession, where the consumption of incense signalling the victory of the imperial other becomes the sign of Christ's victory over death and of the spread of the gospel by 'slaves' of Christ (2.14). While the imagery of victory, slavery and universal evangelization reinvokes a colonizing imperial logic, in which the other may be spent, it also unsettles this logic by bringing into Paul's writing an element of resistance. For example, by emphasizing his own humble status and his willingness to be spent for the sake of the gospel, Paul may be responding to a cultural framework in which 'the Corinthians were evaluating Paul according to the self-exalting standards of their secular environment'.[34] In contrast, Paul understands himself summoned by the

32. Elaine Wainwright, 'Anointing/Washing Feet: John 12:1-8 and its Intertexts within a Socio-Rhetorical Reading', in *'I Sowed Fruits into Hearts' (Odes Sol. 17:13)* (Festschrift Michael Lattke; ed. Majella Franzmann, Pauline Allen and Rick Strelan; Early Christian Studies, 12; Sydney: St Paul's Publications, 2007), pp. 203-20.

33. I am aware of critical issues concerning the composition of 2 Corinthians, in particular the authorship and provenance of 6.14–7.1 and the question of the discontinuities which suggest that two or more letters have been combined. See, for example, Murphy-O'Connor, 'Second Letter to the Corinthians', p. 816. On the whole, however, such questions are beyond the scope of this chapter and not directly relevant to its argument.

34. Savage, *Power through Weakness*, p. 187. While one could question the usage of the adjective 'secular' in relation to a first-century CE context, the point of comparison between Paul's self-understanding and the different cultural expectations within which the Corinthians interpret their relationship with him remains valid.

gospel of Christ, viewing 'himself in his apostolic calling not only as one who *preaches* the message of good news to the world, but equally important, as one ordained by God to be an *embodiment* of that gospel, called to reveal the knowledge of God by and through his very life'.[35]

Expressing his experience of embodiment of the gospel, Paul's shifting imagery of fragrance is complicated. The fragrant knowledge of Christ (2.14) becomes a return to God as the pleasing aroma of Paul and his ministry (or the early Christians) (2.15a), perhaps through Christ's and his mirrored sufferings, but perhaps also by his being conformed to the image of Christ (Rom. 8.29). The use of aroma as image conveys Paul's understanding that the Christian participates in Christ, so much so that the matter of Christ returns to God through the Christian embodiment of the gospel in the world.[36]

In a further shift, fragrance serves to symbolize the effect of the gospel. Bultmann argues that rather than referring to the fragrance of life and the stench of death, the odour from life to life and that from death to death stand for the contrasting or dual effect of the gospel (2.15b-16).[37] While well grounded in biblical and rabbinic traditions, Bultmann's interpretation risks effacing the materiality underlying the symbol of scent, which, when paired with life and death respectively, can evoke for the reader, as it does for Lucretius, an association with particular smells.[38] A contrast between the malodour of death and the fragrance of life calls forth the saturation of a doubled death (the odour from death to death of those being lost) and a doubled life (the odour from life to life of those being saved) (2.15b-16). This contrast parallels Paul's understanding of the cross, which is experienced as folly for those who are lost and the power of God for those who are saved (1 Cor. 1.18).[39] Through the imagery of fragrance, Christ, the gospel and Paul are linked. Moreover, smell also provides the imagery for the divergent responses—as toward death or toward life—occasioned by Paul's proclamation of Christ. The multiple usages of the metaphor of smell in 2 Cor. 2.14-16 suggest that Paul's embodiment of the gospel occurs at this nexus of loss and salvation, death and life. The physical saturation of smell matches the saturation of this experience—a counter-experience—that has Paul exclaim, 'And for these things who is sufficient?' (2 Cor. 2.16b).

35. Scott J. Hafemann, *Suffering and Ministry in the Spirit: Paul's Defense of his Ministry in II Corinthians 2:14–3:3* (Grand Rapids: Eerdmanns, 1990), p. 16.

36. Cf. J.-F. Collange, *Enigmes de la deuxième épître de Paul aux Corinthiens: Etude exégétique de 2 Cor. 2:14–7:4* (Cambridge: Cambridge University Press, 1972), p. 33.

37. Bultmann, *Second Letter to the Corinthians*, p. 68.

38. Classen, Howes and Synnott, *Aroma*, p. 44.

39. Collange, *Enigmes*.

As indicated earlier, 'smell'—as the matter emitted from a thing, its being sensed, and the sensory communion of smelling—links self and other, in such a way that the fragrant or odorous other gives of its essence and is taken into the body of the self. Because it is already a phenomenon of physical saturation that writer and reader experience through the embodied sense, smell can give itself to writer and reader as symbol for the counter-experiential excess of the Pauline vocation. In the imagery of 2 Cor. 2.14-16, the evocation of smell presses writer and reader toward a counter-experiential moment of answerability in the face of the Christian gospel. Is this also a moment of answerability in the face of the spending of Earth others whose being-given forms part of the background to the imagery of smell: namely, the animal or thing consumed in sacrifice or poured forth in anointing, and the enslaved captives whose defeat the triumphal procession celebrates? The saturated communion of smell evoked in 2 Cor. 2.14-16 and situated at the nexus of self and other, loss and salvation, life and death embeds the gospel Paul proclaims in the materiality of the Earth community.

## *Scenting Scenes in the Gospel of Luke*

In the Gospel of Luke, there is no similar saturated imagery of scent. However, four settings associated with scent suggest points of entry for considering the materiality of smell, and its association with life and death, even in its effective absence. They are (i) the Temple , where smell is associated with both incense and whole burnt offerings; (ii) the household, where fragrances were used for the purposes of health and hygiene, for example, for healing ointments and for cleaning; (iii) the burial, where spices and ointments were used for embalming; (iv) the banquet, where perfumes were used regularly as part of the overall experience of the sociality of the meal. I will consider some Lukan examples of these settings: (i) the incense offering in Lk. 1.9-11; (ii) the anointings in Lk. 7.38-50 and 10.25-37; (iii) the preparations for burial in Lk. 23.55–24.3; (iv) the Last Supper in Lk. 22.7-23.

### *The Incense Offering in Luke 1.9-11*

The Lukan infancy narrative begins in the Jerusalem Temple:

> [Zechariah] was chosen by lot, according to the custom of the priesthood to enter the sanctuary of the lord and offer incense. Now at the time of the incense-offering, the whole assembly of the people was praying outside. There appeared to him an angel of the lord, standing at the right side of the altar of incense (Lk. 1.9-11 NRSV).

Harvey comments, 'Within the cultic system proper, the Jerusalem Temple itself could not operate as required without [incense]. Incense offering demarcated temple space as sacred, yielding fragrance unique to the God whose temple it was.... The mere scent of incense could image the cultic traditions as a whole.'[40] Although Luke does not specifically refer to the sense of smell, Lk. 1.9-11 mentions incense or the incense-offering three times. In a cultural context where smell was ubiquitous, the repetition of reference to incense in the setting of this episode is evocative of the fragrance of the incense used in the Temple incense offerings. In this space saturated by scent, an angel appears. As commentators have frequently noted, the Temple setting situates this episode in the space of early-first-century CE Jewish cultic practice.[41] With the allusions to characters from the Hebrew Bible, such as Abraham and Sarah, Elkanah and Hannah, the setting situates the episode in the traditions of the Jewish Scriptures.[42]

Zechariah is chosen by lot according to custom to burn incense θυμιᾶσαι εἰσελθὼν εἰς τὸν ναὸν τοῦ κυρίου ('entering into the sanctuary of the lord', 1.9). The word order in Luke suggests not only that the incense offering occurs in the sanctuary, but that the country priest, Zechariah, who with Elizabeth, his wife, is righteous *before* God (1.6), enters the divine presence in the consummation of the incense. It is as if the transformation of the incense into airborne particles and the fragrance that would accompany this transformation express the orientation of Zechariah before God.

The second reference to incense introduces a temporality—the time/hour of the incense offering (1.10)—and expands the setting to include the whole assembly of the people, on whose behalf Zechariah makes the offering; they are described as praying outside the sanctuary. It is likely that in practice the fragrance of incense served to connect the priest in the sanctuary with those outside as it flowed across the boundary separating the sanctuary from the people assembled. In the third reference, the division between earth and heaven is breached when the angel appears on the right-hand side of the altar of incense (1.11). The references to incense not only serve to situate the appearance narrative at the heart of Jewish religion, but also offer a repeated allusion to the crossing and diffusion of boundaries between earth and heaven, human and divine, death and life. In the tradition of special births, Elizabeth is barren (1.7); the angel appears with a promise of unexpected life (1.13).

### *The Anointings in Luke 7.38-50 and 10.25-37*

In the setting of a meal in a house, a woman's use of fragrant ointment also signals unexpected life:

40. Harvey, *Scenting Salvation*, p. 17.

41. See, for example, Raymond E. Brown, *The Birth of the Messiah: A Commentary on the Infancy Narratives in Matthew and Luke* (Garden City, NY: Doubleday, 1977), p. 267.

42. Brown, *Birth of the Messiah*, p. 269.

> And a woman in the city, who was a sinner, having learned that [Jesus] was in the Pharisee's house, brought an alabaster jar of ointment. She stood behind him at his feet, weeping, and began to bathe his feet with her tears and to dry them with her hair. Then she continued kissing his feet and anointing them with the ointment ...
>
> You did not anoint my head with oil, but she has anointed my feet with ointment (Lk. 7.37-38, 46 NRSV).

Elaine Wainwright argues that the materiality of the woman's touch as she bathes Jesus' feet with her tears and massages them with the ointment (μύρον) signal an erotic action which calls forth a response in him.[43] The forgiveness the Lukan Jesus affirms the woman has already received, and which enables her free act of love, is expressed erotically.[44] Together with her unbound hair, her tears and kisses, the fragrant ointment evokes the excess of the woman's action at the point where the hospitality of forgiveness has called forth an outpouring of love that matches the outpouring of the scent of the ointment. While Luke does not describe the fragrance filling the house as John does (Jn 12.3), like the incense offering in Luke 1 the fragrant ointment in Luke 7 appears in the text at a moment when boundaries are crossed.

An unnamed woman crosses the social boundary of Simon's house and the corporeal boundary of Jesus' body (7.37-38). Simon is locked within the boundaries of his understanding of divine hospitality (7.39). Jesus appeals to the woman's action, her erotic anointing of his feet with ointment, as evidence that the supposed limits of divine hospitality have been crossed (7.44-48). Divine hospitality flows like the ointment with which the woman anoints Jesus. She is able to perform this action because she has already experienced the overflow of divine hospitality as forgiveness.[45]

Boundaries concerning who is neighbour, who calls forth and who offers the divine hospitality of compassion are at issue in Lk. 10.25-37 when a Samaritan acts as neighbour where the religious leaders could not cross the boundary (represented by the road) to do so. The compassion of the Samaritan is in part expressed through the materiality of the oil and wine with which he cleanses and anoints the wounded person (10.34). The scent of the road, of the bloody wounds, and of the wine and oil are absent from the story, but sit in the background where once again a boundary, between

43. Elaine M. Wainwright, 'Unbound Hair and Ointmented Feet: An Ecofeminist Reading of Luke 7.36-50', in *Exchanges of Grace* (Festschrift Ann Loades; ed. Natalie K. Watson and Stephen Burns; London: SCM, 2008), pp. 178-89.

44. Wainwright, 'Unbound Hair', p. 185.

45. The parallel with the parable of 7.41-42 implies that she acts in response to a forgiveness already experienced. See Byrne, *Hospitality of God*, p. 75; Marshall, *Gospel of Luke*, pp. 306-307; Neale, *'None but the Sinners'*, p. 146.

seeing and acting with openness to the other, is traversed. At the nexus of death and life, neglect or compassion, is the fragrance of healing and cleansing oil and wine, diffusing the boundary between self and other.

*The Preparations for Burial, Luke 23.55–24.3*

In Lk. 23.55–24.3, at a boundary between death and life, women enter the narrative with spices and ointment to anoint a body that is absent (23.55). The absence of the living Jesus signalled by the burial of his dead body (23.53) becomes the absence of the corpse itself (24.3) and the presence elsewhere, implied in the question, 'Why do you look for the living among the dead?', and accompanied in some versions by the explicit claim: he 'has risen' (24.5).

The descriptions of the preparation (23.55a) and bringing of the spices (24.1b) also mark a temporality. The Sabbath comes between the women's preparation of the spice and ointment and their use of these fragrant materials to anoint the corpse in the customary manner. The women keep the observance of Sabbath as Torah commands (23.55b) and return at early dawn on the first day of the week (24.1a). With this indication of a world of Torah observance, we are returned to the world of the Lukan infancy narratives, where incense hung in the Temple . With the reference to the first day of the week, we are reminded of Genesis 1 and the beginning of creation, when God separated light from darkness, day from night, when the boundaries between the waters had not yet been set up (Gen. 1.1-8). At this heightened moment in Luke, the customary labour of women as ministers to the dead and the cultic observance of the Sabbath encounter the divine activity of creation. But as the icon *Myrrh Bearers* suggests, the flasks of fragrance remain closed, because as indicated in the previous chapter the body absent from the tomb is with the living.

As I argued there, the appearance narratives continue an engagement with an absent/present body. Gradually, however, the focus shifts from body to word. The focus on touching the body—'Touch me and see; for a ghost/spirit does not have flesh and bones as you see that I have' (24.39)—turns to a recollection of speech and writing: 'These are my words that I spoke to you while I was still with you—that everything written about me in the law of Moses, the prophets and the psalms must be fulfilled' (24.44). The absent/present body gives way to the interpretation of the Scriptures through the lens of the Lukan divine necessity. As considered in Chapter 3, in these Scriptures/writings is the echo of the absent/present place of their writing (the scrolls of the law, prophets and psalms, and the material artefact/s of Luke's own writing). This absent/present materiality also stands behind the commandment of Scripture that authorizes the Sabbath observance (23.56b), creating a space between the women's preparation (23.56a) and their proposed use of the spices and ointment (24.1). This becomes a space between death and life signalled by the closed flask and a body that is not with the dead (24.5).

*The Last Supper in Luke 22.7-23*

The body is both central and displaced in the Lukan Last Supper, where Jesus taking, giving thanks, breaking and giving bread, says, 'This is my body, which is given for you. Do this in remembrance of me' (22.19). Set in the Jewish context of a Passover meal, the Lukan Last Supper also displays aspects of the symposium, a context in which scents were used to enhance the experience of the meal and the conversation thereafter.[46] As elsewhere in the text, reference to scent is absent. Here, Jesus is the host, and one might expect that, where in 7.46 he comments that his host Simon failed to anoint his head with oil, he would not also fail to ensure that his own guests were anointed. But there is no mention of this.

In descriptions of the use of fragrant spices and oil at symposia such as those found in Athenaeus of Naucratis's *Deipnosophists*, servants or slaves were usually the ones who performed such service to the guests (Athenaeus, *Deipn.* 15). Presenting himself as servant (22.27), the Lukan Jesus might be expected to perform this role. Indeed, John 13 has Jesus perform the related foot-washing role as the focus of the supper. The key focus of the meal in Luke 22, however, is the body of Jesus that will be given and the blood poured out in covenant, the betrayal and suffering, the approaching death and the promise of life in the eschatological banquet (22.15-23).[47] If Jesus anoints the disciples who are his guests, it is to share in his role as servant ruler (22.24-30). If he does not anoint them, and the text is silent on this point, perhaps the reason is that for Luke Jesus is the anointed one (2.11, 26; 3.15; 4.41; 9.20; 20.41; 22.67; 23.2, 35, 39; 24.26, 46).

In the absence of descriptions of smells and smelling, fragrant oil and ointment remain in the background of the designation of Jesus as the Christ, the anointed one. For Luke, that Jesus is the Christ is not primarily a matter of anointing, but of proclamation concerning the time of salvation (the Lukan today, 2.11), expectation (2.26; 3.15) and knowledge or recognition (4.41; 9.20), occasioning conflict, including false testimony and abuse (20.41; 22.67; 23.2, 35, 39), as a matter of divine necessity (24.26, 46).

46. See Eugene LaVerdiere, *The Eucharist in the New Testament and the Early Church* (Collegeville, MN: Liturgical Press, 1996), p. 83; Dennis Edwin Smith, *From Symposium to Eucharist: The Banquet in the Early Christian World* (Minneapolis: Fortress Press, 2003), esp. pp. 222-23, 253-66; Harvey, *Scenting Salvation*, pp. 39-40; Wainwright, *Women Healing*, pp. 133-34.

47. John Paul Heil, *The Meal Scenes in Luke–Acts: An Audience-Oriented Approach* (Atlanta: Society of Biblical Literature, 1999), esp. p. 173.

Luke has no one anointing Jesus on the head with fragrant ointment (cf. 7.37-38, 46; Mt. 26.7; Mk 14.3). The Lukan Jesus is anointed not with the materiality of fragrant oil, but is proclaimed as anointed one (Christ/Messiah) through words in a writing that both recalls and conceals its place in a material artefact.

### *Between Life and Death: Smelling, Speaking, Writing*

Although ubiquitous in the ancient world, smell rarely attracts comment in the Second Testament. Where it does, smell often figures at a nexus of death and life. For Paul, in 2 Cor. 2.14-16, smell marks the space from death to death and from life to life evoking an eschatological Christian time that saturates the present time with the consummation of past promise and future expectation. Smell evokes a counter-experience of the embodiment of the gospel. For Luke, smell is effectively absent. Where fragrant materials receive mention, they appear where boundaries between self and other, life and death are crossed, particularly where this crossing is occasioned by a divine visitation. This association is not coincidental.

Smell (as matter and sense) crosses boundaries between self and other. Moreover, smell mediates between different states of matter, from solid or liquid to gas. Smell evokes a temporality: one smells the fire after it has occurred, the rain before it comes. Smell allows the other to enter us minutely and intimately. When a writing refers to fragrance, aroma or odour, the reader can imagine the matter that smell mediates through the medium of air: the lamb whose flesh is cooking, the incense burning, the oil poured out (and the plants from which it has been extracted). With regard to scent, the reader can ask: What is consumed in the production of a scent? What other is inhaled in its smelling?

By analogy, the reader can also ask, What is consumed in the production of a text? What others do I consume when I read? What sorts of consumption occur in the act of interpretation? The Second Testament is sparse in its reference to smell, despite the ubiquity of odour and aroma in its world. In a similar way, the biblical text is sparse in its reference to the material artefacts in which its writings present themselves to readers, and through which Earth is spent and spends itself materially. This materiality intrinsic to the senses, bodies and texts is an absent presence in the Lukan scenes of scent, the depictions of the body of the Lukan Jesus, and the references to the writings, each of which in a different way underscores the Lukan narrative and its invitation to respond to a divine visitation.

# 6

## '... THE STONES WOULD SHOUT OUT' (LUKE 19.40): HEARING AND VOICE

> Hear, O Israel ...
>
> Deut. 6.4 NRSV
>
> And as he said this, he called out, 'Let anyone with ears to hear listen!'
>
> Lk. 8.8b NRSV
>
> Then from the cloud came a voice that said, 'This is my Son, my Chosen; listen to him!'
>
> Lk. 9.35 NRSV
>
> When Elizabeth heard Mary's greeting, the child leapt in her womb...
>
> 'For as soon as I heard the sound of your greeting, the child in my womb leapt for joy.'
>
> Lk. 1.41a, 44 NRSV

The command Hear! Listen! saturates the Bible, not only alluding to its relation to oral tradition and its being read aloud, but also describing an orientation to its God, an orientation demanded of a people who have become people of the book. This imperative links the biblical word with both the voice and the material text. In the paradigmatic *Shema*, the command to hear is a command to keep; here hearts and houses are inscribed and bodies bound with writing:

> Hear, O Israel: Yhwh is our God, Yhwh alone. You shall love Yhwh your God with all your heart, and with all your soul, and with all your might. Keep these words that I am commanding you today in your heart. Recite them to your children and talk about them when you are at home and when you are away, when you lie down and when you rise. Bind them as a sign on your hands, fix them as an emblem on your forehead, and write them on the doorposts of your house and on your gates (Deut. 6.4-9 NRSV modified).

The material artefact in which the writing presents itself is bound to the body (the hands and the head) and the home. The voice with which the words are to be recited as instruction to children and training of memory across place and time (at home and away; evening and morning) is in a sequence with the tefillin/phylacteries that in miniature stand for the material artefact, in which the written command presents itself to reading and remembering. The key element of this hearing-voice-material artefact sequence is the relationship with Israel's God, who visits and withdraws in the writings/Scriptures.

This divine visitation and withdrawal appears in Victor Majzner's painting *Vayeitzei* (Jacob's Ladder/Dream), which depicts a ladder formed of Hebrew letters on which angels/white birds ascend against the landscape of the Flinders Ranges in Australia, which the artist also associates with the Negev.[1] The ascending letters spell the word חלם, dream, associated for Majzner with prophecy. The descending letters spell the word לחם, bread, and for the artist situate the event in the earth/land that sustains. At the base are twelve coloured stones, for the twelve tribes of Israel. In the sky behind the ladder is an open book, black to denote the absence of a God who withdraws in order that the Torah might come into being. This divine absence is not only the absence of the signified in the signifier, but it is also an absence that defines the Torah as a gift that gives a people of the book to itself. In this book, Jacob is Israel and his sons, the twelve tribes. In the narrative to which the painting responds, Jacob says of Bethel, 'How awesome is this place! This is none other than the house of God, and this is the gate of heaven' (Gen 28.17).

Majzner's painting transfers Jacob's affirmation of place to the Australian landscape, with all the associations of colonization, migration and seeking of asylum that accompany a transferral of peoples of the book to Australia. Perhaps the many coloured stones refer not only to the twelve tribes but also to this multicultural transferral of peoples. The book in the sky, like the place Bethel and the Australian land, is a doorway. The open space of the book is a threshold of relationship between a people, land and God, opened by the withdrawal of God in the text.[2]

1. Victor Majzner's *Vayeitzei* can be viewed in colour at http://www.studio-international.co.uk/studio-images/Majnzer/vayeitzei_LR_b.asp; see further Richard McBee, 'Majzner's Illuminated Torah', *The Jewish Press* (January 27, 2010; http://www.jewishpress.com/pageroute.do/42371) and Janet McKenzie, 'Victor Majzner, *Painting the Torah*, Melbourne 2008' (http://www.studio-international.co.uk/painting/Victor_Majzner.asp).

2. In the preceding two paragraphs, my comments on the painting are drawn both from Victor Majzner's notes, received by e-mail 6 February 2010, and my own observations.

This chapter focuses on hearing and voice, situating the material artefacts that are Bibles at the intersection of speech and writing, mediated by the voice. In the command to listen, the voice crosses with the written word. I draw on the work of Jean-Luc Nancy, who suggests that in listening, the self comes into being through self-withdrawal, through being sounded by an other. A text carries a voice that can resound in its reader/hearer. The story of the visitation in the Lukan infancy narrative offers a model for considering the agency of the voice that is sounded in the body. I take the textual imperative to listen to a written voice as prompt for exploring the sounding of the voice of the stones in Lk. 19.40. The stones cry out of matter and grief, resistance and praise.

This material voice echoes in the materiality of a text that, like the divine in Majzner's painting, withdraws to allow the other to be. The sounding of, and being sounded by, the materiality of the voice requires not only the self-withdrawal that is a coming to self of the reader/hearer/listener, or the withdrawal of the divine in the Scriptures, but also the withdrawal of matter in the text. The pattern of withdrawal is part of a material intertextuality, where in language the maternal withdraws and in writing the material artefact withdraws to allow the other to come to voice. As argued in Chapter 2, what is withdrawn nevertheless remains, as an unsettling trace in texts. In Majzner's painting, the withdrawal is also a threshold of relationship.

## *Hearing and Voice*

In the Hebrew Bible, the relationship between people, land and God is marked by an imperative—Hear! Listen! Give ear!—written at the threshold of body and home. The command to hear is linked with the voice, שׁמע קל. 'Hear her [Sarah's] voice', God says to Abraham (Gen. 21.12). 'Hear my voice', Rebekah says three times to her son Jacob (Gen. 27.8, 13, 43). 'Hear the voice of the people', Yhwh commands Samuel (1 Sam. 8.7, 9, 22). Moses prays, 'Yhwh, hear the voice of Judah' (Deut. 33.7). Samuel exhorts Saul, 'Hear the voice of the words of Yhwh' (1 Sam. 15.1). The psalmist cries, 'Hear, Yhwh my voice I cry' (Ps. 27.7); 'Hear the voice of my supplication' (Ps. 28.2); 'Hear my voice, God, in my complaint' (Ps. 64.1). Alongside שׁמע is the verb אזן, which has the same consonantal form as the noun 'ear'; so, Give ear to, Listen, Attend! For example, in Isaiah, the prophet proclaims, 'Listen (האזינו) and hear my voice (ושמעו קולי)/pay attention (הקשׁיבו) and hear my speech (ושמעו אמרתי)' (Isa. 28.23; see also Isa. 32.9; Ps. 130.2).

One can speak a word in someone's ear (Gen. 44.18). The ears and the eyes can stand in parallel as associated senses of attention and understanding (2 Kgs 19.16; Neh. 1.6; Job 13.1; 29.11; 42.5; Ps. 94.9; Prov. 20.12; Isa. 64.4). In prayer, the supplicant calls on God to have attentive ears and open

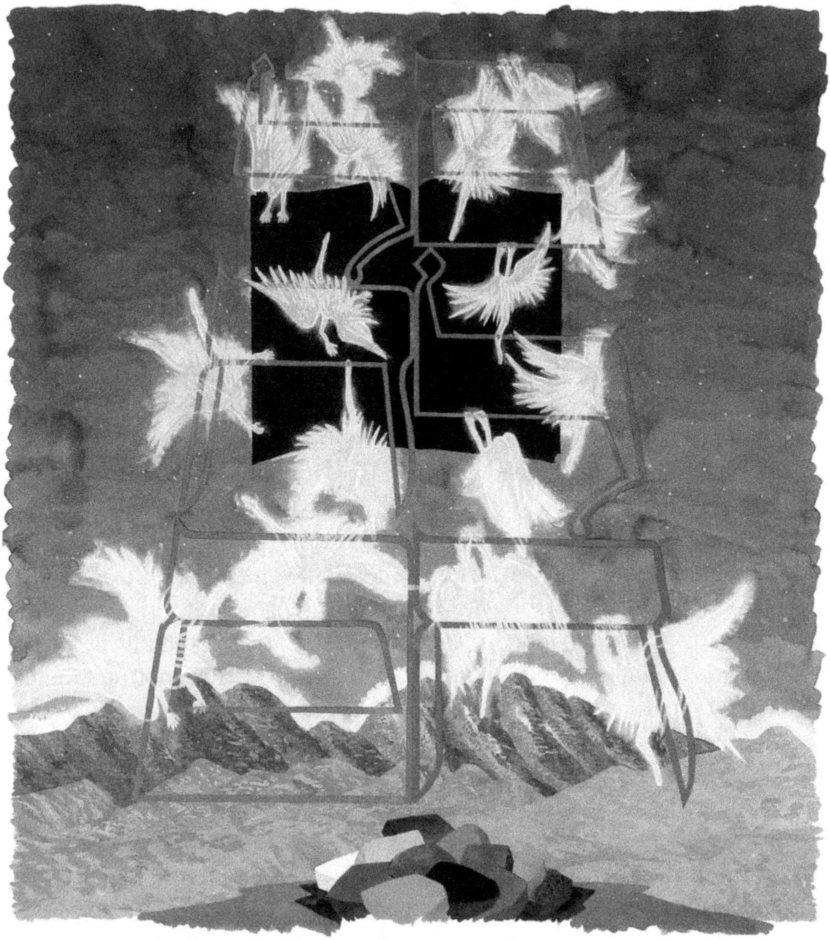

Fig. 3. Victor Majzner, *Vayeitzei* (Jacob's Dream).
Copyright © Victor Majzner/ Licensed by Viscopy, 2010.

eyes (Neh. 1.6; 2 Chron. 6.40; see also 2 Chron. 7.15). The ear tastes words as the mouth tastes food (Job 12.11; 34.3). From the mouth issues the cry to which the ears are given (Gen. 24.57; 2 Sam. 17.5; 18.25; 1 Kgs 13.21; 22.13; Isa. 34.16; 62.2; Jer. 36.4, 6, 18; 44.26; Ps. 66.17; Job 19.16; Prov. 18.6; 2 Chron. 18.12). The mouth speaks wisdom in association with ears oriented toward wisdom (Ps. 49.1-4; Prov. 5.1-2). Stones can cry out (Hab. 2.8), skies give ear and earth hear the words of the mouth (Deut. 32.1).

Like the eyes and the mouth, the ears can open or otherwise (פתח) (Isa. 48.8; cf. Isa. 35.5). An ear is like a doorway (פתח), a threshold where cry or call, word and voice, can enter. Just as in the Lukan usage, the entry of the word into the open ear signifies a welcoming of word, wisdom and understanding in the heart (Ps. 49.3-4; Lk. 8.4-15). As discussed in Chapter 2, there is a metonymy in Luke between ear, heart and earth as places of receptivity to the word/seed (Lk. 8.4-15). Moreover, these places are imaged as storehouses or treasuries (Lk. 2.19, 51).[3] Such storehouses have doors or gates.

In Jewish Scriptures, the skies are divine storehouses which Yhwh can open or shut (Deut. 28.12; see also Jer. 10.13; 51.16; Job 38.22-23; Pss 33.7; 135.7). At the baptism of Jesus, the sky opens (ἀνεῳχθῆναι τὸν οὐρανόν), and a voice comes (or comes into being) from the sky (φωνὴν ἐξ οὐρανοῦ γενέσθαι): 'You are my son the beloved, in you I am well pleased' (Lk. 3.21-22). When in the transfiguration episode a voice comes from the cloud (φωνὴ ἐκ τῆς νεφέλης), the baptismal address to Jesus echoes in the address to the disciples, Peter, John and James: 'This is my son the chosen', with the added command: αὐτοῦ ἀκούετε, 'listen to him!' (Lk. 9.35).

The voice from the skies comes into the world at the threshold of the divine realm, the open door or gate of the divine storehouses, from which also come rain and snow (Job 38.22). At this threshold, the voice affirming Jesus as beloved, chosen kin, does not say 'Listen to me', but rather 'Listen to him'. This command echoes not only in the ears of Peter, John and James, as characters in the narrative, but also in the ears/hearts of the hearers/readers, who themselves can become storehouses of a divine word/thing. It also echoes Jesus' own cry at the end of the parable of the sower and the seed, 'Let anyone with ears to hear listen!' (Lk. 8.8b; see also 14.35).

The command to listen issues from a heavenly threshold (that is, in the ancient biblical world, the materiality of sky) and the divine realm opens into, and onto, a human, and arguably more-than-human, world. The gate or doorway stands for the threshold of divine call and human response. Lady Sophia cries out at the city gates (Prov. 8.3; cf. 24.7). After Elijah experiences a voice of thin/powdery/material silence (קול דממה דקה), he waits at the opening of a cave (1 Kgs. 19.12-13). In the ears of all the people, Baruch reads from the scroll of Jeremiah, at the New Gate of Yhwh's house, that is, the Temple (Jer. 36.10). The material artefact (scroll), the organ of hearing (ears) and the gate of the house of God come together in this passage from Jeremiah to suggest a movement across openings: corporeal, inscribed, built, and divinely ordered. In Majzner's painting of Jacob's ladder, the book-shaped absence in the sky over Bethel (the house of God) marries the book to the heavenly storehouses from which rain, snow and divine voice issue. In the metaphor of the threshold, gateway or opening, the material

3. See Elvey, *Ecological Feminist Reading*, pp. 145-51.

text itself becomes the opening from which issues a divine voice. But in Majzner's painting, this event of divine vocation occurs in the withdrawal of the divine, a withdrawal shaped to the material artefact itself.

### *Sound and Hearing*

The material artefact is dependent on the human body and the embodied sense of hearing as much as sight. As Thomas Staubli and Sylvia Schroer indicate, ancient writing depended on the attentive listening of the scribe to whom the text was dictated.[4] At the interface of oral and written word is the body of the scribe, the sensory engagement of hearing and sight, and the touch of hand on stylus on skin: skin to skin. While one skin folds around the thresholds of ears and eyes, another forms the threshold of the text, where matter opens to writing. At this threshold, writing becomes again voice in the ears/heart of the hearer/reader invited to listen.

Jean-Luc Nancy makes a distinction between hearing and listening. He understands listening to be an intensification of hearing.[5] In listening, one extends one's ears. This notion of extension is found in the Hebrew idiom אטה ... אזני, 'I will incline (stretch out or bend) my ear' (Ps. 49.5 MT). In listening, one extends oneself toward another and toward meaning. For Nancy there is a two-way movement between sound and sense, where sense refers not only to the senses such as hearing but also to sense as meaning, such that through listening, meaning 'is sought in sound' and 'sound, resonance, is sought in meaning'.[6] In the act of listening, one inhabits a margin, or stands at a threshold, between sound and sense.

Sound signals participation or sharing that is of a different quality to the sensation of the visible through sight.[7] In some respects, Nancy's description of the relation of the body to sound parallels the description I gave in the previous chapter of the relation of the body to smell, where I noted the way in which smelling unsettles the boundary between self and other, when the body takes in the essence of the other.[8] However, sound does not produce a particulate intake of the other as an odour does when inhaled through the nose; instead sound sets up a resonance in the body, through the ear but not only the ear, so that the sound sounds, or resounds in, the body. In listening, the body is sounded by something other, and the listener is returned to her- or himself through being sounded.[9]

4. Staubli and Schroer, *Body Symbolism*, pp. 123-24.
5. Nancy, *Listening*, p. 5.
6. Nancy, *Listening*, p. 7.
7. Nancy, *Listening*, p. 10.
8. Nancy, *Listening*, pp. 14-15.
9. Nancy, *Listening*, p. 12.

This notion of being sounded, which can be understood as a corporeal internal resonance in 'the sonorous cave we become',[10] offers a basis for understanding the Lukan crossing between ear and heart. This internal resonance, characteristic of the inner sense of which I wrote in Chapter 3, parallels the receptivity of the heart to which Luke appeals (2.19, 51; 6.45; 8.15). For Nancy, receptivity to being sounded by the other distinguishes the listening self as a self-presence marked by self-withdrawal.[11] A pattern of return to self through the self-withdrawal of being sounded by the other has echoes in the Lukan reference to the necessity for the disciple to gain her or his life through its loss (9.24). This Lukan pattern of self-abandonment is a participation in the divine necessity that describes Jesus' journey toward his passion and execution (9.22-23). Participation in this divine necessity has the force of a call requiring a response. Mary of Nazareth is for Luke a paradigm of faithful responsiveness to such a call (see esp. 1.38). Her responsiveness has the character of an internal resonance (2.19, 51) and, as Simeon prophesies, becomes a participation in the self-abandonment and suffering of the Lukan Jesus (2.34-35).

Mary's fiat stands in the frame of call and response, for which the biblical 'here I am' is paradigmatic. For Jean-Louis Chrétien, the call to which one might answer 'here I am' comes into a self already 'here', whose presence is unsettled by an address.[12] The unsettling occurs, however, in the context of a self that, like the Lukan Mary, when called into presence is already present: 'I have already come forth when I come forth, I have already responded when I respond.'[13] Parallel to Nancy's evocation of self-withdrawal, this self-presence has the character of an absence: 'nothingness alone is what comes to the call and thus listens to it'.[14]

Further, Chrétien claims, 'the call is heard only in the response'.[15] But this response is one in which what cannot be heard, an excess within the call—to borrow Marion's term, a 'saturation' of the audible with the inaudible—both gives speech (or voice) and exceeds the possibility of response.[16] Because the response always includes both the call and the impossibility of response to the call (see, for example, 1.34), the response has a 'choral character'.[17] For example, in the Lukan annunciation to Mary (1.26-38), Mary's 'here I am' (1.34, 38) holds the impossible possibility (1.34, 37)

10. Nancy, *Listening*, pp. 25, 31-32, 37, 67.
11. Nancy, *Listening*, p. 12.
12. Chrétien, *Call and the Response*, p. 19.
13. Chrétien, *Call and the Response*, p. 19.
14. Chrétien, *Call and the Response*, p. 22.
15. Chrétien, *Call and the Response*, p. 30.
16. Chrétien, *Call and the Response*, p. 31.
17. Chrétien, *Call and the Response*, p. 32.

to which she is called. The outer chorus, with which the inner choral character of her response resonates, includes not only the visiting angel, Mary of Nazareth and God, but also a world of Jewish history and expectation (see esp. 1.32) that shapes the meaning both of the divine call and Mary's response. Moreover, the choral character of Mary's response overflows in the visitation scene, where her voice is central in its effects in the pregnant body of Elizabeth (1.40-41, 43), her song (1.46-55) and the world of liberation her song calls forth.

Being sounded by a call, the self is called in its world, as a voice in a chorus, self and world together in one sounding that is plural, if not always harmonious:

> ... by calling me as a person, it calls me not as an isolated and abstract being but calls the totality of the world in space and time along with me, in the inexhaustible chorus of which I am only one voice enduring a perpetual inchoation.[18]

In his poem 'On a Forestry Trail', Robert Gray expresses the experience of response as choral in a more-than-human setting. The poem begins, 'A choir/of eucalyptus saplings' and concludes with the speaker ...

> having awakened in the shape of a man,
> and having a stick with which
> to poke,
> and an old dog,
> and such rare colour
> beside me here; and all of us are
> a choir.[19]

Rather than being transformed, the poet is awakened as what he already is: a human in a more-than-human community where the response of the person is part of the choral response of a more-than-human world. Drawing on Walter Brueggemann's work on the role of the cry in the prophetic imagination, Janet Morgan extends the notion of cry to Earth's cry.[20] The cry arrives in the voices of those humans who break the silence concerning the contemporary ecological crisis. But the Earth community is already resonant with sound—birdsong, trees shushing in the wind, the rumble of oceans, rain, thunder, and cars, trains, sheep, dogs, people in conversation and argument—a whole concatenation of sounds sounding a person in a here and now, in a world.

18. Chrétien, *Call and the Response*, p. 19.

19. Robert Gray, *Certain Things* (Port Melbourne: William Heinemann Australia, 1993), pp. 50-52.

20. Janet Morgan, *Earth's Cry: Prophetic Ministry in a More-than-Human World* (DminStuds; Melbourne College of Divinity, 2010), pp. 44-63.

For Michel Serres, the sounding of a person in a world has three aspects, or three kinds, of audible. They are the body, whose sounds he links with illness and health; Earth and cosmos, from the singing of birds to the noise of distant galaxies; and human society, which he tends to register as disturbance.[21] To the myriad sounds that address the human body, the body adds the feedback of its own voice.[22] In this ubiquity of sound, where even what we call silence is interrupted by the rhythm of a heartbeat, the scurry of a mouse and the breath of wind in a tree, the written text can be conceived as an instrument through which to play a particular series of sounds.[23] The word, written as well as spoken, is 'soundful', and this soundfulness is essential to the play of call and response that sounds a person as its reader/hearer.[24]

In its relations to bodies and a more-than-human sociality (which includes the world-shaping sociality of humans), sound participates in a 'sonorous' materiality.[25] Moreover, sound is one mode of the materiality of words.[26] As in listening to music, in reading/hearing a text, one touches and is touched by a work.[27] For this reason, the material artefact does not exhaust the materiality of a text. The writing in a place in an artefact has another register of materiality in the sound of its words, and this sound-matter acts materially on, and in, the bodies of the readers/hearers of the text, just as Mary's greeting acts on, and in, the pregnant body of Elizabeth (1.40-41, 43).

## *Greeting*

> In those days Mary set out and went with haste to a Judean town in the hill country, where she entered the house of Zechariah and greeted Elizabeth. When Elizabeth heard Mary's greeting, the child leaped in her womb. And Elizabeth was filled with the Holy Spirit and exclaimed with a loud cry, 'Blessed are you among women, and blessed is the fruit of your womb. And why has this happened to me, that the mother of my lord comes to me? For as soon as I heard the sound of your greeting, the child in my womb leaped for joy. And blessed is she who believed that there would be a fulfillment of what was spoken to her by the lord' (Lk. 1.39-45 NRSV modified).

21. Serres, *Five Senses*, pp. 106-11.

22. Serres, *Five Senses*, p. 111.

23. Don Idhe, *Listening and Voice: Phenomenologies of Sound* (Albany: State University of New York Press, 2nd edn, 2007), p. 4.

24. Idhe, *Listening and Voice*, p. 4.

25. Nancy, *Listening*, p. 40, draws on Antoine Bonnet to situate this materiality in the notion of 'timbre'.

26. Nancy, *Listening*, pp. 15, 27, 29.

27. Nancy, *Listening*, p. 65.

In a scene traditionally described as the visitation, Mary's greeting occurs at a number of thresholds. First, the greeting occurs at the threshold of the house of Zechariah. Second, the greeting occurs at the threshold of new life the pregnant body represents. Third, the greeting comes in a passage from sight to hearing. Where in the annunciation to Zechariah the emphasis is on the vision of the angelic messenger (1.12, 22), even to the extent that Zechariah loses his voice (1.20), in the annunciation to Mary the emphasis turns to hearing. Rather than the sight of the angel, the greeting she hears prompts Mary's initial response (1.28-29). Then in the following episode Mary's own greeting, which unlike the angel's goes unrecorded, is pivotal. Referring three times to Mary's greeting, the visitation highlights the agency of the voice (1.40, 41, 44). Both the narrator and Elizabeth herself describe the effect of the voice in the body as a quickening accompanied by joy (1.41, 44).

Artists frequently depict the greeting as conveyed as much by touch and sight as by voice, with the women looking into each other's eyes as if the greeting passes through the gaze.[28] Frequently, the women touch arm to arm or embrace. In several paintings, a hand of one or both women touches or hovers over the womb of the other woman.[29] Of Jacopo Pontormo's *Visitation*, from the parish church of Carmignano, Tuscany, Nancy writes, 'These wombs touch without touching.'[30] The greeting in the space between voice and hearing is a touch, at the threshold of two bodies, voice to ear, body to body, skin to skin.

Mary greets Elizabeth on entering Zechariah's house, that is, at the threshold of the house (1.40). In artwork, often the women appear outlined by an arch or doorway.[31] Frequently, the countryside figures when the

28. See, for example, the paintings of *The Visitation* by Fra Angelico (from *The Annunciation* altarpiece, Cortona, Museo Diocesano; http://www.casasantapia.com/art/fraangelico/annunciation.htm); Jacopo Pontormo (http://www.andrewgrahamdixon.com/archive/readArticle/275), and the Jamb figure sculpture at Chartres cathedral (http://www.artbible.net/3JC/-Luk-01,39_Mary%20visits%20Elizabeth_La%20visitation/slides/13%20CHARTRES%20JAMB%20FIGURE,%20PORTAL%20VISITATION.html).

29. See, for example, the paintings of *The Visitation* by Jacques Daret (http://www.wga.hu/html/d/daret/stvaast2.html) and Jacopo Tintoretto (http://www.artbible.net/3JC/-Luk-01,39_Mary%20visits%20Elizabeth_La%20visitation/slides/16%20TINTORETTO%20THE%20VISITATION.html), and Rogier van der Weyden (http://www.artbible.info/art/large/484.html).

30. Jean-Luc Nancy, *The Ground of the Image* (trans. Jeff Fort; Perspectives in Continental Philosophy; New York: Fordham University Press, 2005), p. 111.

31. See, for example, the paintings of *The Visitation* by Dieric Bouts the Elder (from the winged altarpiece, Museo del Prado, Madrid; http://www.wga.hu/html/b/bouts/dirk_e/altar/index.html); El Greco (Dumbarton Oaks; http://museum.doaks.

domesticity of the women's encounter is framed by the wildness of the hill country of Judah, or its transferral to the countryside of the artists' experience and imagination. In a fresco attributed to Giotto, the women meet and the greeting passes between them outside the doorway of the house, with hills and a single tree in the background.[32] A number of other women look on. The tree grows on a ridge directly above the space between the faces of the two women. The tree, which may recall both the tree of life and the tree of the cross, appears to grow from the space of encounter between Mary and Elizabeth. In this encounter, Mary's greeting prompts the response both of and to the Spirit in Elizabeth (1.41), and Elizabeth's beatitude (1.45) prompts an inspired response in Mary, the Magnificat (1.46-55).[33]

Occurring in the context of the wider Lukan theme of divine visitation, the visitation of Mary and Elizabeth takes place not only at a threshold of human and other-than-human space—the touch of bodies at the house of Zechariah in the hill country of Judah—but also at the threshold of human and divine space. Where in the annunciation to Mary the heavenly divine agent Gabriel arrives with a word, in the visitation the human agent Mary of Nazareth arrives prompting an inspired response in the body of Elizabeth. Elizabeth's response is both quickening and cry of blessing (1.41-42, 44-45). Through the agency of the voice, words resonate in bodies in a moment visual traditions depict as a synaesthesia.

Three aspects of this agency of the voice are important for my consideration of hearing and the material artefact in Luke. They are first, the movement from the agency of voice to the agency of keeping in the characterization of Mary; second, the role of the voice as mediating the word; and third, the role of the cry in giving voice to the other than human.

### *The Agency of Keeping*

Having spoken the Magnificat, left the house of Elizabeth and returned to her home, Mary speaks once more (2.48b), after which she is silent in the Lukan narrative.[34] But she is not without agency. Although silent in the birth narrative itself (2.1-7), Mary acts to give birth to the child, wrap him in

org/Obj823?sid=292&x=80978&port=2625); Domenico Ghirlandaio (Louvre; http://cartelen.louvre.fr/cartelen/visite?srv=car_not_frame&idNotice=13692); and Andrea Pisano's bronze on the southern doors of the baptistry, Florence.

32. See the *Visitation* fresco in the north transept of the lower church of the Basilica of St Francis in Assisi (http://www.artbible.net/3JC/-Luk-01,39_Mary%20visits%20Elizabeth_La%20visitation/slides/14%20GIOTTO%20THE%20VISITATION.html).

33. Mark Coleridge, *The Birth of the Lukan Narrative: Narrative as Christology in Luke 1–2* (Sheffield: Sheffield Academic Press, 1993), p. 79.

34. For a careful exploration of the silence and silencing of women in the Gospel of Luke, see Dowling, *Taking Away the Pound*, pp. 119-85.

bands of cloth and lay him in a manger (2.7). At the conclusion of both the narratives of annunciation to the shepherds (2.8-21) and of finding Jesus in the Temple (2.41-52), Mary acts to keep or store and ponder πάντα ... τὰ ῥήματα ταῦτα (all these things/words/deeds) in her heart (2.19, 51). As I have argued elsewhere, after the birth of Jesus, which is also a transformation of the mother, Mary becomes keeper of all these things, 'the stuff of the narrative or gospel itself, the connectedness of all these things'.[35] In the representation of the Lukan Mary, the agency of the voice in the visitation episode becomes an agency of listening—an inner hearing that stores the narrative, the gospel, and works to understand its meaning.

Through this agency of listening, Mary becomes a paradigm of those who hear, keep and do the word of God (8.19-21; 11.27-28).[36] But Luke dismisses the maternal body in his affirmation of hearing, keeping and doing the word (8.19-21; 11.27-28). Nonetheless, keeping (or storing) is part of a wider Lukan imaginary where the womb becomes identified metonymically with the ear, the heart and the earth as sites of receptivity to the word/seed; the notion of keeping as storing links these sites of receptivity with the Lukan image of a treasury or storehouse.[37]

Storing was the work of the scribe whose occupation was to keep accounts.[38] The authorial voice of the Lukan narrator presents the narrative as an 'account' (1.1), a 'keeping' work. Mary's work of keeping πάντα ... τὰ ῥήματα ταῦτα both parallels and offers a model for the keeping work of the Lukan text. The agency of Mary's keeping is the agency of a body that is open to being sounded by a word. In a parallel manner, through listening in order to write, the scribe is open to being sounded by an account that will become a writing. As part of a network of agency, the scribe produces *a writing in a place in a material artefact*, that is, a text. At thresholds of matter and word, scribe and writing, artefact and reader, a text is open to being sounded in reading or proclamation.

### *Mediating the Word*

For Luke hearing mediates the word, so that through listening the word is properly embodied in action (6.47, 49; 8.21; cf. 10.38-42). Jesus listens and asks questions (2.46); hears and responds (7.9; 8.50; 18.22). Jesus reads from a scroll of Isaiah in the hearing of those assembled in the synagogue at Nazareth (4.16-21). Jesus speaks in the hearing of the people (7.1; 20.45).

35. Elvey, *Ecological Feminist Reading*, p. 135.

36. Elvey, *Ecological Feminist Reading*, pp. 153-55.

37. See Elvey, *Ecological Feminist Reading*, pp. 145-63.

38. This link between storing and keeping account occurs both in characterizations of the Sumerian goddess Nisaba and Lady Sophia in Ben Sira (Elvey, *Ecological Feminist Reading*, p. 152).

'All who heard' forms a kind of refrain (1.66; 2.18; 2.47; 7.29) accompanied by a response (pondering, amazement, acknowledgment). This pattern begins in the infancy narratives and calls to the reader/hearer, as the Lukan Jesus does in the vocations, 'you who listen' (6.27); 'let these words sink into your ears' (9.44). Often what is heard is Jesus' immediate words or teaching—the Pharisees heard all this (16.14); when the rich ruler heard this (18.23); those who heard (18.26); when they heard (20.16)—occasioning a response.

Sometimes, the response is a refusal (4.21; 7.30; 16.14), an expression of dismay (18.23, 26; 20.16) or rage followed with violence (4.28). Having already executed John the Baptist, Herod is perplexed and fascinated by what he hears about Jesus (9.7, 9; 23.8). But hearing also relates to healing. The crowd presses in to hear the word of God (5.1); the crowds gather to hear Jesus and be cured (5.15; 6.18); a centurion hears about Jesus and sends Jewish elders to ask him to heal his slave (7.3; cf. 7.7); tax collectors and sinners come near to hear Jesus (15.1). There is a force to the desire of the people to hear him: all the people are intent on what they hear (19.48); the people would get up early in the morning to listen to him in the Temple (21.38).

The force of this desire is echoed in the movement between hearing, keeping and doing the word; the word prompts a response that in keeping and doing is also a kind of obedience, a coming under what is heard. The verb to obey, ὑπακούω, includes the verb 'to hear', ἀκούω. In Luke, ὑπακούω is used only in relation to responses from other-than-human characters: the winds and the waters (8.25) and a mulberry tree (17.6). Matter, too, can hear and respond—perhaps even the matter of the text. Reading from a scroll of Scripture is both vocalization and vocation, coming into the ears of its hearers (4.21). To the extent that a scroll, book or screen can be open to being read, the material artefact is also obedient to a voice, the inscribed voice and the voice of its reader. Is the material artefact also obedient to the divine word/matter?

A number of Lukan references to the word, words and writings need to be read together:

1. the word (λόγος) and the thing or matter (ῥῆμα) of God (2.29; 3.2; 5.1; 8.11, 21; 11.28);
2. the word/or words and thing/or matters the Lukan Jesus and other agents of God speak, or are reported as speaking, within the narrative (Jesus: 2.50; 4.32, 36; 5.1; 6.47; 9.28, 44-45; 10.39; 18.34; 20.26; 22.61; 24.8; other divine agents: 1.20, 29; 2.15, 17);
3. the word about Jesus (5.15; 7.17; 24.17, 19, 44);
4. the matters and words that are heard and kept in the heart (1.37-38; 2.19, 51; 7.1; 8.11-15, 21; 11.28; 24.32);

5. the writings (on scrolls) to which Jesus refers (3.4; 4.4, 8, 10-11, 12; 4.16-22; 7.27; 10.26; 18.31; 19.46; 21.22; 22.37; 24.27, 32, 44, 45, 46 );
6. the word and words of the gospels (1.1, 4); and
7. the Lukan Gospel itself, which comes to us in a variety of material artefacts.[39]

These references form a network of relations linking human and divine words with writings that include the Jewish Scriptures, early Christian accounts about Jesus, and the Gospel of Luke itself. Luke links the Jewish Scriptures (what is written/the writings) with the word of God, particularly through the motif of the divine necessity. Luke's own writing is an account, the business of which is the words about Jesus. Luke's writing becomes an interpretation of the Jewish writings and the word of God. The words of the Lukan Jesus and Luke's words about Jesus resonate, without being fully identified, with the word of the Lukan God. Through this resonance, when the material artefact mediates a Lukan writing it both gives itself to the agency of the voice of its reader/proclaimer and gives voice to a certain understanding of the word of God. To this extent, the material artefact mediates a divine voice. But there are other voices to which the text also pertains.

*The Cry*

In the visitation narrative, Elizabeth refers to the voice, φωνή, of Mary's greeting (1.44). Earlier, Elizabeth herself exclaims/gives voice with a loud cry (ἀνεφώνησεν κραυγῇ μεγάλῃ, 1.42). The voice (φωνή of the prophet calls out from, and is a trope in, the scroll of Isaiah—a voice calling out both in the desert and in the texts of Isaiah and Luke (3.4). As noted earlier, in the baptism and transfiguration accounts, a voice φωνή comes from the sky (3.22; 9.35-36). Like Elizabeth, who cried out a blessing, a woman lifts her voice (φωνήν) to speak a beatitude (1.42; 11.27).

From the underworld, the rich man calls out to Abraham for pity (16.24). The lepers give voice (φωνήν) to their plea to Jesus for mercy (17.13); on seeing he is healed, one returns to glorify God with a loud voice (μετὰ φωνῆς μεγάλης, 17.15). As Jesus approaches Jerusalem, the 'whole multitude of the disciples' begins to praise (αἰνεῖν) God in a loud voice (φωνῇ μεγάλῃ, 19.37). A person with a spirit of an unclean demon shouts out in a loud voice (ἀνέκραξεν φωνῇ μεγάλῃ, 4.33). The Gerasene demoniac is portrayed shouting out (ἀνακράξας) in a loud voice (φωνῇ μεγάλῃ, 8.28). In Jesus' passion, the people 'kept urgently demanding with loud shouts (φωναῖς μεγάλαις) that he should be crucified; and their voices (αἱ φωναὶ αὐτῶν) prevailed' (23.23; see also 23.18). As he is dying, the

39. Note, too, that in Luke 16.2, λόγος refers to an account.

Lukan Jesus cries out (voices) in a loud voice (φωνήσας φωνῇ μεγάλῃ, 23.46).

To call or voice (φωνέω) is to summon and command (16.2; 19.5), but also to invite (14.12). Jesus calls/voices (ἐφώνει), 'Let anyone with ears to hear listen!' (8.8) He calls (ἐφώνησεν) to the daughter of Jairus, 'Child, arise!' (8.54). In the passion narrative, a cock calls/voices:

> Jesus said, 'I tell you, Peter, the cock will not crow (φωνήσει) this day, until you have denied three times that you know me' (22.34 NRSV).
>
> At that moment, while he [Peter] was still speaking, the cock crowed (ἐφώνησεν). Then Peter remembered the word of the lord (τοῦ ῥήματος τοῦ κυρίου), how he had said to him, 'Before the cock crows (φωνῆσαι) today, you will deny me three times' (22.60b-61 NRSV modified).

Into the relationship between Peter and Jesus comes an other-than-human voice, that of a cock, as a sign both of the separation Peter has effected through his denial and the connection Jesus maintains through his foresight. Through the agency of the voice of a rooster, Peter remembers this connection and is moved to tears (22.62).

Like the other-than-human voice of the rooster, the voice of stones in Luke 19 is compelling. Jesus says, 'I tell you, if these [namely the multitude of disciples voicing praise of God in 19.37-38] were silent, the stones would shout out (οἱ λίθοι κράξουσιν)' (19.40). That the voices of roosters and stones can have agency suggests an interconnectedness between the Lukan Jesus and the more-than-human world he inhabits. In the next section, I will explore the possibility of listening for the voice of stones at the textual threshold of matter and word, material artefact and writing.

### *Conclusion*

In the visitation episode, the voices of women mediate an interconnectedness, the interconnectedness of self and other in the pregnant body and the interconnectedness of two kinswomen meeting at a threshold of divine and human space in a more-than-human context. With its emphasis on the agency of a voice uttered at a threshold, the visitation becomes a model not only of the divine visitation as a narrative trope, but also of the visitation that is the writing/reading–hearing of a gospel narrative, conveyed in a Lukan voice. Concerning Pontormo's *Visitation*, Nancy writes that the painting 'is seeking ... the mutual visitation of a spectator and a painting, or a *subject* of painting'.[40] Does Luke's Gospel, likewise, seek the mutual visitation of a reader/hearer and a writing, where the reader becomes a *subject* of the text (a writing in a place in a material artefact)? A material

40. Nancy, *Ground of the Image*, p. 112.

artefact, in this case a version of the Lukan narrative, is a presence that conveys an absence the reader/hearer touches with the senses.[41] This touching and being touched by the text registers in the inner sense where the reader/hearer listens to, and is sounded by, the text. In the encounter with the text, the reader/hearer is visited not only by a present absence of the divine visitor but also by the present absence of the materiality that underlies the artefacts in which the Lukan writing of divine visitation presents itself to reading.

Bearing the voice of its author, mediating a divine voice through a particular interpretative lens, and voiced by a reader, a writing is multi-vocal in at least two further ways. As argued in Chapter 2, a text emerges in a context of multiple positions as an intertext or transposition, and carries the multiple voices of the socio-cultural worlds and traditions in which the text is produced, which it interprets and in turns shapes. Further, the text gives voice to certain characters within its writing and elides or suppresses others. For example, although the paradigm of the agency of the voice occurs in a narrative in which the divine agency passes between women in what is in effect a mutual visitation, women seem to be increasingly silent and silenced in the Lukan Gospel, as Elizabeth Dowling has shown.[42] From an ecological feminist perspective, the silencing of women sets up a destructive resonance in the more-than-human sociality of the text, as, too, does the language of mastery. But, as Turid Seim argues, Luke's message concerning women is not univocal.[43] Nor, as I argued in Chapter 1, is Luke's appeal to the imagery of master and slave. Without denying the force of colonizing usages of master–slave imagery, a reading of a pattern of compassionate responsiveness in the Gospel of Luke offers an alternative paradigm to their violent legacies, as I proposed in Chapter 4. Similarly, the agency of the voices and bodies of Mary and Elizabeth in their visitation offers an alternative paradigm to the silencing of women.

This co-agency of women occurs in a more-than-human sociality often taken as background. Attention to a pattern of call and response signalled in the visitation, voices and bodies of two women can suggest that we also pay attention to the voices of other-than-human characters, particularly those whose voices appear to have agency within the narrative. If the voice of Mary sounds in the body of Elizabeth, in what way do the voices of other-than-human characters, such as the stones of Lk. 19.40, sound in bodies?

41. See similarly Nancy on the encounter with the present absence in the painting (*Ground of the Image*, p. 122).

42. Dowling, *Taking Away the Pound*, pp. 119-85.

43. Seim, *Double Message*.

*'and the stones would shout' (19.40)*

In Luke, Jesus' saying, 'if these were silent, the stones would shout out' (19.40), appears at the end of his processional and prophetic entry into Jerusalem (19.28-40) and in reference to the vocal praise of God by a multitude of Jesus' disciples (19.37-38). It comes as exclamation or rebuke to the complaint of some Pharisees in the crowd (19.39). The saying also comes immediately before Jesus' weeping over the coming destruction of the city, when one stone will not be left upon another, as a consequence, according to Luke, of a refusal or inability to 'recognize the time of your visitation' [most translations add, 'from God'] (19.41-44). The saying also has echoes of a prophetic oracle in Habakkuk, who warns of stones crying out from the wall, perhaps in judgment on the city (Hab. 2.9-12).[44] Noting these contexts, David Horrell and Dominic Coad suggest that both 'the themes of praise and protest or rebuke' need to be taken into account when we consider the agency of the stones as having the capacity for voice in this text.[45] They note also that 'the combination of praise and critique is evident elsewhere in Luke, not least in Mary's Magnificat (Lk. 1.46-55)'.[46] In attending to the shout of the stones in the following sections, I consider stones under the themes first of matter and grief, then resistance and finally praise.

This hermeneutic attentiveness to more-than-human voices has parallels with the ecopoeisis of which Kate Rigby writes.[47] Rigby analyzes two modes of ecopoeitic writing about nature. The first endeavours to evoke the 'thinginess'—a kind of material transcendence—of things, and to celebrate the plural otherness of an Earth community that has being, sociality, purposes and agencies that are more than human. The second sets out to grieve ecological losses, past, present and those anticipated in the future, especially those losses predicated on human action and inaction. Drawing on, but going beyond, Martin Heidegger's notion of dwelling, Rigby sees both forms of writing as simultaneously possible and impossible for our dwelling in this moment of ecological loss, when we need to call to consciousness the inestimable worth of what is and to be moved to compassion to nurture what may be no longer.[48] Thus, ecopoiesis—as writing, art and action—must be an embodied practice that embeds writers and readers more surely

44. E. Earle Ellis, *The Gospel of Luke* (NCBC; Grand Rapids: Eerdmans, 1981), p. 226.

45. David G. Horrell and Dominic Coad, '"The Stones Would Cry Out" (Luke 19.40): A Lukan Contribution to a Hermeneutics of Creation's Praise', *Scottish Journal of Theology* 64 (2011), pp. 29-44 (36).

46. Horrell and Coad, '"The Stones Would Cry Out"', p. 37 n. 32.

47. Rigby, 'Earth, World, Text', pp. 427-42.

48. Rigby, 'Earth, World, Text'.

within a more-than-human Earth community from which certain rationalistic philosophies and economics have separated us. To this extent there is an (im)possible ecopoiesis of writing and reading that endeavours to hear or recover both the 'thinginess' of matter and grief for its loss.

A third ecopoietic moment in writing and reading also needs to be accounted for, namely the ecopoiesis of resistance. In the ecojustice principles informing the Earth Bible project, the principle of resistance reads, 'Earth and its components not only suffer from injustices at the hands of humans, but actively resist them in the struggle for justice'.[49] Underlying this principle of resistance is recognition of the agency of the Earth community. Such recognition of Earth's agency is fundamental to an ecopoeisis. Finally, Horrell and Coad identify an important fourth ecopoeitic moment when they consider a hermeneutics of creation's praise.[50] In the shout of stones, can we hear these ecopoeitic moments of matter, grief, resistance and praise as evocative of a material intertextuality that assists us in approaching the intertextual materiality of the text?

### *Stones as Intertext*

How are we to read stones as intertext? In *The Fundamental Concepts of Metaphysics,* Heidegger claims:

> The stone is worldless, it is without world, it has no world.... Worldlessness ... is constitutive of the stone in the sense that the stone *cannot even be deprived* of something like world.[51]

Explaining what he means by this, Heidegger argues:

> The stone is without world. The stone is lying on the path, for example. We can say that the stone is exerting a certain pressure upon the surface of the earth. It is 'touching' the earth. But what we call 'touching' here is not a form of touching at all in the stronger sense of the word. It is not at all like *that* relationship which the lizard has to the stone on which it lies basking in the sun. And the touching implied in both these cases is above all not the same as that touch which we experience when we rest our hand upon the head of another human being.[52]

Heidegger understands 'world as the accessibility of beings' and argues that the stone has 'no access to those beings (*as* beings)' among which the stone is stone.[53] In this account 'access' relates to a capacity to possess

49. Habel (ed.), *Readings from the Perspective of Earth*, p. 24.

50. Horrell and Coad, '"The Stones Would Cry Out"'.

51. Martin Heidegger, *The Fundamental Concept of Metaphysics* (trans. William McNeill and Nicholas Walker; Bloomington: Indiana University Press, 1995), p. 196.

52. Heidegger, *Fundamental Concept of Metaphysics*, p. 196.

53. Heidegger, *Fundamental Concept of Metaphysics*, pp. 197-98.

and, I would argue, a capacity for agency. In contrast to the lizard, the stone appears in a particular here and now without apparent volition.[54]

Nancy takes up Heidegger's claim concerning the stone and the world.[55] He argues that Heidegger's stone is an abstraction; but the concrete stone that a lizard warms itself on, or a human person throws or stubs a toe against, is within a world. It does not *possess* a world, but nor does a lizard (or a human being). Nancy writes that the stone 'is a world', and as such is liable to sense.[56] He affirms the stone as something 'worlded' because it is always already in contact with and shaping the worlds of more-than-human, including human, others.[57] The contact of stone and world occurs 'in the mode, to be sure, of the wound for a foot and the barrier for an insect or for a stream, but also in the mode of a mere occupied place on the earth, of shadows cast, or of an ornamental cut incised in space, an unassignable gift'.[58] The qualities of stone as stone, moreover, give particular contours *or voice* to its world-shaping capacity, which is a kind of agency.

In his poem 'A Critique of Pure Representation', Jesper Svenbro writes of the obstinacy of stone; of stone as something that can be touched; of the way the word 'stone' rolls on the tongue.[59] He asks to what extent the word 'stone' can express the matter of stone.[60] In 'Material for a Geological Theory of Language', he writes further of stone, ice and water as ancestral to the Swedish language; they are teachers from which humans learned the shape of words.[61] Yet, he is aware, too, that language is arbitrary. 'Stone' is not stone. Indeed, the Hebrew אבן and the Greek λίθος are neither hard nor obstinate. Nevertheless, as argued earlier, language is material. Its abstraction is embedded in the materiality of the human body, the embodied mind.[62]

54. Heidegger, *Fundamental Concept of Metaphysics*, p. 197.

55. Nancy, *Sense of the World*, pp. 59-63.

56. Nancy, *Sense of the World*, p. 62.

57. Nancy, *Sense of the World*, pp. 60-61.

58. Nancy, *Sense of the World*, pp. 60-61. I take issue with Nancy's qualification of an 'occupied place' with 'mere'. In the framework of the ecological humanities, place and human relations to place, the occupation in place of people and things is hardly insignificant. In relation to the current discussion of the shouting stones of Luke, the place the stones occupy in the text and in relation to the road and the Jerusalem Temple is crucial.

59. Jesper Svenbro, *Three-Toed Gull: Selected Poems* (trans. John Matthias and Lars-Håkan Svensson; Evanston, IL: Northwestern University Press, 2003), p. 5.

60. Svenbro, *Three-Toed Gull*, p. 5.

61. Svenbro, *Three-Toed Gull*, p. 6.

62. This claim parallels that of Lakoff and Núñez concerning mathematics and the uses of metaphor therein (George Lakoff and Rafael E. Núñez, *Where Mathematics Comes from: How the Embodied Mind Brings Mathematics into Being* [New York: Basic Books, 2000]).

Exploring relationships between the materiality of stone and human experience, anthropologist Christopher Tilley takes a phenomenological approach where 'a dialectical exchange between the embodied structures of the engaged perceiver and the structures of that which is perceived ... involves an opening of my body to things', a mutual touching and being touched.[63] This mutuality of contact nevertheless involves a chiasm, where inside and outside 'mediate each other but never totally fuse'.[64] In this participatory relatedness, experience is potentially animistic.[65]

Rather than denying an animism underlying Lukan representations of other than humans—such as the winds and waters, the mulberry tree and the stones that can be responsive to, and co-agents with, human and divine actors (8.25; 17.6; 19.40)—can we understand their capacity for obedience and voice as part of a tradition of biblical animism? In this tradition, not only humans but also, more particularly, the whole creation is capable of responding to God, and by extension to each other.[66]

Christopher Tilley reminds us of the implications of human embodiment and embeddedness in an Earth community, where 'social relations are simultaneously relations between material forms' and stones are partners in a world that is more than human.[67] As an emblem of our struggle to engage with the communicative otherness of 'mute' things, Annie Dillard writes of 'teaching a stone to talk'.[68] Val Plumwood describes stones that teach her.[69] She sets out to 'reinvest with speech, agency and meaning the silenced ones, including the earth and its very stones, cast as the most lifeless and inconsiderable members of the earth community'.[70] Under the heading 'speaking stone', Plumwood writes:

63. Christopher Tilley, *The Materiality of Stone: Explorations in Landscape Phenomenology* (Oxford: Berg, 2004), pp. 29-30.

64. Tilley, *Materiality of Stone*, p. 30.

65. Tilley, *Materiality of Stone*, p. 30.

66. See Walsh, Karsh and Ansell's comments on the way in which we have 'disenchanted' the biblical tradition by ignoring this aspect of its cultural worldview (Brian J. Walsh, Marianne B. Karsh and Nik Ansell, 'Trees, Forestry, and the Responsiveness of Creation', in *This Sacred Earth: Religion, Nature, Environment* (ed. Roger S. Gottlieb; New York: Routledge, 1996), pp. 423-35 (425-27). I am grateful to Deborah Rose for the challenge to biblical ecological theologians to engage with animism.

67. Tilley, *Materiality of Stone*, pp. 31, 217.

68. Annie Dillard, 'Teaching a Stone to Talk', in *This Sacred Earth: Religion, Nature, Environment* (ed. Roger S. Gottlieb; New York: Routledge, 1996), pp. 32-36.

69. Val Plumwood, 'Journey to the Heart of Stone', in *Culture, Creativity and Environment: New Environmental Criticism* (ed. Fiona Becket and Terry Gifford; Amsterdam: Rodopi, 2007), pp. 17-36.

70. Plumwood, 'Journey to the Heart of Stone', p. 19.

> My house walls are made from a special kind of sandstone, a conglomerated sandstone into which are kneaded occasional small round river stones, like raisins in bread. My local stone is lightly conglomerated compared to the coarse, soft conglomerate of the mountains to my north, a wild, complicated landscape of hidden caves and valleys where romantic walkers like me love to wander. These coarse conglomerates tell a story that refutes our illusion of stone as silent and static, a complicated, amazing but quite readable story of the weathering of hard bedrock into rounded river stones, later compressed with finer weathered materials as sand beneath an ocean, then lifted up and exposed as soft conglomerate. Conglomerate, like so much else, is built up from those who went before, those we count for nothing.[71]

With these evocations of stone in mind, I turn to Lk. 19.40, where we find stones already invested with the possibility of speech and agency. Rather than being 'dead matter' stones carry a variety of meanings in Luke 19–20, through metaphor and metonymy. Stones are not only part of a world in the text, as potential speakers in the narrative (19.40). Nor are they simply part of a world behind the text, where the stones to which the Lukan Jesus refers have their material counterpart beside the road or in the Temple walls. In significant part, stones also produce the worlds of the text, quite literally as they lay down the bones of a place long before plants, animals, humans and language come to inhabit it.[72] They, too, tell a story.

In the Gospel of Luke, the motif of stones calling or crying out appears in complex interplay with a number of other textual stones (Lk. 19.28–20.19). For Luke the play on the word 'stone' is not accidental. Three, possibly four, of the five references to stone (λίθος) or stoning (καταλιθάζω) are specific to Luke (19.40; 19.44; 20.6; possibly 20.18). Elsewhere in the Gospel of Luke, references to stone and stoning have parallels in the Gospels of Matthew, Mark or both (Lk. 3.8//Mt. 3.9; Lk. 4.3//Mt. 4.3; Lk. 4.11//Mt. 4.6; Lk. 13.34//Mt. 23.37; Lk. 17.2//Mt. 18.6; Lk. 21.5//Mk 13.1; Lk. 21.6//Mt. 24.2//Mk 13.2; Lk. 24.2//Mt. 28.2//Mk 16.3-4). Luke 20.1-8 has parallels in Mt. 21.23-27 and Mk 11.27-33, but Lk. 20.6 is specific to Luke. Luke 20.18 may have a parallel in Mt. 21.44, but this parallel is attested in only some manuscripts and may be an addition. The quotation from Ps. 118.22 in Lk. 20.17, however, has parallels in Mt. 21.42; Mk 12.10; and Acts 4.11. In the references specific to Luke are stones that would shout (19.40); the stones of city and Temple (19.44); stones through which corporal and capital punishment is carried out (20.6); the rejected stone (20.17); and the traumatic intersection of the hardness and sharpness of stone with the softness and vulnerability of flesh (20.18).

71. Plumwood, 'Journey to the Heart of Stone', pp. 35-36.

72. Tilley, *Materiality of Stone*, p. 31, Mark Tredinnick, *The Blue Plateau: A Landscape Memoir* (St Lucia: University of Queensland Press, 2009), pp. 147-48.

Apart from these explicit references, in the appeal to what is written (19.46), we can hear the divine writing on stone; for example, the Torah written on tablets of stone (Exod. 34.1), sometimes by the finger of God (Exod. 32.15; Deut. 9.9-11). These inscribed stones are among a range of biblical associations with stone. Stones appear as witness and boundary markers (Gen. 31.43-54); standing stones (Josh. 24.26); foundation stones (Isa. 28.16); stones quarried to build Solomon's Temple (1 Kgs. 6.7); stones mined deep in the earth (Job 28.1-11). Stones are thrown in punishment (Lev. 24.23); stones fell giants (1 Sam. 17.49); stones cry out (Hab. 2.11). One stone has a name ('the stone Zoheleth', 1 Kgs. 1.9). In Lk. 3.8 and the parallel saying in Mt. 7.9, stones appear as potential ancestors, children of Abraham. Remembering the dependence of humans on the long world-shaping history of stone, we may hear these stones as ancestral to the people, perhaps also as ancestral witnesses to the liberating acts of God (Josh. 4.20-24).[73]

In the ancient Near East, stones were sometimes venerated[74]; the prophet Habakkuk denounces this practice:

> What use is an idol
> once its maker has shaped it—
> a cast image, a teacher of lies?
> For its maker trusts in what has been made,
> though the product is only an idol that cannot speak!
> Alas for you who say to the wood, 'Wake up!'
> to silent stone, 'Rouse yourself!'
> Can it teach?
> See, it is gold and silver plated,
> and there is no breath in it at all (Hab. 2.18-19 NRSV).

Despite the earlier prophecy that 'the very stones will cry out from the wall' (Hab. 2.11), Habakkuk characterizes stone as silent. But the following verse reads:

> But Yhwh is in his holy temple;
> let all the earth keep silence before him! (Hab. 2.20 NRSV modified).

Silence is not always the muteness Habakkuk ascribes to a stone god; a more-than-human silence can both respond to and mediate the presence and voice of God (1 Kgs. 19.12-13). The materiality of stone gives itself to an image of silent stone, but it also resonates in the motif of stones that shout. Drawing on C.F. Evans, Horrell and Coad note that in apocalyptic writing the motif of stones crying out is 'reasonably well-established, and not to

73. Ringe, *Luke*, p. 241.

74. Horrell and Coad, '"The Stones Would Cry Out"', p. 33.

be seen as merely a hyperbolic image' (see, for example, *4 Ezra* 5.5; *Liv. Proph.* 10.10-11).[75] The stones matter.

*Matter*

To what stones does the Lukan Jesus refer in 19.40 when he answers, 'I say to you, if these will keep silent (σιωπήσουσιν), the stones will shout (οἱ λίθοι κράξουσιν)'? There are two key candidates for 'the stones'. First are the stones of, and beside, the path down from the Mount of Olives at the approach of which 'the whole multitude of the disciples began to praise God joyfully with a loud voice for all the deeds of power they had seen' (19.37). Second are the stones of the city of Jerusalem and the Second Temple, of which the Lukan Jesus prophesies, 'They will not leave within you one stone upon another' (19.44). Apart from the stones to which the Lukan narrative refers, the setting relies on the matter of other stones and the worlds to which they give substance. These include the stoniness of the Mount of Olives; the soil formed there from weathered stone; the trees that draw minerals from the soil; the readers and writers who eat the olives and drink their oil. There are also the stones of the city and the quarries from which they came.

For many interpreters, the stones of Lk. 19.40 are the stones of city and Temple of which Jesus says, 'they will not leave within you one stone upon another' (19.44; 21.6). Joseph Fitzmyer writes:

> *the stones will cry out!* This is possibly an allusion to Hab 2:11, 'For a stone will cry out from a wall, and a beam from the wood-paneling will answer it,' i.e. a threat uttered against a nation which plunders people and acquires gain by violence. Now in God's plan of salvation-history the arrival of Jesus in Jerusalem would make Jerusalem's stones cry out to acclaim him as the agent of it, if his disciples did not.[76]

Immediately following Jesus' claim that the stones will shout (19.40), Luke refers to the stones of the city (19.41-44) and in the next episode makes the accusation that the Temple has become a refuge of robbers (19.45-46). These aspects of the text support the case for a link with Hab. 2.11. Earlier the Lukan Jesus longs to nurture the city that 'kills the prophets and stones those sent to it' (13.34). Brendan Byrne reads in 19.40 a reference to the stones of the city longing for the advent of the messianic king whom the disciples proclaim (19.35-38).[77] Stones are not incidental to Luke's Jerusalem.

75. Horrell and Coad, '"The Stones Would Cry Out"', p. 34.

76. Joseph A. Fitzmyer, *The Gospel according to Luke X–XXIV: Introduction, Translation, and Notes* (AB; New York: Doubleday, 1985), p. 1252.

77. Byrne, *Hospitality of God*, 156. See also Fitzmyer, *Gospel according to Luke X–XXIV*, p. 1251; Ringe, *Luke*, p. 240; Charles H. Talbert, *Reading Luke: A Literary*

Not only does Luke 19–20 refer to the stones of the Temple and city, but also the threat of stoning arises in Jerusalem. As Jesus teaches in the Temple, the religious leaders fear the possibility that the people will stone them if they deny the authority of John the Baptist (20.6). In the Acts of the Apostles, Luke sets the narrative of Stephen's stoning between two presentations of Jerusalem: first as locus of a spread of the 'word of God' and the 'obedience to the faith' of a 'great many priests' (Acts 6.7) and then as the site of a severe persecution of the church (Acts 8.1). Stoning relies on the sharpness of stone and the vulnerability of flesh. Both the building stones and stones used in punishment have certain material characteristics that support the uses to which they are put.

Josephus tells that 'the temple was built of stones that were white and strong', probably meleke limestone, quarried from the vicinity of Jerusalem (*Ant.* 15.11.392). This porous white limestone has a 'chalky appearance' and is wet and friable within an underground quarry, hardening from the 'outside inward' when exposed to air.[78] In describing the siege of Jerusalem, Josephus writes of the intransigence of these stones (*War* 6.220-24). Of the stones of the Temple, the Babylonian Talmud has:

> It was said that he who had not seen the new Temple of Herod had not, in all his life, seen a fine building. 'With what material did he build it?' asked Rabha. With ornamented marble stone of different colors, the stones being not in a straight line, but alternately projecting and receding, the gaps being intended to receive the lime. He intended to cover it with gold, but the rabbis advised him not to do so, because as it was it looked as effulgent as the waves of the sea (*B. Bat.* 1).

Extrabiblical texts from the Second Temple period and later, describing the construction of the First Temple, give an indication of the variety of materials and labour involved in the reconstruction of the Second Temple under Herod. The *Testament of Solomon,* a pseudepigraphal Christian text probably dating between the first and third centuries CE, has quarried stone, marble, wood, hemp and fired bricks used in the construction process; the labourers, including paid human workers and conscripted demons, work both day and night (*T. Sol.* 1.1-2; 2.5; 4.12; 6.9; 10.7-8; 14.8).[79] *Eupolemus,*

*and Theological Commentary on the Third Gospel* (New York: Crossroad, 1988), p. 179.

78. Zeev Lewy, 'Short Contribution: Geological and Religious Factors for Subsurface Quarrying That Formed the Zedekiah Cave in Jerusalem', *Israel Geoarchaeology: An International Journal* 21.2 (2006), pp. 187-96 (187, 191-92).

79. Given the dating of the *Testament of Solomon,* I think it reasonable to assume some conflation of First and Second Temples in the mind of the author. The *Testament* is thought not to be of Palestinian provenance, and this would perhaps explain why some of the stone is described as coming across the Arabian Sea and from Thebes, rather than from the traditional King Solomon's quarries in the vicinity of Jerusalem.

a Hellenistic Jewish history written prior to the first century CE, lists the construction materials for the First Temple as 'gold, silver, bronze, stones, cypress and cedar trees' (*Eupol.* 30.6; cf. 1 Chron. 22 and 28). The descriptions of the vast amounts of metals, stones, trees, other plants and animals, and human labour required for the construction of the First Temple and the institution of Temple sacrifice (see also 1 Kgs. 5–7; 8.62-64; 2 Chron. 2.1–7.12) reflect the extensive indebtedness of Temple construction and reconstruction projects to the Earth community. The importance of demons in the construction process described in the *Testament of Solomon* suggests an animistic understanding of the elements, particularly of sea and wind, and a sense, too, that the work with stone to construct a temple required more than human labour. Similarly but more modestly, the book of Ezra describes the building of the Second Temple, and in this, too, can be read an indebtedness to a more-than-human Earth community.

The stones of Jerusalem were material artefacts when they became parts of roads and buildings; as such they were invested not only with their own material qualities, such as porosity and hardness, but with the more-than-human (including human) labour and the social, cultural and political meanings of those who collaborated in their construction and use. If as readers we listen for the materiality of stone in the stones of Luke 19–20, can we hear the voices of a more-than-human network of materials, labour and meaning that situate these stones in Jerusalem's roads and buildings?

*Grief*

After Jerusalem is laid siege and the Second Temple destroyed, the stones remain stones, but as tumbled memorials of what once stood, and as a Temple wall still standing, the Western wall, a Wailing wall, a place for prayer and longing. Josephus describes the destruction of the Second Temple as cause for lament and a sign that the transience of constructed works parallels the mortality of living creatures (*War* 6.267-68). His narration of reluctance on the part of the Romans to destroy the Temple—a reluctance some commentators read as ironic—suggests something of the grief that followed its destruction (*War* 6.249-66).[80] For Luke, too, this destruction is cause for grief.

Three times the Lukan Jesus is associated with mourning in relation to Jerusalem (13.34; 19.42-44; 23.28-30). Grief for the execution of Jesus is not so much conflated with, but rather gives way to, grief for destruction of

80. I am grateful to James McLaren for pointing out the probable irony in Josephus. Jonathan Price concludes that Josephus is wrong in his assertion that Titus tried to avoid destroying the Temple (Jonathan J. Price, *Jerusalem under Siege: The Collapse of the Jewish State 66-70 C.E.* [Leiden: E.J. Brill, 1992], p. 945).

Temple, city and people (see, for example, 23.28-31). This tragic destruction is enfolded with a divine necessity that informs the passion, death and resurrection of the Lukan Jesus (9.22; 17.25; 22.37; 24.7, 26). As noted earlier, suffusing events, this necessity (δεῖ) is not quite the fate of Greek tragedy nor the election of Hebrew theology, but has elements of both.[81] The failure of the Jewish leaders to recognize Jesus, and so to welcome the divine visitation, is identified in the city of stone. For Luke this city stones those sent, including Stephen (13.34a; Acts 7.58-59). Here Jesus will be executed not by stoning but by crucifixion.[82]

The prophetic lament of 19.41-44 implies that the city's fall is consequent on a tragic refusal written in bodies and stone (see Jer. 9.1; 13.17; 14.17; Amos 5.1-3).[83] Several Lukan references to stones and stoning accompany narrative dramatizations of the tension between John the Baptist and the crowd (3.7-8) and between Jesus and the Jewish leaders and sometimes the city itself (19.39-40, 41-44; 20.1-8, 17-19). Meron Benvenisti writes, 'The chronicles of Jerusalem are a gigantic quarry from which each side has mined stones for the construction of its myths and for throwing at each other.'[84] The tragedy of the Roman siege of Jerusalem and the destruction of the Second Temple is part of a story of imperialist violence, of which stones are part. Judith Lieu holds that '[l]ater Christian writers saw that destruction as divine judgment on the Jews' refusal to recognize Jesus; Luke does not do this'.[85] For the contemporary reader the tragedy is, in addition, that Luke's linking the city's fall to what he reads as Jewish rejection of Jesus, even if Luke makes this link in hope, becomes part of a climate of Christian anti-Judaism that among other things made possible the immense horror of the Shoah.

Although the death of the Lukan Jesus is the result of human actions that unwittingly serve a divine necessity, for Luke these human actions and the consequent fall of the city are not inevitable in the way Oedipus's fate is for Sophocles. There is always and repeatedly the possibility of welcoming the divine visitation.[86] But where the visitation is unwelcome, the divine necessity reshapes the tragedy of refusal and its consequences from within, *without taking away the grief that accompanies the tragic.* More than 'a

81. Cosgrove, 'Divine Δεῖ', pp. 168-90.

82. Robert C. Tannehill, 'Israel in Luke–Acts: A Tragic Story', *JBL* 104 (1985), pp. 69-85; Tannehill, *Narrative Unity,* I, p. 159; Robert C. Tannehill, *The Narrative Unity of Luke–Acts: A Literary Interpretation.* II. *The Acts of the Apostles* (Minneapolis: Fortress Press, 1994), pp. 90, 93-96.

83. Green, *Gospel of Luke*, p. 688; cf. Lieu, *Gospel of Luke*, pp. 157-58.

84. Meron Benvenisti, *City of Stone: The Hidden History of Jerusalem* (trans. Maxine Kaufan Nunn; Berkeley: University of California Press, 1996), pp. 3-4.

85. Lieu, *Gospel of Luke*, pp. 157-8.

86. Byrne, *Hospitality of God.*

warning of judgment', Jesus' prophetic lament over the city (19.41-44) is not only attended by 'a vision of what might have been', as Ringe suggests, but also by hope for restoration.[87] When as readers we listen for the voice of the stones in Luke 19–20, can we hear this story of grief? The stones do not so much join in Jesus' lament; they accompany it as part of the grief world of the story, which is also a world of hope.

*Resistance*

For Luke, this hope is the basis for a kind of resistance. Describing Lukan style, Bruce Longenecker suggests that in his writing, Luke is averse to 'humps and hollows' in the text, favouring instead a kind of narrative enchainment.[88] This enchaining includes subtleties that leave room for interpretation. For example, there are links between the infancy narratives and Lk. 19.28-44.[89] In particular, the disciples' proclamation of peace in 19.38 parallels the angels proclamation to the shepherds (2.14). But the locus of messianic peace has shifted from earth to skies. Is this a recognition that temporarily at least the falling stones signify no peace for Jerusalem?

Jerusalem and the Temple are key features of Luke's narrative chains.[90] In the Acts of the Apostles, Luke depicts the early Christian communities in Jerusalem as faithful Jews praying in the Temple. His infancy narratives begin and end in the Temple.[91] His Gospel concludes with the eleven and their companions 'continually in the temple blessing God' (24.53). In contrast to Mark's version, in Luke the Temple curtain is torn (23.45; Mk 15.36) just prior to the death of Jesus (23.46; Mk 15.37). While this may signal that in a certain non-temporal sense the destruction of the Temple precedes, rather than proceeds from, the death of the Lukan Jesus, it also suggests an opening out in which the Lukan Jesus is 'in communion' with and reveals the God of the Temple.[92] Ringe writes:

87. Ringe, *Luke*, p. 241. See also Pheme Perkins, 'If Jerusalem Stood: The Destruction of Jerusalem and Christian Anti-Judaism', *BibInt* 8 (2000), pp. 194-204. Perkins writes of the possibility of a different relationship between Christian anti-Judaism and the destruction of Jerusalem. See also Brent Kinman, 'Lucan Eschatology and the Missing Fig Tree', *JBL* 113 (1994), pp. 669-78 (678).

88. Bruce W. Longenecker, 'Lukan Aversion to Humps and Hollows: The Case of Acts 11.27–12.25', *NTS* 50 (2004), pp. 185-204.

89. Tannehill, *Narrative Unity*, I, p. 159; Robert C. Tannehill, *Luke* (Abingdon New Testament Commentaries; Nashville: Abingdon Press, 1996), pp. 284-85.

90. On the centrality of Jerusalem for Luke, see Kitchen, 'Good News of Restoration', pp. 160-63.

91. See Dennis M Hamm, 'The Tamid Service in Luke–Acts: The Cultic Background behind Luke's Theology', *CBQ* 65 (2003), pp. 215-31.

92. Tannehill, *Luke*, p. 284.

> Not merely the stones (19:40), but the whole cosmos has taken up the cry from the silenced disciples and the dying Jesus. God no longer dwells in the thick darkness of the temple's holiest center, but rather in the darkness that covers the whole earth.[93]

This opening out is part of a Lukan divine necessity that resists human violence or destructiveness by offering a possibility of life not beyond but through the consequences of this violence. One aspect of the stones' cry is protest, judgment on the violence that brings the death of Jesus and the destruction of Temple and city.[94]

Can we hear the protest of stones in their materiality? Josephus describes the hardened resistance of stone to Roman battering. Luke 19.43 may refer to the resistant stone of Roman battlements when during the siege of Jerusalem Titus erected a stone wall around the city, reportedly in three days (Josephus, *War* 5.499-501).[95] Witness to so much human aspiration, violence and possibility, the Western wall still standing in Jerusalem is testament not only to the resistance of stone, but also to the apparent passivity of stone, its capacity to be cut and brought and raised into structures of human design. In the Lukan allusions to stoning (13.34; 20.6) and being crushed by stone (20.18), passive resistance becomes a force that presses into and damages the less resisting matter of flesh and bone. Listening for the resistant properties of Luke's stones, can the reader hear in the matter of stone the voice of their protest?

The Lukan reference to stones that will shout also signifies divine (and sometimes human) mastery over nature within a framework of command-obedience in which trees can be uprooted and thrown into the sea by a faithful word (17.5-6), stormy seas stilled (8.22-25), and stones recognize the divine visitation even when humans fail to do so (19.40-44). In affirming the potential for stones to recognize the divine visitation, Luke sets the divine necessity in a more-than-human framework in which the matter of stone participates in the resistance that registers as hope in the midst of tragedy and grief. While Luke's is a dangerous story because of its own violent legacies, it also offers a pattern in which grief and resistance work together, where resistance is enchained with grief. The materiality of stones that are both porous and hardened parallels the textual interweaving of grief with resistance.

There is a sense, however, in which the materiality of stone is resistant to the word, even the words of Luke's narrative. Writing of trees, Judith

93. Ringe, *Luke*, p. 179.

94. Horrell and Coad, '"The Stones Would Cry Out"', p. 37.

95. H. Jagersma, *A History of Israel from Alexander the Great to Bar Kochba* (trans. John Bowden; London: SCM Press, 1985), p. 144.

Wright says, 'Words are not meanings for a tree.'[96] Although words may not be meanings for a stone, in the framework of a biblical animism, stones may shout. Can we as readers allow ourselves to be sounded by the otherness of Luke's stones that do not cry in a human voice but speak through their materiality of a resistance that registers both in a wall that remains standing and in their foreignness to human meaning?

*Praise*

In the Lukan framework, both stones and humans are subject to a divine call. The shout of Luke's stones parallels the praise of the crowd of disciples (19.37-40). For Horrell and Coad this parallel inserts praise as the primary mode of the shout the stones will make, should the crowd of disciples be mute, as Zechariah once became (19.39-40; cf. 1.20).[97] In the flow of the narrative, Jesus' answer, 'I say to you, if these will keep silent (σιωπήσουσιν), the stones will shout (οἱ λίθοι κράξουσιν)', comes as a rebuke to some of the Pharisees in the crowd who ask that Jesus order his disciples to stop crying out praise. The echo of Hab. 2.11 and the reference to the fall of the stones in the fall of Jerusalem in 19.41-44 suggest that, as Horrell and Coad argue, praise functions here as rebuke.[98] The combination of rebuke with praise implies that the shout of the stones has a critical and corrective function in relation to the praise, or failure to praise, of humans. Does the creation praise God simply by being itself or is this praise 'an eschatological goal'? Horrell and Coad tend to opt for the latter:

> The (potential) cry of the stones in Luke 19 does not consist of a continuation of what the stones have always done, in their very existence as stones, but rather of a dramatic and eschatological cry of praise, which at the same time protests against the failures of humanity to recognise God's anointed.[99]

There is an alternate way of understanding the cry of praise of the stones. Drawing on Chrétien's understanding of call and response, the potential voicing of praise by stones can be understood as a response to a call.

Already present in the stones being stones (and not humans or trees), their response comes into being in their being called. The stones—porous and hardened; incorporated into material artefacts that are roads, walls and the Second Temple—accompany the Lukan enchaining of grief and resistance with a (potential) voice of recognition at the threshold of Jesus' entry

96. Judith Wright, 'Gum-Trees Stripping', in *Collected Poems* (Pymble, NSW: Angus & Robertson, 1994), p. 133.

97. Horrell and Coad, '"The Stones Would Cry Out"', pp. 36-37.

98. Horrell and Coad, '"The Stones Would Cry Out"', esp. pp. 37, 42.

99. Horrell and Coad, '"The Stones Would Cry Out"', p. 40.

to Jerusalem and his teaching in the Temple in the time leading to his death. Like Mary's greeting at the threshold of Zechariah's house, like Elizabeth's shout of recognition, the stone's cry of praise occurs at a threshold of relationship, between God and humans; between Romans and Jews, imperial occupiers and their subjects; between men and women; Jews and Gentiles. In carrying the threads of grief and resistance, it is a properly stony praise, porous and hardened.

In the context of grief over the destruction of the Second Temple, the stony praise also echoes not only the prayer and praise of the early communities of believers in Acts (2.46-47) but the praise of other-than-human creatures who may inhabit the Temple itself:

> How lovely is your dwelling place,
> Yhwh of hosts!
> My soul longs, indeed it faints
> for the courts of Yhwh;
> my heart and my flesh sing for joy
> to the living God.
> Even the sparrow finds a home,
> and the swallow a nest for herself,
> where she may lay her young,
> at your altars, Yhwh of hosts,
> my King and my God.
> Happy are those who live in your house,
> ever singing your praise (Ps. 84.1-4 NRSV modified).

Luke's depiction of the early Christians, written after the destruction of the Second Temple, presents praise as an eschatological hope of habitation with God such as that represented by the psalmist. From an ecological perspective, such eschatological hope need not be otherworldly; rather, like the cry of the stones, it comes as critique of a human failure to recognize the time of our visitation, especially as it arrives in the call of a more-than-human community to which we might find in ourselves a response, 'Here I am'.

## *Conclusion*

Toward the end of the Lukan Gospel, the women who come with spices and ointment to anoint Jesus' corpse find the stone rolled away from the entrance to the tomb (24.1-2). The stone at the threshold of the empty tomb signals an absence. The women enter the tomb and do 'not find the body' (24.3). Like the 'two men in dazzling cloths' who appear beside the women and speak (24.4-7), the stone proclaims that the body of Jesus is elsewhere. As I argued in Chapter 4, this elsewhere is characterized by a corporeality that in Luke is touchable and by a movement from body to word, where the writings that are the Jewish Scriptures and the Lukan narrative itself give witness to an absent presence.

As in Majzner's depiction of 'Jacob's Ladder', the material artefacts of Scripture also give witness to this divine absence. Underlying these artefacts are the skins (of papyrus, parchment, paper, screen) that give themselves to writing, and the stones that are the bedrock of Earth. The stones of Jerusalem not only support the construction (and destruction) of temples and early writing, and the soils from which writers and readers draw sustenance, but also give themselves to the metaphors and metonymy that a writing weaves around the material qualities of stone. Stones are only mute insofar as humans are listening for something human in them.

While stone may give itself as stone, the world of stone is not wholly our world. Stone gives itself to the miner's cut, not without resistance; to flesh, which erupts in bruises and blood; to the hand that places a prayer inscribed on paper drawn from trees into a crevice in a wall, left standing, when not one stone was left upon another; and to language and thought. As stone presses against flesh, the material artefact sounds in writing; and the text, like Mary's greeting, sounds in the body of its reader/hearer.

Nevertheless, the foreignness of stone to the word also echoes in the elision of the material artefact in writing. In the complex relations of material artefact, writing and reading, can the text—like Luke's stones—shout praise that is also rebuke? To what kind of visitation might we also then exclaim, 'Here I am'? Can we approach the present-absence of the materiality of the text through a giving ear to a cry, such as the cry of stones within the Lukan Gospel?[100] In the long history of world making, stones are part of a community of more-than-human agency, active in building construction and textual production. Keeping this material agency in mind, with what other-than-human voices may we be sounded when we read and hear and respond to the textual imperative to listen? In the next chapter, I explore ways in which the text resounds in the body through the sense of sight as a visible voice.

100. David Rhoads suggests that on the basis of the principle of interconnectedness, when we read with Earth 'in mind' our readings can mediate the voice of a wider Earth community. See David Rhoads, 'Who Will Speak for the Sparrow? Eco-Justice Criticism of the New Testament', in *Literary Encounters with the Reign of God* (Festschrift Robert Tannehill; ed. Sharon H. Ringe and H.C. Paul Kim; Harrisburg, PA: Trinity Press International, 2004), pp. 64-86.

# 7

## The Visible Voice and the Dust of Things

> Now about eight days after these sayings Jesus took with him Peter and John and James, and went up on the mountain to pray. And while he was praying, the appearance of his face changed, and his clothes became dazzling white. Suddenly they saw two men, Moses and Elijah, talking to him. They appeared in glory and were speaking of his departure, which he was about to accomplish at Jerusalem. Now Peter and his companions were weighed down with sleep; but since they had stayed awake, they saw his glory and the two men who stood with him. Just as they were leaving him, Peter said to Jesus, 'Master, it is good for us to be here; let us make three dwellings, one for you, one for Moses, and one for Elijah'—not knowing what he said. While he was saying this, a cloud came and overshadowed them; and they were terrified as they entered the cloud. Then from the cloud came a voice that said, 'This is my Son, my Chosen; listen to him!' When the voice had spoken, Jesus was found alone. And they kept silent and in those days told no one any of the things they had seen.
>
> Lk. 9.28-36 NRSV

The first extant visual representation of the transfiguration can be found in the Monastery of St Catherine on Mount Sinai, in the mosaic of the apse.[1] Christ is 'inscribed in a blue mandorla', a focus of light with rays emanating from him.[2] The images surrounding the mosaic situate the transfiguration at the axis of relationship between divinity and humanity. Portraits of Moses before the burning bush and receiving the law place the transfiguration in particular relation to the mountain on which the image itself is situated. An

1. Maria Giovanna Muzj, *Transfiguration: Introduction to the Contemplation of Icons* (Boston: St Paul Books & Media, 1991), p. 120; Solrunn Nes, *The Uncreated Light: An Iconographical Study of the Transfiguration in the Eastern Church* (Grand Rapids: Eerdmans, 2007), p. 56. See also 'Mosaics', The Holy Monastery of the God-trodden Mount Sinai, St Catherine's Monastery, http://www.sinaimonastery.com/en/index.php?lid=112.
2. Nes, *Uncreated Light,* p. 68.

interpolation of the emperor Justinian as David locates the image at a nexus of political and religious power. While the three stripes of colour representing the land on which the transfiguration occurs minimize the importance of place, the place of the mountain on which the monastery is situated is present in the references to Moses and the Torah.[3] Later icons of the transfiguration, of which that attributed to Theophane the Greek from the Cathedral of the Transfiguration in Pereslavl is representative, give much greater emphasis to the mountain. The mountain is 'the meeting place' of earth and heaven. Maria Giovanna Muzj argues with reference to the fifteenth-century transfiguration icon of Novgorod school that Jesus is identified with the mountain, 'as the absolute meeting place between God and his people'.[4] Further, in the transfiguration icon the relationship between vision and the image is particularly close.[5] As in the Lukan account, the sense of sight is paramount; it is as if the narrator like the iconographer (and through the narrator, the reader/hearer like the one who contemplates an icon) is a witness.

Even before we read that Peter, John and James *saw* two men talking with Jesus (9.30), we as readers/hearers 'see' the transformation of 'the appearance of his face' (9.29). The sense of sight and the impact of light on the eyes (even the eye of the imagination of the reader/hearer) are aligned; we are invited to be dazzled when his clothes become 'dazzling white' (9.29). The two men, namely Moses and Elijah, whom the disciples see, appear 'in glory' (9.31). Although 'weighed down with sleep', as they will be again in the Garden of Gethsemane because of their grief (22.45), the three disciples awaken to see 'his glory and the two men who stood with him' (9.32).[6] While the Lukan narrator describes Moses and Elijah in conversation with Jesus, no direct speech is reported. The focus is on the visual. With Peter's comment to Jesus, 'Master it is good for us to be here ...' (9.33), voice and vision become interwoven. No longer focused on a vision of light, the reader's gaze turns toward shadow and cloud (9.34). The overshadowing is also a manifestation of the divine, as the voice from the cloud attests (9.35).

3. Nes, *Uncreated Light*, pp. 56-73.

4. Muzj, *Transfiguration*, p. 122. This icon can be viewed at http://www.icon-art.info/masterpiece.php?lng=en&mst_id=125.

5. Muzj, *Transfiguration*, p. 122.

6. The verb διαγρηγορέω occurs nowhere else in the Second Testament or in the Septuagint. Based on other Greek literature, there are two possible translations of the aorist active particle διαγρηγορήσαντες in this verse, either 'since they had kept awake ...' or 'when they were fully awake ...' (BAGD, 182). While the NRSV translators opt for the former, John Paul Heil argues for the latter (John Paul Heil, *The Transfiguration of Jesus: Narrative Meaning and Function of Mark 9:2-8, Matt 17:1-8 and Luke 9:28-36* [AnBib, 144; Rome: Editrice Pontificio Istituto Biblico, 2000], p. 266). The parallel with the agony in the garden suggests the latter, although the former is equally possible as a point of contrast.

After the voice affirms the divine election of Jesus (9.35) and the disciples find themselves alone with him, the narrator reminds us of the visual, by commenting that they were silent about 'the things they had seen' (9.36). The movement between sight and voice, from the appearance of the face to the divine command 'listen to him!' suggests that, in the glorified Jesus, the face calls.[7]

In the context of the Lukan narrative, this is a call to receptivity, to participation in the hospitality of God, to recognition (seeing and knowing) of the time of visitation (1.68-79; 19.42, 44). That Jesus' heavenly interlocutors, namely Moses and Elijah, speak to him of his exodus in Jerusalem (9.31), the city toward which he will soon set his face on the journey toward his passion and death (9.51), suggests that Jesus' glorification is not separate from his passion.[8] As Dorothy Lee argues, the use of the verb 'fulfil' (he is to fulfil, πληροῦν, 9.31) in relation to this exodus implies that the meaning is 'primarily Christological'.[9] For the Lukan Jesus, 'his path through life and death ... is the path of God's visitation'.[10] This visitation encompasses a fullness of life. Muzj describes the structure of the transfiguration icon—the circle over the triangle, and the rays emanating from the vertical axis bisecting the circle—and notes that the 'first message conveyed by this structure is that the fullness of life (the circle), manifested as light radiating from the figure of Christ does not remain enclosed in itself but includes all creation in its movements, especially humanity'.[11]

The appearance beside Jesus of both Moses and Elijah connects two material sites of divine–human encounter: the mountain and the text. In Moses the reader/hearer/viewer is reminded of the Sinai covenant and the Torah, the books of the Law. Elijah calls to mind the moment of encounter in the empty wind/small voice on Horeb and the Navi'im, the scrolls of the prophets. In icons of the transfiguration, Moses is usually depicted holding a book. The Lukan reference to these two key scriptural figures speaking about the exodus Jesus is to fulfil in Jerusalem (9.31) recalls the fulfilment of a writing, which Jesus locates in a place in a scroll and of which he proclaims, 'Today this writing/scripture (ἡ γραφὴ αὕτη) has been fulfilled in your ears' (4.21). When the Lukan Jesus, himself the agent of divine visita-

7. Westphal, 'Transfiguration', p. 30. See also Marion, *In Excess*, pp. 116, 119.

8. See, for example, Heil, *Transfiguration of Jesus*, pp. 278-79. For Thomas Martin, in the Lukan Transfiguration account, 'glory is humiliation, not exaltation' (Thomas W. Martin, 'What Makes Glory Glorious? Reading Luke's Account of the Transfiguration over against Triumphalism', *JSNT* 29 [2006], pp. 3-26 [6]); cf. Westphal, 'Transfiguration', esp. p. 31.

9. Dorothy A. Lee, *Transfiguration* (New Century Theology; London: Continuum, 2004), p. 73.

10. Lee, *Transfiguration*, p. 73.

11. Muzj, *Transfiguration*, p. 122.

tion, is transfigured on the mountain—a meeting place between creator and creation—the reader/hearer/viewer is reminded, albeit indirectly, of another mode of encounter, namely the material artefacts that give themselves to the Scriptures (writings).

As I work with the transfiguration episode, I return several times to the thin pages of my Greek New Testament and the thinner pages of my NRSV to check a word or a translation. I rely on my eyes and my reading glasses to assist me in listening for the traces of the materiality of a text in writing.[12] In the previous chapter, I considered the materiality of the voice as part of the materiality of the text. In this chapter, I appeal to Jean-Louis Chrétien's description of a visible voice to describe, first, a Lukan appeal to the sense of sight, for which the transfiguration episode provides a paradigm in a face that calls; second, the text itself, where the material artefact opens to an interplay between sight and hearing in the act of reading. Around the middle of Luke's narrative of divine visitation, the transfiguration account presents a vision that becomes a command: Listen! This crossing between sight and hearing offers a paradigm of Chrétien's 'visible voice' that is encountered as a command to hospitality.[13] The importance of the theme of hospitality and the divine visitation in the Gospel of Luke has been well established.[14] Through a consideration of the dust shaken off (Lk. 10.11) as a sign of failure of receptivity of the divine visitation, signalled by the imminence of the βασιλεία of God, I take up an understanding of material agency introduced in Chapter 1. The materiality of Earth, texts, humans and their voices share a community of agency that gives itself to the visible voice of the text.

## *The Visible Voice*

Jean-Louis Chrétien writes of the gaze as already given 'to the possibility that something could appear' prior to 'any apparition, darkling or luminous'.[15] Just as, in his understanding, a call is a calling forth of an already-available (or, perhaps more strongly, already-given) response or responsiveness, seeing involves a givenness to the possibility that something will be, or become, visible. In Chapter 3, I considered Jean-Luc

12. Others with more serious visual impairments than long-sightedness might rely on their hands rather than their eyes to hear what the text is saying. I am not in a position to address the different ways in which this literal touching the text to read might inform a reader's engagement with its materiality, although this would be an interesting investigation.

13. Although not making explicit reference to the transfiguration, Chrétien's introduction of the 'visible voice' in several places echoes the transfiguration episode (Chrétien, *Call and the Response*, p. 33).

14. See Byrne, *Hospitality of God*; Heil, *Meal Scenes*.

15. Chrétien, *Call and the Response*, p. 33.

Marion's concept of a saturated phenomenon as a basis for my describing reading as a saturated communion. An experience such as that narrated in the Lukan transfiguration narrative offers one paradigm of a saturated phenomenon, which dazzles by over-fulfilment of expectation and sense.[16] Drawing on Shane Mackinlay's reading of Marion, I suggested in Chapter 3 that saturation is less a characteristic of a phenomenon in its own right, although it is also this, than a mode of hermeneutic encounter with a thing. For Marion, a saturated phenomenon appears in excess of the possibility of its being grasped through intuition and, in this sense, can be understood to be an appearance prior to the gaze. In contrast, for Chrétien a thing appears to a gaze that is given to its appearance. In being given to a thing's appearing, the gaze is also (as in Marion's terms) gifted. The gaze is given to itself by, and receives itself from, the thing that appears. Thus, there is a two-way movement between the gaze and the thing that appears. In this movement, when the thing appears gifting a gaze, which is already given to the appearance of the thing, the visible calls.[17] The visible has a voice to which the gaze responds.

Beauty, such as that encountered in the transfiguration event—experienced as καλός by the disciples in Luke's account (9.33)—is a paradigm of the visible that speaks a word that can take one's breath away, claiming one's own voice, as the disciples were rendered silent after what they had seen (9.36).[18] Chrétien claims a mutuality of response between sensed and sense. 'Things of themselves call us and invite us to interrogate them. Their beauty calls by responding and responds by calling.'[19] For Chrétien there is an interplay between word and gaze that implies what might be called a hermeneutics of sight that destabilizes the notion of a proper sensible with the possibility of an eye that listens.[20]

The eye listens not only to beauty but also to suffering: 'To see the suffering and beauty of the visible in the form of voice is to be dedicated to providing it forever with the asylum of our own voice. When the eye listens, we must answer what we hear and answer for what we will hear.'[21] The eye listens to a visible voice, and this visual listening resounds as asylum. The asylum of our own voice is that of a body and a subjectivity, which has been, to borrow Nancy's term, 'sounded' by the visible. Through this

16. On the transfiguration as saturated phenomenon, see Marion, 'They Recognized Him', p. 148; Mackinlay, *Interpreting Excess*, pp. 184, 188, 255-56 n. 17; Westphal, 'Transfiguration', esp. pp. 31-32.

17. Chrétien, *Call and the Response*, p. 33.

18. Chrétien, *Call and the Response*, pp. 33, 35.

19. Chrétien, *Call and the Response*, p. 36.

20. Chrétien, *Call and the Response*, pp. 33-34, 37, 43.

21. Chrétien, *Call and the Response*, p. 43.

sounding, the one sounded proffers, and provides the conditions for, hospitality. Luke offers a model for such a sounding by the visible. As I argued in Chapter 4, a pattern exists across Lk. 7.11-17; 10.25-37; 15.11-24, in which seeing the other's need is prompt for a compassionate responsiveness mediated by touch, a compassion that is one mode of the hospitality of God. In this seeing, the protagonist listens to the visible voice of the other and responds with the hospitality of a compassionate touch that consents to the body, even to the point of the body's being toward death, that is, mortal. This being subject to decay is a characteristic not only of human and other animal bodies, but also of things, including the material artefacts that are Bibles.

Chrétien does not limit his notion of the visible voice to human bodies, but describes it as an effective property of things that call us, inviting us to respond. Applying the concept of the visible voice to a text, that is, a writing as it appears in a particular material artefact, I want to suggest that a text addresses its reader in the mode of a visible voice. This is quite literally the case if one considers reading aloud from, or at a place in, a material artefact as an instance of the eye listening. The material artefact itself opens to a writing that is a visible voice, to which one listens with one's eyes and towards which one might respond with what Edith Humphrey describes as 'a hermeneutics of welcome'.[22] Humphrey intends that an interpreter should welcome a biblical writing on its own terms across its myriad material appearances. In contrast, I envisage welcoming the text as a writing in a particular material artefact before me in a particular here and now, for example, the CD-ROM on which is encoded the Nestle–Aland Greek New Testament with which I happen to be working away from my usual desk today. What this hermeneutic hospitality to the text as a material thing means for a practice of biblical interpretation is difficult to identify. The Gospel of Luke, where hospitality is a major theme, offers a point of conversation for exploring the possibility of such a hermeneutics.

In Luke, one can read a narrative hermeneutics of divine welcome. Reading from a place in the scroll of Isaiah, the Lukan Jesus proclaims a divine responsiveness to suffering. Poverty, captivity, blindness and oppression appear in the mode of a prior call on the one who anoints, which becomes a commissioning of the anointed one:

> he has anointed me
> to bring good news to the poor.
> He has sent me to proclaim release to the captives
> and recovery of sight to the blind,
> to let the oppressed go free,
> to proclaim the welcome year of the lord (4.17-18 NRSV modified).

22. Humphrey, *And I Turned to See*, p. 29.

The movement from oppression to freedom, from captivity to release, is a proclamation of good news and divine visitation. As Chad Hartsock notes, the restoration of sight (ἀνάβλεψις) is a key element of this proclamation.[23] After the Lukan Jesus reads the passage and rolls up the scroll, the narrator reports, 'The eyes of all in the synagogue were fixed on him' (4.20). The next section takes up the theme of blindness and sight in the Gospel of Luke.

### *Sight and Blindness in Luke*

The prologue to Luke's Gospel refers in the NRSV translation to 'eyewitnesses and servants of the word' (1.2). 'Eyewitnesses' translates the Greek αὐτόπται, the plural of αὐτόπτης, a word occurring only here in the Second Testament and not at all in the Septuagint. In classical Greek, αὐτόπτης refers to an eyewitness, and the related verb αὐτοπτέω means to see with one's own eyes, especially a divine manifestation (LSJ).[24] The relatively frequent use of αὐτόπτης in Polybius's *Histories*, from the second to first centuries BCE, offers some helpful insights into the tenor of the term. Polybius uses the term to refer to a superior way of understanding something (*Hist.* 1.4.7; see also 12.28a.4). For example, when one sees a living, dynamic and beautiful creature rather than the disparate parts of its body, however beautiful they may be, one sees for oneself the whole in its context and so has a better knowledge of the thing (*Hist.* 1.4.7). Nevertheless, a universal history cannot be extrapolated perfectly from isolated cases (*Hist.* 1.4.7).

If one is an eyewitness, one can be more confident in one's knowledge than if one has only heard a report (*Hist.* 20.12.II frag.). A nobleman offers to run a Roman blockade at Lilybaeum to bring an eyewitness account to the Carthagian government concerning the situation there (*Hist.* 1.46.4). Later Polybius compares the experience of a generation who have been eyewitnesses of war with that of the succeeding generation, which is less appreciative of a hard-won peace (*Hist.* 2.21.2). Further, he claims himself to be eyewitness, actor and occasionally director of the events he is to narrate concerning the rule of the Roman conquerors (*Hist.* 3.4.13; see also *Hist.* 10.11.4; 25.6.5). However, on occasion, seeing for one's self proves difficult in a foreign environment (*Hist.* 3.58.8).

Polybius also refers to the desire to be an eyewitness of spectacular places, such as the city of Byzantium (*Hist.* 4.38.12). Polybius quotes Herodotus's 'eyewitness' account of the lotus (*Hist.* 12.2.1). In his criticism of

23. Chad Hartsock, *Sight and Blindness in Luke–Acts: The Use of Physical Features in Characterization* (Leiden: E.J. Brill, 2008), pp. 173-79.

24. 2 Peter 1.16 refers to ἐπόπται, lookers-on or spectators.

Timaeus, he argues that given the impossibility of being an eyewitness to events and things in multiple places and times, one ought seek the advice of as many people as possible (*Hist.* 12.4c.4; cf. 12.4d.2). Eumenes' speech to the Romans appeals to those who have been eyewitnesses, knowing that what he has spoken of is true (*Hist.* 21.21.1). Polybius comments that the course of his writing (γραφή) brings him to the time of the destruction of Macedonia concerning which he, having been an eyewitness (*Hist.* 29.21.8), must offer a fitting word/report (λόγος). Being an eyewitness—seeing with one's own eyes—involves knowledge based on first-hand experience, for which the sense of sight is a paradigm, and the accompanying assurance of veracity in speaking and writing.

Considering the meaning of αὐτόπται καὶ ὑπηρέται in Lk. 1.2, Karl Kuhn links the notion of eyewitness principally to the notion of witness.[25] Joseph Fitzmyer reads Lk. 1.2 in the light of Acts 1.21-22, which states that, in fulfilment of the Scriptures,

> one of the men who have accompanied us through the time that the lord Jesus went in and out among us, beginning from the baptism of John until the day when he was taken up from us—one of these must become a witness with us to his resurrection (Acts 1.21-22 NRSV modified).[26]

In the experience of being with Jesus from the beginning of his ministry to his ascension, this seeing for oneself becomes for Luke in Acts 1 a basis for witnessing to the resurrection. Joel Green argues that for Luke witnessing is not a 'graduation' from earlier eyewitnessing; rather an eyewitness, αὐτόπτης, is a witness, μάρτυς.[27] For Kuhn, however, the terms αὐτόπται and ὑπηρέται refer not only to the disciples who will witness Jesus' ministry, passion and death, but also to key characters in the infancy narratives, such as Zechariah and Elizabeth, Mary, the shepherds, Simeon and Anna, whose being eyewitnesses calls forth proclamation.[28] For example, the shepherds respond with praise, which for Kuhn is a form of proclamation, to what they have seen and heard (2.20).[29] Their praise is a response of witness to the visible voice of the birth event they have seen with their own eyes. The interplay between sight and hearing in the birth account (esp. 2.15-20) is a dramatic rendering of the visible voice of a divine visitation.

25. Karl A. Kuhn, 'Beginning the Witness: The αὐτόπται καὶ ὑπηρέται of Luke's Infancy Narrative', *NTS* 49 (2003), pp. 237-55. While there is evidence from Greek literature for linking the notion of eyewitness (αὐτόπτης) with that of witness (μάρτυς) (Demosthenes, *Andr.* 22:22), there is a difference.

26. Fitzmyer, *Gospel according to Luke I–IX*, p. 294.

27. Green, *Gospel of Luke*, p. 41.

28. Kuhn, 'Beginning the Witness', pp. 242-43.

29. Kuhn, 'Beginning the Witness', p. 247.

While the link between eyewitness and witness is important, other aspects of the pair αὐτόπται and ὑπηρέται need to be read more closely. Luke refers to a tradition handed on by those who became from the beginning eyewitnesses and attendants of the word.[30] The only other place in the Gospel of Luke where ὑπηρέτης occurs is in 4.20, where the word refers to the synagogue attendant to whom Jesus returns the rolled scroll after his reading from Isaiah. As Fitzmyer explains:

> In itself *hypēretēs* means 'a servant, helper, assistant,' and it designated assistants to physicians, kings, courts, the Sanhedrin, and in a synagogue (Luke 4:20). In Acts 13:5 John Mark is called an 'assistant' of Barnabas and Saul, precisely in a context in which they announced 'the word of God' in a Jewish synagogue at Salamis in Cyprus.[31]

To be a servant of the word, therefore, has a material basis in being an attendant responsible for the scrolls kept in a synagogue, where the writings to which Luke refers on many occasions, as I showed in Chapter 3, could be physically located. In the parallel between αὐτόπται and ὑπηρέται is a potential interplay between the visible voice of an event to which an eyewitness witnesses and the visible voice of the material artefact. The visible voice of the scrolls of Isaiah or the Psalms, for example, is literally proclaimed in the human voice of a reader (such as the Lukan Jesus in Luke 4) translating visual codes (letters) into the sound of words. For Luke, the visible voice is also the fulfilment of these writings in the events seen and heard by their eyewitnesses.

A further aspect of Luke's reference to eyewitnesses in the prologue is significant. Where Polybius's *Histories* and Acts 1.21-22 privilege the experience of the eyewitness, the tenor of the Lukan prologue is not to do so. Luke does not propose a lesser account for its being secondary to that provided by eyewitnesses.[32] Rather, Luke promises an account that does what Polybius claims for the writing of a good eyewitness. Luke offers his reader accuracy (adv. ἀκριβῶς) and assurance (ἀσφάλεια), and parallels the tradition handed on by those who were from the beginning (ἀπ᾽ αρχῆς) eyewitnesses with his careful investigation from the first, or for a long time (ἄνωθεν) (Lk. 1.2-4). Rather than devaluing or displacing the sense of

30. In coherence with Greek usage, I am taking the view that γενόμενοι relates both to αὐτόπται and ὑπηρέται, not simply the latter, as it regularly appears with αὐτό πτης in the literature. See further Fitzmyer, *Gospel according to Luke I–IX*, p. 294; Green, *Gospel of Luke*, p. 41.

31. Fitzmyer, *Gospel according to Luke I–IX*, p. 294.

32. 1 John 1.1 explicitly expands the privileging of the eyewitness to include the witness of the senses of hearing and touch as well as sight. This first-hand sensory experience, which includes touch and hearing, is implied in the notion of eyewitness.

sight, this understanding of what can be assured in writing is accompanied by a sustained use of sight as symbol.

As noted in Chapter 6, the focus in Lk. 1.5-25 is on the visual. A shift occurs in 1.26-38, where hearing receives greater emphasis. By Lk. 2.1-18, there is a synaesthesia between sight and hearing. In the programmatic scene of Lk. 4.16-30, where likewise sight and hearing are interwoven, the Lukan Jesus proclaims restoration of sight to the blind as a key element of the divine visitation of which he is the commissioned and anointed agent. In the verses from Isaiah that Jesus proclaims in the Nazareth synagogue, good news, restoration and release are promised to the poor, captives, the blind and the oppressed. Hartsock notes that while release for captives and the oppressed is not explicitly mentioned again in Luke, references to the poor and the blind occur in several places.[33] Luke, Hartsock argues, refers to both physical and spiritual blindness; the reference to blindness in Lk. 4.18-19 signals not simply that the 'healing ministry of Jesus typified by healing of the blind' (see 7.21-22) is programmatic, but so too is 'the healing of spiritual blindness'.[34]

Hartsock bases his analysis of references to blindness and sight in Luke–Acts on his exploration of the literary trope of physiognomy and its role in the ancient Greek-speaking world. Physiognomy refers to a practice of characterization in which physical features convey moral meaning.[35] He identifies four layers to the meaning and representation of blindness in Greek literature: (i) blindness is a negative condition, associated with helplessness and dependence, and is a sign of divine disfavour; (ii) blindness is a (divine) punishment for crimes, whether intentional or unintentional; (iii) blindness is equivalent to ignorance; (iv) in contrast, the blind (for example, blind prophets) are those who see truly.[36] These representations also form a basis for understanding blindness metaphorically, for example, the Lukan Jesus plays on the trope of ignorance when he gives the example of blind guides (Lk. 6.39). Arguing that restoration of sight to the blind 'becomes an interpretive heuristic' for Luke–Acts, Hartsock shows that physical and spiritual blindness are mutually interpretative, especially, for example, when 'Saul's physical condition [becoming blind] is made to match his spiritual condi-

33. Hartsock, *Sight and Blindness*, p. 175.

34. Hartsock, *Sight and Blindness*, p. 176.

35. Hartsock, *Sight and Blindness*, p. 7.

36. Hartsock, *Sight and Blindness*, pp. 63-64. Hartsock suggests that Luke uses physiognomy subversively in several episodes (Lk. 13.10-17; 19.1-10; Acts 3.1-10; 8.26-40); however, his conclusions concerning the gait of the person at the Temple in Acts 3 are not established as surely as he suggests.

tion' (Acts 9.1-9).[37] Conversely, the healing of the physical blindness of the beggar near Jericho matches his spiritual sight, that is, his faith (Lk. 18.35-43).

Hartsock also describes three ancient theories of vision that underscore the representations of blindness and sight: (i) intromission, where light is understood to enter the eyes to produce images; (ii) extramission, where light is emitted or channelled by the eye in order to see; (iii) a combination of intromission and extramission.[38] The sense of sight was understood variously as receiving and giving light (and, in its absence through blindness, darkness). Hence, the Lukan Jesus speaks of the eye as a lamp:

> No one after lighting a lamp puts it in a cellar, but on the lampstand so that those who enter may see the light. Your eye is the lamp of your body. If your eye is healthy, your whole body is full of light; but if it is not healthy, your body is full of darkness. Therefore consider whether the light in you is not darkness. If then your whole body is full of light, with no part of it in darkness, it will be as full of light as when a lamp gives you light with its rays (Lk. 11.33-36 NRSV).

Using the image of a lamp, Luke develops the metaphor of sight and blindness in terms of the related symbols of light and darkness. Just as a body can be sounded by a voice, the body can be filled with light or darkness. A healthy eye is a conduit for light; an unhealthy, or blind, eye (though the Lukan Jesus does not refer directly to blindness in this passage) is a conduit for darkness. If the eye is a lamp, it not only casts light into the body, but also casts light outward from a whole body full of light.

These sayings about the light of the body appear in Luke between two passages concerning failures to recognize Jesus. As such, the passage stands out in the text as itself a lamp putting into sharper focus the condemnation of 'this generation' (11.29-32, 37-52, esp. 50-52). Their failure to see what is in their midst is taken up again in 19.41-44, when the Lukan Jesus on seeing the city of Jerusalem speaks of a failure to recognize (or know) 'the things that make for peace' (19.42) and 'the time of your visitation' (19.44). Is Jesus addressing the Pharisees named in 19.39, or the city itself, and implicitly its leaders and people, 'this generation' (see also 13.34-35)? As in Lk. 11.37-52, it seems likely that the response of the scribes and Pharisees, which Luke sets up earlier as a paradigm of failure to accept God's purpose (7.29-30), and the response of 'this generation' are interwoven. A failure to receive the divine visitation is metaphorically signalled by dark-

37. Hartsock, *Sight and Blindness*, pp. 172, 179. It terms of voice, Zechariah's muteness may perform a similar function (Lk. 1.20). Does Zechariah's being silenced reflect his inability to speak knowledgeably about his vision and the promise given him, because he has failed to believe the words spoken by the angel?

38. Hartsock, *Sight and Blindness*, p. 144.

ness; by implication, the body illumined by the healthy eye recognizes and welcomes the divine visitation.

This use of the metaphor of the eye as a lamp is dangerous because it contributes substantially to an identification between darkness and the people of Jerusalem that is anything but benign (see also Acts 2.22-23). In considering the possibility that the text, as a writing in a particular material artefact, can be understood as a visible voice to which the reader might respond hospitably, we need to be aware the writing itself opens not only to hospitality but also to its opposite, when it opens to the possibility of interpretations that promote violence against the other.

### *Hospitality: Receiving and Not Receiving*

Although the Lukan narrative does not deal with its own potential for interpretations that prove inhospitable to some, perhaps against the intention of the author, the narrative does deal with the issue of failure of hospitality to Jesus and his disciples.[39] Luke 10.1-12 offers a particular case:

> After this the lord appointed seventy others and sent them on ahead of him in pairs to every town and place where he himself intended to go. He said to them, 'The harvest is plentiful, but the workers are few; therefore ask the lord of the harvest to send out workers into his harvest. Go on your way. See, I am sending you out like lambs into the midst of wolves. Carry no purse, no bag, no sandals; and greet no one on the road. Whatever house you enter, first say, "Peace to this house!" And if a daughter or son of peace is there, your peace will rest on that person; but if not, it will return to you. Remain in the same house, eating and drinking whatever they provide, for workers deserve their wages. Do not move about from house to house. Whenever you enter a town and its people welcome you, eat what is set before you; heal the sick in it, and say to them, "The βασιλεία of God has come near to you." But whenever you enter a town and they do not welcome you, go out into its streets and say, "Even the dust of your town that clings to our feet, we wipe off against you. Yet know this: the βασιλεία of God has come near." I tell you, on that day it will be more tolerable for Sodom than for that town' (Lk. 10.1-12 NRSV modified).

39. Robert Tannehill argues that Luke presents a tragic history of Israel that is open to hope. It is not Luke's intention to incite violence against Jews. Others have made the case that Luke's presentation of the Pharisees and scribes is itself multivalent. See, for example, Tannehill, 'Israel in Luke–Acts', pp. 69-85; Gowler, *Host, Guest*. We need to read Luke on his own terms, however, and note where his own metaphor of hospitality fails, particularly in relation to his characterization of Jerusalem and its people. See, for example, Sanders, *Jews in Luke–Acts*; Elvey, 'Legacies of Violence', pp. 21-34.

The passage comes within the context of the journey to Jerusalem, which begins in earnest with Jesus setting his face toward Jerusalem (9.51). For Luke, Jerusalem is the site not only of the impending death of Jesus but also of the later destruction of Temple and city in 70 CE. Within the context of this orientation toward Jerusalem, the theme of response to the divine visitation is paramount (9.52-56; see also 19.41-44). Attendant on this theme of response to the divine visitation is a question of judgment, prompting a sense of urgency concerning discipleship (9.57-62). Following 10.1-12, the theme of judgment continues in 10.13-16 before the disciples return to report their success (10.17).

In Lk. 10.18-23, a congregation of sight language occurs. Following the disciples' jubilant return from their mission (10.17), for which they are commissioned in 10.1-12, the Lukan Jesus reports a vision: 'I watched Satan fall from the sky like a flash of lightning' (10.18). The report of the disciples' success is particularly striking for the reader, coming as it does immediately after the woes of 10.13-15, which dramatically announce a failure of receptivity to the divine visitation.[40] The reiteration in 10.16 of the cases set out in 10.8-12, concerning welcoming and not welcoming the disciples, ends on rejection, setting up a contrast with the disciples' positive report (10.17). Of a piece with the dramatic shift from unwelcome (10.13-16) to welcome (10.17) is the tenor of the vision report (10.18). Almost midway between Satan's departure (4.13) and return (22.3) in the Lukan Gospel, Jesus reports Satan's downfall, and thus Luke points ahead to the ultimate success of Jesus' mission, which is already present in the disciples' success.

The Lukan 'Jesus is both seer and interpreter'.[41] He explains to the disciples 'both what he has seen (the downfall of Satan) and what they have seen (the banishing of illness and evil), for the vision and the mission are one'.[42] But he points them away from their immediate success: 'Do not rejoice at this, that the spirits submit to you, but rejoice that your names are written in the skies (ἐγγέγραπται ἐν τοῖς οὐρανοῖς)' (10.20). In the worldview of the Lukan narrative, the skies hold a divine register, a material artefact (whether scroll or book), that is probably understood like the heavens/skies themselves as a physical site.[43] The shift of focus is not from material earth to spiritual heaven; the two are physically connected. The shift from their

40. Humphrey, *And I Turned to See*, p. 107.

41. Humphrey, *And I Turned to See*, p. 113.

42. Humphrey, *And I Turned to See*, p. 111.

43. I am grateful to Dr Catherine Playoust for conversations about the way in which in the Second Testament and Second Temple literature heaven was understood as a physical place to and from which seers could journey. A register held in heaven would likewise be understood as a physical thing.

immediate success is followed by another that elaborates on the meaning of the first.

In what many read as a Johannine interpolation or echo, the narrative changes tone:

> At that same hour Jesus rejoiced in the Holy Spirit and said, 'I thank you, Father, lord of heaven and earth, because you have hidden these things from the wise and the intelligent and have revealed them to infants; yes, Father, for such was your gracious will. All things have been handed over to me by my Father; and no one knows who the Son is except the Father, or who the Father is except the Son and anyone to whom the Son chooses to reveal him' (Lk. 10.21-22 NRSV).

Like the earlier shift, this solemn prayer and proclamation is intended to train 'the gaze of the disciples' and by extension Luke's readers/hearers ... 'so that their attention can be redirected and deepened'.[44] The blessing on the eyes that follows signals the orientation of this redirected attention. When Jesus says to the disciples in private, 'Blessed are the eyes that see what you see!' (10.23), and continues with reference to the longing of the prophets to see and hear (10.24), the reader is returned to the prophet Simeon, who longed to see (2.25-26).

When Simeon takes the Lukan Jesus in his arms, he praises God (2.28). Using the language of a slave to a master, Simeon proclaims his release in peace according to God's word (2.29). Given the earlier remark of the narrator that 'a response or transaction had been made with him by the Holy Spirit, that he would not see death (ἰδεῖν θάνατον) before he had seen (ἴδῃ) the lord's Christ' (2.26), the release refers to his death. In this context, where seeing the Christ comes before his seeing death, Simeon's speech brings together several elements related to the sense of sight and vision in Luke: the eyes as the organ of sense, seeing as the act of sensing, the face, the related medium of light, and the manifestations of revelation and glory. He acclaims:

> my eyes have seen (εἶδον οἱ ὀφθαλμοί μου) your salvation,
> which you have prepared in the face (κατὰ πρόσωπον) of all the peoples,
> a light for revelation (φῶς εἰς ἀποκάλυψιν) of the Gentiles
> and glory (δόξαν) of your people Israel (Lk. 2.30-32; NRSV modified).

There are three important parallels of identification operating in this segment. First, salvation is identified as a light for ('to give') revelation and glory (the preposition εἰς governs both ἀποκάλυψιν and δόξαν).[45] The sense of εἰς here is difficult to translate. The sense is that light which can enter and/or be emitted from the eyes either makes it possible for salvation

44. Humphrey, *And I Turned to See*, p. 111.
45. See Fitzmyer, *Gospel according to Luke I–IX*, p. 428.

as revelation and glory to be seen, or results in its being seen. In either case, salvation becomes visible to Simeon in the infant Jesus.

In the second identification, together the Gentiles and the people of Israel represent all the peoples.[46] A light making visible revelation belonging to the nations is a light making visible glory belonging to Israel.[47] The third parallel between revelation and glory shows these to be equivalent manifestations of the one light rather than separate aspects belonging properly to the Gentiles and Israel respectively. As Simeon's address to Mary indicates, this light for revelation and glory is also infused with suffering (2.34-35).

In this narrative encounter, Simeon responds to the visible voice of the infant and his mother, who together call forth from him a voice of praise and prophecy. The focus on the salvation made visible in the child prompts the reader to listen to the visible voice of the Lukan Jesus, as the disciples and the reader will be commanded explicitly in the transfiguration narrative (9.35). The themes of seeing, the face, and glory infused with suffering, associated with this visible voice, also occur in the transfiguration account. Unlike the earlier prophets who for Luke did not see and hear (10.24), Simeon saw in the visible voice of the infant Jesus the salvation for which he longed. The disciples and Luke's readers/hearers, who are like infants themselves (10.21), are called to see (and hear) the visible voice of the Lukan Jesus, who is no longer an infant. Responding to this visible voice, like Simeon, the disciples and the reader see and have their seeing blessed (10.23).

In the flow of the narrative of Luke 10, the parable of the Good Samaritan (10.25-37) dramatically depicts the hospitality of compassion as a responsive listening to the visible voice of the suffering other. Jesus prompts the lawyer to move from his initial question, 'What must I do to inherit eternal life?' (10.25), to the question 'Who is my neighbour?' (10.29). The former question concerns how the lawyer's name might be assured entry in the divine register (see 10.20). But the Lukan Jesus turns the gaze away from heaven (the skies) (cf. 10.18, 20) to the Torah—a material text that is written and can be read (10.26)—and to a road from Jerusalem to Jericho (10.30). The focus is neither on Jesus nor solely on the suffering other. The gaze is directed to the other who is unexpectedly, even excessively, compassionate.[48] The multiple meanings of the parable signalled by the difference between the questions, 'Who is my neighbour?' (10.29) and 'Who acted as neighbour?' (10.36), are mediated by shifts in focus from the man who has been attacked (10.30) to those who see him and their subsequent actions

46. See discussion in Brown, *Birth of the Messiah*, p. 459.

47. See discussions in Fitzmyer, *Gospel according to Luke I–IX*, p. 428, Marshall, *Gospel of Luke*, p. 121.

48. Elvey, *Ecological Feminist Reading*, pp. 237-43; Elvey, 'To Bear the Other'.

(10.31-35). In its entirety, the parable itself can be said to be a thing that presents with a visible voice to which the lawyer, and by extension the reader, must respond.

The narrative of sending seventy (or seventy-two) disciples (10.1-12) occurs in this wider context of response to the visible voice of the Lukan Jesus and of the Lukan Gospel as together they call to the reader/hearer to see and listen. There are partial parallels to Lk. 10.1-12 in Lk. 9.1-6; Mt. 9.37–10.1; 10.7-16; and Mk 6.7-13. The passage begins by referring to the Lukan Jesus as 'lord' (10.1). Jesus speaks of the 'lord of the harvest' (10.2). Luke associates Jesus with the lord or master of the harvest. The term 'lord' suggests hierarchy and dominion of the human and the divine over the non-human. The lord of the harvest is the master who oversees the crops and whose task it is to employ workers to sow the seed, tend the growing plants and then harvest the ripened crops. He is an image of human agricultural intervention in natural processes of growth and reproduction, for the sustenance of human beings. The focus on his role of management and mastery tends to hide the processes of growth and reproduction of plants—the Earth work that makes possible a harvest.

In the Lukan narrative, the harvest itself is a symbol of urgency. Extra workers are needed without delay because there is only a limited time in which a ripe crop can be harvested. The word for harvest, θερισμός, occurs only here in Luke, but the verb θερίζω, 'to harvest or reap', occurs in 12.24 and 19.21-22. The metaphor of harvest, based in the separation entailed in the act of harvesting, relates to judgment.[49] The urgency of the harvest and its relation to judgment echo in the 10.3-12. As lord of the harvest, the Lukan Jesus sends out seventy or seventy-two disciples. Lambs and wolves appear in a metaphor for the experience of the disciples (10.3). This metaphor of prey and predator goes back at least to Homer. In Luke 10, it suggests the vulnerability of the disciples.[50] It allies the disciples with the vulnerable prey and their oppressors/enemies with the predator, echoing both the separation and judgment signalled by the idea of harvest.

The Greek word ἀρήν (plural ἄρνας), 'lamb' or 'lambs', occurs only here in the Second Testament. Matthew has πρόβατον, 'sheep'. In the Septuagint, ἀρήν or ἄρνας and λύκος or λύκοι 'wolf' or 'wolves' occur together in the Isaian depictions of the peaceable kingdom: 'even a wolf will feed together with a lamb' (Isa. 11.6) and 'at that time wolves and lambs will be nourished/fed at the same time' (Isa. 65.25). With the Lukan emphasis on peace in 10.5-6 and the imminence of the βασιλεία of God

49. F. Hauck, '*Therismós*', in *The Theological Dictionary of the New Testament, Abridged in One Volume* (ed. Gerhard Kittel and Gerhard Friedrich; Grand Rapids: Eerdmans, 1985).

50. Green, *Gospel of Luke*, p. 413.

in 10.9 and 11, the reader is invited to hear an echo of the Isaian peaceable kingdom motif.[51] In Lk. 10.5, peace is more benediction or blessing than greeting. An effective gift, peace can rest on its recipient or return to the giver (10.6). Fitzmyer writes, 'Peace is not to be understood in this context as merely the opposite of war, but in the OT sense of šālôm, the root of which is šlm, "completeness, wholeness." It expresses rather the comprehensive bounty of God's salvific presence and activity.'[52] The blessing of peace and the exercise of hospitality co-occur (10.6).

The image of wolves and lambs feeding together in the peaceable kingdom can inform Luke's picture of hospitality, with a recollection of the more-than-human (including human and divine) providers of sustenance (see also 12.24). Although the Isaian image suggests as ideal a problematic homogenization of predator and prey, its echo in Luke 10 may also unsettle the harsher images of judgment with the hope that disciples and their opponents might in the βασιλεία of God be nourished together.[53] This nourishment relies in Luke 10 on human hospitality.

In 10.4, the Lukan Jesus commands the disciples: Take nothing. In comparison with Lk. 9.3, Mt. 10.9-10 and Mk 6.8-9, the text does not list what the disciples are to refrain from carrying with them. Rather, in contrast to Lk. 12.22-31, where the emphasis is on human dependence (like the ravens) on God's providence, the focus in 10.5-8 is on their dependence on the hospitality of other humans. While the disciples will be dependent on the hospitality of those who receive the peace they bring, the peace-sharing household participates in divine bounty through the hospitality they give (10.7). Not only is this hospitality underwritten by the Earth community that makes it possible, but also (perhaps problematically) by the image of lambs and wolves eating together. Yet from the perspective of the interconnectedness of the Earth community, this peaceful hospitality also suggests a deliberate openness to, and sharing in, the wholeness of the entire Earth community.

When in 10.8-11 the Lukan Jesus speaks of the ways in which the disciples are to respond to their reception or otherwise, the earthiness of this whole community appears in the symbol of dust (κονιορτός). In 10.8, the

51. Robert Karris, 'The Gospel according to Luke', in *The New Jerome Biblical Commentary* (ed. Raymond E. Brown, Joseph A. Fitzmyer and Roland E. Murphy; London: Geoffrey Chapman, 1991), p. 701.

52. Fitzmyer, *Gospel according to Luke X–XXIV*, p. 848.

53. On the problems with the peaceable kingdom motif, see Anne Elvey, 'Desiring the "Peaceable Kingdom"? Use/Respect Dualism, the Enigma of Predation and Human Relationships to Other Animals', *PAN: Philosophy Activism Nature* 3 (2005), pp. 31-40. Further, from the perspective of human interdependence with and in a wider Earth community, we need to recognize that the Earth community is necessary for the exercise of both human hospitality and divine providence.

passage shifts focus from the hospitality of the household to that of town or city. When the disciples do not find a welcome, they are to go out into the wide dusty streets of the city or town and prophetically wipe the dust from their feet against the inhabitants of the town (10.11). The action of removing the dust is a claiming of separateness from those whose hospitality has failed. If the disciples had been welcomed into a house in a town, it is likely they would have had the dust washed from their feet by their host or by the household slaves on behalf of the host. Not to provide this service to a guest is a failure of hospitality on the part of the host (see 7.44).[54]

Shaking, or perhaps scraping, the dust from one's feet is also an act of separation from the dust. But what is this dust? In the Septuagint, κονιορτός does not translate earth or land, ארץ, nor the ground/dust, אדמה, from which the human, אדם, is formed. Rather, κονιορτός is the dust kicked up by the horses, elephants, chariots and human feet of approaching armies (Ezek. 26.10). It is the swirling dust picked up by storm winds (Job 21.18; Isa. 17.13). In one instance, clouds are the dust an angry God kicks up as he strides about the skies (Nah. 1.3). It is the dust that appears on the horizon before one sees approaching crowds of friends or enemies (2 Kgs. 9.17). Dust, therefore, can act as a sign of what is to come.

κονιορτός can also be both the opposite of fragrant perfume, thus an odorous dust (Isa. 5.24), and a powder that has been perfumed (Song 3.6). In several cases, κονιορτός appears in the Septuagint in association with judgment. The plague of dust will cause boils (Exod. 9.9). The Golden Calf is ground to dust (Deut. 9.21). God will change the rain of the land to dust (Deut. 28.24). The flower of the people will go up like dust (in this instance, like the rising cinders from a fire) (Isa. 5.24). The people will be trodden down like dust in the street by Assyria as instrument of divine judgment (Isa 10.6).

Isaiah presents the imagery of dust as both contrast and precursor to a divine visitation:

> But the multitude of your foes shall be like small dust (κονιορτός),
> and the multitude of tyrants like flying chaff.
> And in an instant, suddenly,
> Yhwh of hosts will make a visitation (ἐπισκοπή)
> with thunder and earthquake and great noise,
> with whirlwind and tempest, and the flame of a devouring fire
> (Isa. 29.5-6 NRSV modified with reference to LXX).

54. I am grateful to Merrill Kitchen for alerting me to this point, and also to other participants at the Baptists Today conference in 2005, held at Amberley in Melbourne, Australia, for their welcoming of this discussion of the dust in Luke 10.11.

In Lk. 9.5 and the parallel in Mk 6.11, the shaking of dust (or in Mark soil, χοῦς) is a witness (μαρτύριον) against the people of the place. Mark's use of χοῦς links the action with the ground from which the human was formed in Gen. 2.7, whereas Luke's use of κονιορτός suggests more strongly the link with judgment. Although Luke does not repeat μαρτύριον in 10.11, the sense of witness is also evident there, as also in Acts 13.51. The action of removing the dust from one's feet is a visible sign to the people of the town, both something they can witness and a witness against them for their failure of hospitality.

In this sign, the commanded action involves not only the intentional act of the disciples but also the qualities of fine dust that clings to feet sweaty from walking. Dust clings to the feet of the disciples, suggesting their connectedness with the ground. Some commentators read the admonition not to carry sandals as an indication that the disciples should here go unshod.[55] They are in direct contact with the dust of the roads and streets they travel. This dust must be wiped, not shaken, off. It will not easily let go. In the context of Luke, removing the dust is closely related to the imminence and immanence of the βασιλεία of God, the visitation that is upon the people (10.11), as hospitality and judgment. Therefore, the symbolic act also echoes other qualities of dust that underscore its use as a visible sign in the Septuagint both of judgment and of what is on the horizon.

Taken together, the human action of shaking, or scraping, off the dust and the characteristics of dust itself—as both a thing that clings to feet and a thing that can be seen from a distance—form a community of agency. This community of agency is a material witness to both the impending visitation of God and the failure to receive this visitation. In Lk. 9.1-6, Jesus directs the twelve in the third person concerning removing the dust, 'Wherever they do not welcome you, as you are leaving that town shake the dust off your feet as a testimony against them' (9.5; see also Mt. 10.14; Mk 6.11). In Lk. 10.11, Jesus directs the disciples to pronounce in the second person a sign against the inhabitants of the town. They are to say, 'Even the dust clinging to us from your city, to the feet, we wipe off against you' (10.11a, literal translation). The *verbal witness* of this proclamation in the second person makes explicit the *voice* of the *visible sign* of a more-than-human community of agency that comprises the action of wiping off the dust.

### *The Verbal Icon*

The participation of the dust with the disciples in a community of agency that has a visible voice offers a model for thinking of the agency of matter

55. Ellis, *Gospel of Luke*, p. 156.

in relation to the visible voice of a biblical text. Represented by papyrus, tree, used paper, sheep, goat or calf skin, fossils, and the minerals, metals, and ochres for ink, and by the material artefacts of scroll, codex, illuminated manuscript, printed book, CD-ROM, computer into which these materials have been formed, matter is part of a community of agency with writer, reader and hearer of the text. The community of agency that presents in a biblical text open to reading is in the mode of hospitality, the hospitality of the visible voice of a writing to interpretation. This mode of hospitality is interdependent with a prior mode of corporeal hospitality in which the embodied senses, of which sight is for Chrétien the model, open to the sensible. For example, as noted earlier, sight opens to the visible. The visible has a voice to which the eye listens.

In Chapter 1, I suggested that the Bible as a material artefact (or many of these) could be imagined as a 'verbal icon'. The concept of a verbal icon suggests a visible voice. As noted in Chapter 1, the transfiguration forms a basis for iconography. As Solrun Nes writes of the transfiguration icon attributed to Theophane the Greek, 'the combination of gold leaf and transparent egg tempera colour creates the impression that light penetrates matter and in this way makes the entire landscape shine from within'.[56] The material light of the icon enacts an affirmation that 'the Creator of matter ... became matter' and refers both to the incarnation and the transfiguration.[57] There is a two-way movement between creator and creation in which matter and God are interconnected. Moreover, while 'the icon expresses visually what the gospel proclaims verbally', the separation between sight and hearing this implies is not absolute.[58] The transfiguration narrative offers a paradigm of the visible voice. The disciples and the reader/hearer/viewer can only witness the transfiguration to the extent that they heed the command to listen. The transfiguration offers a model for understanding the biblical text, a writing in a place in a material artefact, as a verbal icon that is a visible voice. In the transfiguration account, the face of Jesus calls not only to the three disciples but also to the reader to witness a material light, and to listen to what they see.

The Lukan transfiguration account continually points the disciples and the reader/hearer forward and backward in the narrative. The face of Jesus will be set toward Jerusalem (9.29, 31, 51). The address ἐπιστάτα reminds the reader of the earlier moment when the disciples misread the situation

56. Nes, *Uncreated Light*, p. 107.

57. Nes, *Uncreated Light*, pp. 46-49, quoting from John of Damascus, *On the Divine Images* 1.16.

58. Nes, *Uncreated Light*, pp. 50-51.

in the boat, also a heightened moment when the wind and the waters rouse the lake while the Lukan Jesus sleeps (8.22-26; 9.33). In the transfiguration account, the disciples are weighed down with sleep (9.32), as they will be again in 22.45, when Jesus on another mountain faces his impending suffering. The two episodes mirror each other across Jesus' glory and suffering. The overshadowing cloud (9.34) recalls Mary's being overshadowed by the Holy Spirit (1.35).[59] As Heil argues, the voice from the cloud commanding 'listen to him!' pivots the disciples 'back to the previous teaching of Jesus (8.8, 18), especially his teaching about the necessity for him and his followers to suffer and be put to death (9.21-27) before entering into the heavenly glory of God's kingdom anticipated by Jesus' transfiguration'.[60] This command also pivots 'them forward to the subsequent prediction of the necessity for him to suffer and be put to death as a rejected prophet in Jerusalem (9.44, 51-56; 13.33-35; 18.31-33; 20.9-19; 22.14-23, 39-46; 24.4-7, 25-26, 44-46)'.[61] Included for Heil in this forward movement is a call to compassion and an assurance of being raised and sharing in heavenly glory.[62] The transfiguration thus brings to a focus the Lukan Gospel from the infancy narratives to the resurrection.[63]

Throughout this narrative, the divine visitation is described by way of a divine necessity related to the Jewish writings (see, for example, 24.26-27, 44-47), which for Jesus and his followers, including the author of Luke–Acts, were the Scriptures. Moses and the prophets are synonymous with these writings (24.27). Moreover, the disciples have been witnesses to the working out in the life, death and resurrection of Jesus of this divine necessity fulfilling the Scriptures (24.48). Three disciples are witnesses on the mountain to the transfiguration, where Moses and Elijah stand as figures of the Scriptures. In the working out of the divine necessity in the life, death and resurrection of the Lukan Jesus, there is a community of agency between Jesus, the writings, God, and events that impact on bodies, cities and places, so that disciples and readers are invited to witness and listen to what they see.

Understanding the writings, and Luke's own writing which will become part of the Christian Bible, as a visible voice is not an appropriation of Chrétien to Luke or vice versa. In the First Testament, after God speaks

59. Lee, *Transfiguration*, p. 77.
60. Heil, *Transfiguration of Jesus*, pp. 278-79.
61. Heil, *Transfiguration of Jesus*, p. 309.
62. Heil, *Transfiguration of Jesus*, p. 309.
63. With reference to a Western Ottonian manuscript illumination that juxtaposes the birth of Jesus with his glorification, Solrunn Nes, *Uncreated Light*, pp. 41-54, similarly describes the theological necessity of the incarnation for the transfiguration.

the words of the law at Sinai in Exod. 20.1-17, the narrator relates, 'all the people saw (ראים) the voices (הקולת)' (Exod. 20.18a).[64] The Septuagint has similarly, Καὶ πᾶς ὁ λαὸς ἑώρα τὴν φωνήν. On Horeb, Elijah recognizes Yhwh in 'a voice (of) thin/gauze-like/powdery silence/whisper/wail' (קול דממה דקה), which the Septuagint has as φωνὴ αὔρας λεπτῆς, 'a voice of thin air' (1 Kgs. 19.12b). The voice here is not immaterial, but particulate, powdery, like dust or fragrance (see, for example, Lev. 16.12, where דק is used in reference to a handful of crushed incense). In fact, elsewhere in the Septuagint דק is rendered by κονιορτός (Isa. 29.5). The visible voice can be imaged materially.

No direct link exists between the renderings of a voice materially, as visible in Exodus 20 and powdery in 1 Kings 19, and the witness of which κονιορτός is a material agent in Luke 10. Nevertheless, the visible voice associated with Moses and Elijah can be understood, like κονιορτός, as expressed in a more-than-human community of agency. When this visible voice is a material artefact of a biblical writing, the artefact takes on the characteristic of an icon.

Concerning the icon, Marion writes, 'The icon gives itself to be seen in that it makes me hear its call.'[65] In so doing, it has a face that calls me not only to see but also to be seen.[66] The icon calls forth 'a kind of *kenosis*', in which I am put into question by an irreducible other that gazes on me.[67] The beginning of Luke's Gospel refers to eyewitnesses and attendants of the word (1.2). At the end, the Lukan Jesus speaks of witnesses to the fulfilment of the Scriptures (24.44-48). These Scriptures are writings in places in scrolls that can be held in the hands.[68] If the Scriptures are a verbal icon that faces me with a gaze, their fulfilment cannot be found simply by looking into Scriptures to give meaning, or witness to, the events witnessed by the disciples. Fulfilment is also having these witnessed events and their witnesses looked at by the Scriptures.

If we understand that the writings always come to us as texts that are materially embodied and embedded, and as having a material voice, this being looked at is not only a standing under the word but also a standing under matter. Moreover, the former may be in tension with the latter. Just

64. Rev. 1.12 also refers to seeing a voice.

65. Marion, *In Excess*, pp. 118-19. See also Robyn Horner, 'The Face as Icon: A Phenomenology of the Invisible', *The Australasian Catholic Record* 82 (2005), pp. 19-28 (27).

66. Cf. Horner, 'Face as Icon', p. 23. It should be noted, as Horner points out, that Marion does not completely identify the face and the icon.

67. Horner, 'Face as Icon', pp. 22, 27-28.

68. As Alexander points out, given the materiality of texts and their capacity to decompose or be lost, Luke very likely did not imagine his writing would become Scripture (Alexander, 'What If Luke Had Never Met Theophilus?', p. 162).

as dust that arrives from the Mallee in Victoria, Australia, may speak back to us of topsoil loosed from an overused land, matter may speak back to us of its givenness to writing. This givenness appears in the modes of both hospitality and sacrifice of matter to text. I will take up these two aspects of the relationship between matter and writing in the next chapter.

# 8

## 'So I opened my mouth and he gave me the scroll to eat' (Ezekiel 3.2): The Taste of the Text

*O Taste and See*

The world is
not with us enough.
O taste and see

the subway Bible poster said,
meaning The Lord, meaning
if anything all that lives
to the imagination's tongue,

grief, mercy, language,
tangerine, weather, to
breathe them, bite,
savor, chew, swallow, transform

into our flesh our
deaths, crossing the street, plum, quince,
living in the orchard and being

hungry, and plucking
the fruit.



In Denise Levetov's poem 'O Taste and See', the speaker comes upon a material artefact, a subway Bible poster with the words 'O taste and see', and proffers a 'meaning'. The meaning shifts from an ostensibly religious meaning, 'O taste and see that the Lord is good' (Ps. 34.8a), to 'all that lives/ to the imagination's tongue', followed by a list that moves from 'grief and mercy' through language to the materiality of things and human engagement with them, for which eating and digestion are symbols. With reference to William Wordsworth's 'The world is too much with us', the poem takes us into a world that is 'not with us enough'. The poem progresses from nouns to verbs, from tangerine and weather to the first action 'to breathe them', followed by a list of infinitives, 'to bite,/savor, chew, swallow'. These actions spill into an interpretation of the taking-in of things through breathing and eating: 'to transform//into our flesh'. Immediately, without further punctuation, 'our flesh' flows into 'our/deaths'. The material engagements of tasting and seeing, breathing and eating are reminders of our material embeddedness, our consenting to the body and so to mortality. But the poet does not leave the reader with 'our deaths'. The next phrase, 'crossing the street', enacts a crossing, and the poem draws its reader into an orchard by way, first, of the names of fruit, 'plum' and 'quince', and then by making explicit the shift from 'our deaths' to 'living in the orchard'.

The poet returns the reader to the subway and the unstated poverty associated with the subway in 'being hungry'. The reader is left with a tension between the divine goodness the psalmist enjoins us 'taste and see', and to which the fruit of the orchard and our material engagement with things witness, and the reality of human hunger. Finally, with the reference to 'plucking the fruit', the poems recalls the Bible and the primaeval forest garden of Genesis 2. John Felstiner writes:

> In that closing echo of Eve's fall we can hear a stubborn celebration of earthly sweetness, and throughout 'O Taste and See' we hear—not a rejection of that psalmic metaphor for acknowledging divine goodness, but a furtherance of it. The Christian subway poster tells her what Gerard Manley Hopkins and Walt Whitman and William Carlos Williams told her: to taste and she will see the sacramental sensuousness of 'all that lives to the imagination's tongue.'[1]

The tone of the poem calls into question the idea of a 'fall'. The poem's invitation 'taste and see' evokes the goodness of both God and matter, suggesting that they cannot be fully separated. Is a 'fall' coherent with this shared goodness? By the interplay of nouns and verbs, and by the movement and variation through the list of being and doing and the phrases 'transform// into our flesh our/deaths' and 'living in the orchard', the poem performs the interrelatedness between humans and the Earth community of which we are part and on which we depend for sustenance and celebration. There is an ordinariness to 'being//hungry, and plucking/the fruit' that asks the material embeddedness of human life to speak (or speak back) to the biblical text on a subway Bible poster.

1. John Felstiner, '"O Taste and See": The Question of Content in American Jewish Poetry', *Jewish Social Studies* 5.1/2 (1998–99), p. 117.

This material embeddedness is underscored by the sense of taste. As with smell, taste involves taking in the substance of the other.[2] Like smelling, tasting can mean taking in only a little of the other, for example, when one samples wine. However, as a precursor to eating, taste signifies taking-in, normally through the mouth, and transforming the other into one's flesh and so, in turn, being transformed. We ingest the other through the mouth and the digestive system for nourishment, pleasure and sometimes healing. Further, since tasting requires discerning between things that are good to eat or drink and those that will do us harm, between bread and poison, taste is also a metaphor for judgment.

The tongue in the mouth is the organ of the sense of taste. Moreover, the tongue and the mouth are associated not only with the taste of food and drink but with the production of speech and language. This dual association of tongue and mouth with eating and speaking gives the ground for the metaphors of tasting words and eating scrolls. Eating and speaking are social acts. Even eating on one's own engages one in the wider sociality of the Earth community when one is nourished by more-than-human others.

In Lk. 14.15-24, the parable of the great dinner brings both the sociality of eating and the metaphor of taste to the question of response to the divine visitation, which I discussed in Chapter 7 in relation to Lk. 10.1-12.

> One of the dinner guests, on hearing this, said to him, 'Blessed is anyone who will eat bread in the βασιλεία of God!' Then Jesus said to him, 'Someone gave a great dinner and invited many. At the time for the dinner he sent his slave to say to those who had been invited, "Come; for everything is ready now." But they all alike began to make excuses. The first said to him, "I have bought a piece of land, and I must go out and see it; please accept my regrets." Another said, "I have bought five yoke of oxen, and I am going to try them out; please accept my regrets." Another said, "I have just been married, and therefore I cannot come." So the slave returned and reported this to his master. Then the owner of the house became angry and said to his slave, "Go out at once into the streets and lanes of the town and bring in the poor, the crippled, the blind, and the lame." And the slave said, "Sir, what you ordered has been done, and there is still room." Then the master said to the slave, "Go out into the roads and lanes, and compel people to come in, so that my house may be filled. For I tell you, none of those who were invited will taste my dinner"' (Lk. 14.15-24 NRSV modified).

The final sentence of the parable suggests judgment on those who fail to receive the divine visitation. Their consequent non-participation in the eschatological dinner means they will not taste it. Moreover, their failure to exercise sound judgment in their response to the invitation of the master is a failure of taste. Here tasting refers to the experience not only of sustenance

2. Borthwick, 'Olfaction and Taste', pp. 127-40.

through eating a meal, but more particularly to the experience of participating in the βασιλεία (reign or rule) of God.

For Luke, the breaking of bread is paradigmatic of this experience (9.10-17; 22.14-23; 24.28-31). The breaking of bread signifies a eucharistic materiality where hospitality and sacrifice characterize the gift of 'edible matter'. In this chapter, I focus on a eucharistic materiality as basis for understanding the way in which matter is given, or gives itself, to writing in the material artefacts that are biblical texts. To take a book and eat it (Ezek. 3.2; Rev. 10.9-10), bypassing the eyes and the ears, or rather in a synaesthesia to eat by way of seeing and hearing, is not only to open oneself to being nourished by the text, but also to transforming, and being transformed by incorporating, the text into one's flesh. The metaphor of eating a scroll cannot hold without the Scriptures understood as material artefacts. In this chapter, I allow the links between eating and speaking, food and scroll, to resonate with an understanding of Earth as eucharistic, asking what kind of hospitality does matter give to writing? What are the ethical implications for writers and readers concerning this givenness?

## *Taste and Speech*

In the Septuagint, the sense of taste relates not only to tasting food (1 Kgdms 14.24, 29, 43; 2 Kgdms 3.35; 2 Macc. 6.20)—by humans as well as other animals (Jon. 3.7)—and so eating (Gen. 25.30; Tob. 2.4; 7.12), but also to judgment and pleasure (Job 20.18). The multitalented woman of Proverbs 31 tastes her produce to judge its goodness (Prov. 31.18). Pleasure, perception and judgment are evoked when the psalmist cries, 'O taste and see' (Ps. 33.9 LXX). Taste parallels hearing in Job as a metaphor for discernment: 'for the ears separate words/matters (ῥήματα) as the larynx tastes grain' (Job 12.11) and 'the ears test words (λόγους) as the larynx tastes meat' (Job 34.3). The taste of a thing encompasses not only the experience of its physical taste but also the incorporation of its symbolic meaning; this is especially so of the taste of manna, a divine gift (Exod. 16.31; Num. 11.8). This dual aspect of taste gives itself to taste as a metaphor for experiencing the character of a thing or group of persons (for example, the taste of the daring of the Jews, 2 Macc. 13.18; the taste of Moab, Jer. 31.11). Taste signals a heightened physical experience of the other.

In the Gospel of Luke, γεύομαι, 'to taste', occurs only twice, both times in relation to participating in the βασιλεία of God. The Lukan Jesus proclaims, 'there are some standing here who will not taste death before they see the βασιλεία of God' (9.27). In the context of a parable about the βασιλεία meal, the Lukan Jesus concludes, 'none of those who were invited will taste my dinner' (14.24). Both are solemn proclamations: 9.27 begins λέγω δὲ ὑμῖν ἀληθῶς, 'but I tell you truly' or 'I assure you', and 14.24, λέγω γὰρ ὑμῖν, 'for I say to you'. In these solemn statements, taste functions as a metaphor for experience, in the context of the heightened expectation of the βασιλεία of God. The eschatological banquet, brought about by Jesus' death and resurrection, is characterized by 'joy, nourishment and abundance' (see esp. 9.12-17).[3] The material bases for Luke's use of the metaphor of taste are: (i) the physical incorporation of the other (death or the life of the βασιλεία feast), an incorporation that occurs in gustation; (ii) the discernment, between that which is live-giving or death-dealing, which taste signifies.

In the Lukan narrative, eating occurs in relation to the hospitality of God, which can be experienced in the person of the Lukan Jesus as a divine visitation of compassion and forgiveness, and the associated immanence and imminence of the βασιλεία of God (see esp. 14.15-24; 15.22-24; 22.14-20). That Jesus eats and with whom he eats become issues on which he is judged (5.30; 7.33-34; 15.2). That Jesus eats with tax collectors and sinners is one sign of the divine visitation (15.2). But Jesus also regularly eats with Pharisees (7.36; 14.1), and his eating becomes a moment for tasting and testing whether his hosts understand, and are open to receiving, the divine hospitality that arrives with their guest. In anticipating the eschatological banquet, the meals of Luke–Acts highlight and develop a number of interwoven Lukan themes: repentance, proper leadership, inclusivity, salvation, divine necessity and hospitality.[4]

Eating in Luke relates directly to hunger (4.2; 6.1, 4; 15.16) and is a sign of life (8.55; 24.43). Satisfaction of physical hunger and compassion for social outcasts are essential to the communality of the meal (see esp. Acts 2.43-47).[5] Satiation of hunger, especially for those in poverty, is a promise of liberation and salvation accompanying the divine visitation (1.53; 6.21, 25). Eating rather than fasting is symbolic of the divine visitation in Jesus (5.33). To eat is a sign of hospitality received (10.7-8). But like storing up food unnecessarily, eating can be symbolic of thoughtless or unjust consumption or over-consumption (12.19; 12.45; 17.27-28; see also 8.5; 15.30; 20.47). Nevertheless, food is also a sign of an earthy sustenance that mediates a divine providence (12.22, 29). Provision of food, however, is mediated by slaves, whose needs for sustenance are usually subordinated to those of their masters (17.8; cf. 12.37). But the service of hospitality through which the Lukan Jesus unsettles the master–slave paradigm on which Luke draws is based in physical acts of provision of food, most notably in the feeding and Last Supper narratives (9.12-17; 22.14-27; see also 24.30). In the post-resurrection appearances of the Lukan Jesus, his eating provides an assurance of his corporeality (24.41-43).

3. Heil, *Meal Scenes*, pp. 128, 216.
4. Heil, *Meal Scenes*; Byrne, *Hospitality of God.*
5. Heil, *Meal Scenes*, p. 37.

Like the ancient symposia which they echo, Luke's meals become occasions for discourse (see particularly 14.7-24; 22.14-30). The associations of taste with pleasure and discernment are embedded in this function of the meal as a setting for eating and speaking. The mouth performs a double role as the opening for ingestion of food and declaration of speech. Underlying this double role is biblical imagery depicting a mouth that opens like a door to consume and to speak. The former occurs, for example, when the earth opens to swallow Korah and other rebels (Num. 16.32; 26.10). The latter occurs when the mouth of Balaam's donkey is opened to speak (Num. 22.28); a person speaks out on behalf of the oppressed (Prov. 31.8-9); Zechariah's muteness is relieved (Lk. 1.64). The metaphor extends to consuming a text: 'So I opened my mouth and he gave me the scroll to eat' (Ezek. 3.2; see also Ezek. 3.27; 24.27; 33.22; cf. Ezek. 41.2). God speaks through the mouth of God's prophets (Lk. 1.70); gracious words come from the mouth of Jesus (Lk. 4.22). The mouth opens to wisdom or otherwise: 'Out of the abundance of the heart, the mouth speaks' (Lk. 6.45); 'I will give you a mouth and a wisdom that none of your opponents will be able to withstand or contradict' (Lk. 21.15).[6]

As Staubli and Schroer observe, the mouth is multifunctional; beyond its opening to eat and to speak, the mouth can be full not only of food but of laughter (Job 8.21-22); and the mouth can touch the other with a kiss, even a kiss of betrayal (Lk. 22.47-48).[7] The mouth opens to life-giving sustenance, speech and touch, and its opposites: poison, violent speech and betrayal.[8] A kiss of welcome (7.45) and perhaps laughter, but certainly the opportunity for speech, was part of a culture of hospitality underlying the meal scenes in Luke. From the sensual engagement of the mouth with food and words and skin, I turn to the edible matter (i.e. the food), without which the other aspects of the hospitality of a meal, such as discourse, could not occur because the meal would have no material ground.

## *Material Blessing*

In Luke's version of the feeding of five thousand men (Lk. 9.12-17), Jesus takes five loaves and two fish, looks up to heaven, blesses, breaks and gives (Lk. 9.16). The actions of taking, looking up to heaven, blessing and break-

6. Michel Serres (*Five Senses*, pp. 153-54) also associates taste with wisdom: '... homo sapiens refers to those who react to sapidity, appreciate it and seek it out, those for whom the sense of taste matters—savouring animals—before referring to judgement, intelligence or wisdom, before referring to talking man. . . . wisdom comes after taste, cannot arise without it'.

7. Staubli and Schroer, *Body Symbolism*, pp. 134-37.

8. Staubli and Schroer, *Body Symbolism*, pp. 139-43.

ing occur in the parallel passages in the Gospels of Mark and Matthew (Mk 6.41; Mt. 14.19b). In the Markan Last Supper, four of the actions occur: taking, blessing, breaking and giving (Mk 14.22). The Lukan version has taking, giving thanks, breaking and giving (Lk. 22.19), while the breaking of the bread in the Emmaus narrative is described by taking, blessing, breaking and giving (Lk. 24.30). A second version of the feeding, found in Matthew and Mark but not in Luke, has taking, giving thanks, breaking and giving (Mt. 15.36; Mk 8.6). The feeding narrative in the Gospel of John has the sequence: taking, giving thanks and distributing (Jn 6.11). The first letter to the Corinthians has taking, giving thanks and breaking (1 Cor. 11.23-24). According to Joseph Fitzmyer, both sequences, *taking–blessing–breaking–giving* and *taking–giving thanks–breaking–giving* were probably used in early Christian eucharistic rituals, with the former being the earlier version.[9]

The verb εὐλογέω, 'to bless', frequently refers to a blessing on the divine (for example, Gen. 24.48; Deut. 8.10; Pss. 15.7; 25.12; 33.2 LXX) or a divine blessing (for example, Gen. 1.22, 28; 5.2; 9.1; 12.2; Judg. 13.24 LXX). In the Gospel of Luke, εὐλογέω can refer to human praise of God (Lk. 1.64; 2.28; 24.53) or to an invocation of divine blessing on a human being sometimes as a recognition that a particular person is divinely favoured or blessed (for example, Lk. 1.42; 2.34; 6.28; 13.35; 19.38; 24.50-51; see BAGD, 322). But in the feeding narrative of Lk. 9.10-17, the object of blessing is neither human nor divine; the Lukan Jesus invokes a blessing on bread and fish (9.16). The direct blessing of bread and fish suggests not only a calling down of divine blessing on these foods, offered in response to the need of the crowd for sustenance (9.12-13), but also a recognition that such foods are already divinely favoured or blessed. Moreover, it is not these foods uniquely that are recognized as blessed, but bread (and fish as well in this instance) is blessed inasmuch as it stands for food in general.

Somewhere in the practice of the early church, the verb εὐλογέω, 'to bless', becomes εὐχαριστέω, 'to give thanks', which gives us the word 'Eucharist'.[10] The food necessary to sustain life, declared blessed (Lk. 9.16; 24.30), is subject of thanksgiving. For Paul, blessing and giving thanks were synonymous (1 Cor. 14.16). In relation to Eucharist, blessing suggests a focus on the mediated earthly matter of food and drink as of worth in itself, an Earth gift that mediates a divine gift. Giving thanks suggests a

9. Fitzmyer, *Gospel according to Luke I–IX*, pp. 767-68.

10. Fitzmyer, *Gospel according to Luke I–IX*, pp. 767-68. Unlike the verb εὐλογέω, εὐχαριστέω occurs infrequently in the Septuagint, being found only six times, and those instances are outside what became the canon of the Hebrew Bible (Jdt. 8.25; 2 Macc. 1.11; 12.31; *3 Macc*. 7.16; *Odes* 14.8; Wis. 18.2).

recognition that what is received from the other, from many others, in eating and drinking carries with it a blessing (the blessing of sustenance) that calls forth a response in the recipient (namely gratitude).[11] In Lukan and early Christian eucharistic traditions more generally, there is ground for reading a two-way movement in relation to matter: an acknowledgment of the blessedness of matter and a call to respond to the blessing matter bestows.

In the feeding stories this material blessing is imaged by the abundance of food. This abundance echoes a scriptural tradition of divine blessing of people and land, accompanying a promise of fertility, prosperity and well-being (Deut. 7.12-14; 16.15; 28.3-6). Because of the close verbal links between the feeding and the Last Supper narratives, this abundance is mapped on to Eucharist.[12] While the feeding narratives begin with scarcity, the paradigm shifts to abundance. In the Last Supper narratives, this abundance is bound up with Jesus' impending death. Seen in the light of the blessedness of matter and the call to respond to the blessing matter bestows, Jesus' kenotic self-giving in death is embedded in a eucharistic materiality.[13] In the next two sections, I explore two aspects of a eucharistic materiality important for a consideration of Earth as eucharistic: first, a communion paradigm; and second, the interplay of hospitality and sacrifice. Both aspects can inform an understanding of the relationship between matter and writing in the production and interpretation of biblical texts.

### *A Eucharistic Materiality: A Communion Paradigm*

Teilhard de Chardin's essay 'The Mass on the World' begins:

> Since once again, Lord—though this time not in the forests of the Aisne but in the steppes of Asia—I have neither bread, nor wine, nor altar, I will raise myself beyond these symbols, up to the pure majesty of the real

11. See also Neil Darragh, *At Home in the Earth: Seeking an Earth-Centred Spirituality* (Ponsonby, Auckland: Accent Publications, 2000), p. 163, and discussion in Elvey, *Ecological Feminist Reading*, pp. 281-87.

12. A third-century image in the catacombs of Saint Calixtus depicts this connection with the baskets and fish around the supper table. See *Eucharistic Banquet* (beginning of the third century); Catacombs of Saint Calixtus, Cubiculum of the Sacraments. http://www.aug.edu/augusta/iconography/newStuffForXnCours/catacumbasCristianas/banqueteEucaristico.html.

13. David Toolan (*At Home in the Cosmos* [Maryknoll, NY: Orbis Books, 2003], p. 210, quoted in Mary Grey, 'Cosmic Communion: A Contemporary Reflection on the Eucharistic Vision of Teilhard de Chardin', *Ecotheology* 10.2 [2005], p. 175) imaginatively describes this material embedding of Eucharist in its cosmic context.

> itself; I, your priest, will make the whole earth my altar and on it will offer you all the labours and sufferings of the world.[14]

Teilhard understands Eucharist on a cosmic scale, with Earth not only as the table at which the celebrant gathers other-than-human and human elements, those present in the steppes of Asia that morning and those present to his imagination, but also as itself bread and wine for consecration.[15] Denis Edwards comments that for Teilhard, 'The unique presence of Christ in the Eucharist is extended in the divinizing presence of Christ at work in the whole of creation. The Eucharist is an effective prayer for the transformation of the universe in Christ.'[16] Turning to the theology of John Zizioulas, Edwards writes, 'In the Eucharist, creation is lifted up to God in offering and thanksgiving. ... this "lifting up" ... involves all human interactions with the rest of creation.'[17] In both cases, creation 'lifted up' remains acted on, rather than active, except through the 'God-given' agency of human creatures. Rosemary Radford Ruether argues, 'The blessing and sharing of eucharistic bread and wine should be reembedded in its creational context.'[18] In the light of the Lukan affirmation of matter as blessed, can we re-embed Eucharist in its more-than-human context in such a way that a more-than-human community of agency is affirmed? The understanding of a eucharistic community of material agency may then offer a basis for conceiving the community of material agency that is a text.

The Earth Bible project sets out six ecojustice principles, of which the principle of interconnectedness reads: 'Earth is a community of interconnected living things that are mutually dependent on each other for life and survival.'[19] Beatrice Bruteau describes this interconnectedness and mutual

14. Pierre Teilhard de Chardin, 'The Mass on the World', in *Hymn of the Universe* (trans. Gerald Vann; London: Collins, 1965), p. 19.

15. While it is not a great extrapolation to read in Teilhard's 'Mass on the World' a sense of earthly interconnectedness and interdependence that for him were directed toward an immense evolutionary leap in the cosmic Christ, two threads remain in tension for ecological and feminist readings. On the one hand, 'The Mass on the World' celebrates matter as sacred in a way that is consonant not only with a Christian understanding of sacraments and sacrality but also with much contemporary deep ecological philosophy and spirituality. On the other hand, the whole idea of a mass on the world and the voice in which it is expressed retain strong elements of anthropocentric (and hierarchical) presumption.

16. Denis Edwards, 'Celebrating Eucharist in a Time of Global Climate Change', *Pacifica* 19 (2006), pp. 1-15 (7).

17. Edwards, 'Celebrating Eucharist', p. 9.

18. Rosemary Radford Ruether, 'Ecological Theology: Roots in Tradition Liturgical and Ethical Practice for Today', *Dialog: A Journal of Theology* 42 (2003), pp. 226-34 (33).

19. Habel (ed.), *Readings from the Perspective of Earth*, p. 24.

dependence as eucharistic: 'I want to perceive Earth as a Eucharistic Planet, a Good Gift planet, which is structured as mutual feeding, as intimate self-sharing.'[20] She argues further that a 'sense of the Eucharistic Planet, of the Real Presence of the Divine in the world, is something we need now for the protection of the planet'.[21] A description of Earth as a 'Good Gift planet' may seem overly romantic against the background of extreme weather events such as tsunamis, floods and bushfires. Nevertheless, a focus on the interdependence of Earth—characterized by 'mutual feeding' and 'intimate self-sharing'—as itself sacramental and the basis for the celebration of the sacrament of Eucharist offers participants a vantage from which to re-view their interactions in the Earth community. For Bruteau, such a revision would entail replacing the 'domination paradigm'—of which ecological theologians such as Ruether and philosophers such as Val Plumwood are justly critical—with the 'communion paradigm'.[22]

In the Gospel feeding narratives, Last Supper and Emmaus accounts, the movement between blessing and giving thanks allows for an understanding of matter as blessed, as a material basis for a communion paradigm. This is not to say that Luke or the other evangelists intended a theology of sacrament as it has developed in various Christian traditions over two millennia. Rather, the gospel echoes of the early Christian practice of 'the breaking of bread' present what Jane Bennett calls 'edible matter' as integral to the actions of blessing and thanksgiving.[23] In this respect, 'the breaking of bread' in the context of a meal, which has come to be understood as eucharistic, occurs within a community of more-than-human (including human and divine) agency. More particularly, 'edible matter' acts on, modifying, 'the human matter with which it comes into contact' through ingestion.[24]

An interplay of material capacities contributing to a community of more-than-human agency makes possible the ritual breaking of bread. These material capacities include the capacity of grain to be ground into flour, to be constituted with water, oil, salt and yeast into dough that can be baked as bread; the potentiality of fire; the texture of bread that allows it to be torn. They also encompass the capacities of the human eye and hand to measure, mould, and tear. They include also the way bread tastes in the mouth and acts in the gut; its capacity to be transformed by flesh and to transform flesh

20. Beatrice Bruteau, 'Eucharistic Ecology and Ecological Spirituality', *Cross Currents* 40.4 (1990/1991), pp. 499-514; http://search.epnet.com/login.aspx?direct=true&db=rlh&an=9611263218.

21. Bruteau, 'Eucharistic Ecology'.

22. Bruteau, 'Eucharistic Ecology'; Ruether, *Gaia and God*, pp. 173-201; Plumwood, *Feminism and the Mastery of Nature*, pp. 41-68.

23. Bennett, *Vibrant Matter*, p. 39.

24. Bennett, *Vibrant Matter*, p. 44.

through reactions in the digestive tract; the ability for food to change a human's mood. These aspects of the material agency of bread and humans who make, break and eat it act together with humans who gather intentionally in a material place to share food and discourse in the hospitality of a meal.

Anne Primavesi offers a helpful description of the way we need to account for this community of agency in our thinking about the 'breaking of bread':

> I would suggest that when we reflect on the image of Jesus inviting us to remember him by taking bread and wine, blessing and sharing it, saying: 'This is my body; this is my blood', we look at that image in present time and understand the bread and wine as his body and blood because they sustained his life: just as food and drink now sustain ours. Without them, he would have had no body. Without them, we would not be here to remember his body in the present. The continuity between his life and mine lies ultimately in our shared dependence on the gifts given us by the land. I, like him, depend on earth and its photosynthesizing labours; on water and its cleansing power; on air and the chemicals it transpires; and above all, on the heat of the sun fuelling Gaian biogeochemical cycles. His incarnation, like mine, depended on all of these.[25]

Like Bruteau, Primavesi appeals to the notion of Earth's gifts. She understands the givenness of Earth, 'built up over deep time' and supporting 'countless' more-than-human others, as Earth's gift, which we so often misunderstand.[26] We forget both the conditions for Earth's ongoing sustenance of human life and the many other-than-human lives Earth sustains. Just as parenting labour, especially maternal labour, is often denied and omitted from our economic accounting, particularly in Western societies, the labour of Earth is elided.[27] Redressing this, Primavesi describes Earth's 'photosynthesizing labours' in the context of Eucharist. The words prayed during the celebration of Eucharist to describe the bread and wine—'fruit of the earth and work of human hands'—accord the labour to humans, as if humans are separate from Earth for which all is an easy coming to fruit. From an ecological perspective, bread and wine are the fruit of both other-than-human and human labour. While Eucharist does not involve the consumption of other animals, the celebration of Eucharist relies on at least three more-than-human factors. They are (i) sun's labour, the labour of the whole cycle

25. Anne Primavesi, *Sacred Gaia: Holistic Theology and Earth System Science* (London: Routledge, 2000), p. 174.

26. Anne Primavesi, *Gaia's Gift: Earth, Ourselves and God after Copernicus* (London: Routledge, 2003), pp. 134-35.

27. See, for example, Ariel Salleh on the 'holding labour' of women and Earth, in Ariel Salleh, *Ecofeminism as Politics: Nature, Marx and the Postmodern* (London: Zed Books, 1997), p. 153.

of transpiration, plants' labour, soils' labour and human labour in the growing of grain and grape and then in their mediation into bread and wine; (ii) the provision of an Earth space for gathering; (iii) human bodies and voices, air and breath. Moreover, humans and other Earth beings are interconnected not only in this shared labour but also by the very act of consumption.

The necessity of consumption to our lives, albeit dangerously exaggerated in global consumerist economics, implies that our being is never solely singular but, to borrow a term from Jean Luc Nancy, 'singular plural'.[28] As Angel F. Méndez Montoya argues, food 'displays a complex interrelation between self and other; object and subject; appetite and digestion; aesthetics, ethics, and politics; nature and culture; and creation and divinity'.[29] The interrelatedness characteristic of food implies, as Nancy does in a different context, that being is always co-being, co-existence, being-with-, being-toward-, being-for-the other. Pregnant and nursing women know this in their bodies in a particular way. In a eucharistic context, we can understand this being-for-the-other as a constitutive hospitality.

The Earth community is shaped by hospitality, but being-for-the-other is not without its cost. The other side of hospitality is *sacrifice*. In our eating, drinking, clothing and sheltering ourselves, and in our being food for mosquitoes, lice, and sometimes crocodiles or sharks, we participate in this earthly being-for-the-other that links life and death. For the late Val Plumwood, herself a one-time survivor of a crocodile attack, the link between food and death needs to be recalled so that we can re-imagine 'ourselves ecologically, as members of a larger earth community of radical equality, mutual nurturance and support'.[30] By understanding the interdependence of the Earth community, especially as it arrives in the food–death nexus, as a mode of being-for-the-other, we can both understand Eucharist as a particular expression of the hospitality and sacrifice that underlie that earthy interdependence and consider an earthy materiality as eucharistic.

### *A Eucharistic Materiality: Hospitality and Sacrifice*

The notion of an earthy material as eucharistic relies on an understanding that the interconnectedness and interdependence of the Earth community can be described as in the mode of being-for-the-other. This being-for-the-other is complex in that the necessity of consumption for the survival and flourishing of particular individuals, communities, societies and species

28. Nancy, *Being Singular Plural*.

29. Angel F. Méndez Montoya, *The Theology of Food: Eating and the Eucharist* (Malden, MA: Wiley–Blackwell, 2009), p. ix.

30. Val Plumwood, 'Tasteless: Towards a Food-Based Approach to Death', *PAN: Philosophy, Activism, Nature* 5 (2008), pp. 63-68 (64).

sets up relations of both cooperation and conflict between individuals and groups. Moreover, in contemporary consumer societies, the necessity to consume to survive and flourish has been dangerously exaggerated. Consumption, the eating up of the other, is at issue in all areas of human activity, including the production and reproduction of texts. If matter as part of communities of material agency has a eucharistic character, what might this mean for our understanding of the materiality of texts?

As noted above, when we offer hospitality, when we share meals, there is always a hidden reliance on Earth others.[31] In several ways, Eucharist is a communion without communion. As Anne-Claire Mulder comments, Eucharist is not only a taking part in the body of Christ, but as ritual it constructs 'a' local body of Christ in a way that is both inclusive and exclusive of women.[32] 'They are present at the scene, while the scene re-enacts their exclusion from the scene.'[33] This experience of being simultaneously absent and present makes Eucharist a communion without communion for many women, but not only for women. The eucharistic vision of communion is called into question by human poverty. Pedro Arrupe's much quoted comment—'If there is hunger anywhere in the world then our celebration of Eucharist is somehow incomplete in the world'[34]—reflects the terrible paradox that while the celebration of the eucharistic meal occurs others are without food. William Blake's 1794 poem 'Holy Thursday [II.]' represents the experience of poverty as an 'eternal winter', an image of a more-than-human Earth community out of climatic balance.[35] Not only is winter a time when poverty is felt with particular keenness, but poverty becomes its own winter, a winter that encompasses all who live in 'a land of poverty' not only those who hunger.

In our contemporary world, as Anne Primavesi explains:

> for the hungry, food forces itself on their attention as an insistent symbol of life sustained or destroyed. But our consumer-glutted society keeps us safely at one remove from hunger's savage insistence. Hunger is a forgot-

31. See especially 'Women, the Sacred, Money', in Irigaray, *Sexes and Genealogies*, pp. 73-88. Cf. Dennis King Keenan, 'Irigaray and the Sacrifice of the Sacrifice of Woman', *Hypatia* 19.4 (2004), pp. 167-83. For Carol Adams and Marjorie Procter-Smith, for example, the sacrificial aspect of Eucharist is of particular concern in relation to our treatment of other animals (Adams and Procter-Smith, 'Taking Life', p. 306). Cf. Berkman, 'Consumption of Animals', p. 203.

32. Anne-Claire Mulder, *Divine Flesh, Embodied Word: Incarnation as a Hermeneutical Key to a Feminist Theologian's Reading of Luce Irigaray's Work* (Amsterdam: Amsterdam University Press, 2006), p. 66.

33. Mulder, *Divine Flesh*, p. 66.

34. From his speech given at the Eucharistic Congress, Philadelphia, 1976.

35. William Blake, 'Holy Thursday (II)', in *The Norton Anthology of Poetry* (ed. Alexander W. Allison *et al.*; New York: W.W. Norton, 3rd edn, 1983), p. 504.

> ten feeling. Here to eat well means to eat less. And to live well no longer implies sharing food or hospitality with others, since it is assumed they can provide for themselves or, if not, that there are organizations, state-funded or otherwise, who will look after them.
>
> This has led to a loss of the essential correspondence between the ritual meal of bread and wine and the role played by food, and by its sharing, in our lives.[36]

The ability to share, or refuse to share food, is a theological issue, but our distortion of the necessity of consumption undoes the meaning of eucharistic hospitality.[37] If, for Luke, the βασιλεία of God is imaged by sharing a meal, what might this mean for any process of consumption—for example, of food or texts—that can be described as a community of material agency and conceived as eucharistic?

The parable of the great dinner in Lk. 14.15-24 follows Jesus' challenge to his dinner companions to invite those who cannot repay their hospitality, that is, to leave open the circle of exchange to a kind of unconditional hospitality: 'When you give a banquet, invite the poor, the crippled, the lame, and the blind' (14.13).[38] While the gift of hospitality will not be returned in kind, it returns as eschatological blessing (14.14). Hearing this, one of Jesus' dinner companions says, 'Blessed is anyone who will eat bread in the βασιλεία of God' (14.15). As in 11.27-28, a character's exclamation of blessing prompts Jesus to teach and correct, or deepen, the speaker's point of view. In this case, the teaching is in the form of a parable that has a parallel in Mt. 22.1-14. Where Matthew's Jesus speaks of a marriage feast, Luke's Jesus speaks of a banquet. Although both passages deal with issues of exclusion and inclusion in the eschatological banquet, there are several differences of detail, significantly Luke's sustained metaphor of participating in the meal compared with Matthew's focus on the acts of judgment of the host.

For Luke the hospitality associated with the eschatological feast in Lk. 14.15-24 is fourfold. First, the hospitality of God must be received. Non-reception implies judgment; in failing to receive and respond to the divine invitation one is judged by one's actions (14.17-20). Second, the hospitality of God is inclusive of those who are on the margins, 'the poor, maimed, blind and lame' (14.21; see also 14.13; 15.1-2). Third, the hospitality is characterized by largesse; when those who have been invited from the streets attend, there is room for more (14.22). Fourth, this hospitality entails

36. Primavesi, *Gaia's Gift*, p. 134.

37. Méndez Montoya, *Theology of Food*, pp. 40-41.

38. There is a resonance here with the discussion of hospitality (as unconditional) and the gift as the impossible in Derrida and Dufourmantelle, *Of Hospitality*.

a kind of compulsion, or violence; it is imperative that the banquet be fully attended (14.23; cf. 16.16).

Underlying the image of the hospitality of the βασιλεία meal is a first-century CE Mediterranean concept of balanced reciprocity, in which hospitality needs to be received and returned.[39] The host in the parable seems to unsettle the expectation of the latter while affirming the necessity for the former. The parable ends with the host declaring, 'None of those who were invited will taste my dinner' (14.24). The judgment they have brought on themselves by failing to receive the hospitality offered is precisely the consequence of their refusal, that is, they will not taste the dinner. But the tenor of the declaration, which occurs in the last place of the story, suggests that there is more to this dinner, and their refusal of it, than they suspected. They have not simply offered a social slight to the host. They have missed what was being offered, the inclusiveness and largesse of the βασιλεία meal, which reveals an economy of divine hospitality. This hospitality is characterized not by scarcity or the particularity of relationship to property and kin but by an abundance, such that when one shares in it, one will not want food, clothing, shelter or kin (18.29-30). To what extent is this kind of abundance counter to the false abundance of contemporary consumerist economies?

When we come in the Gospel of Luke to the Last Supper account, we read:

> When the hour came, he took his place at the table, and the apostles with him. He said to them, 'I have eagerly desired to eat this Passover with you before I suffer; for I tell you, I will not eat it until it is fulfilled in the βασιλεία of God.' Then he took a cup, and after giving thanks he said, 'Take this and divide it among yourselves; for I tell you that from now on I will not drink of the fruit of the vine until the βασιλεία of God comes.' Then he took a loaf of bread, and when he had given thanks, he broke it and gave it to them, saying, 'This is my body, which is given for you. Do this in remembrance of me.' And he did the same with the cup after supper, saying, 'This cup that is poured out for you is the new covenant in my blood. But see, the one who betrays me is with me, and his hand is on the table. For the Human One is going as it has been determined, but woe to that one by whom he is betrayed!' (Lk. 22.14-22 NRSV modified).

Jesus' farewell meal occurs in the context of his impending suffering (22.15) and betrayal (22.21), as it has been determined (22.22), that is, as part of a divine purpose that encompasses his passion, death and resurrection (9.22; 17.25; 22.36-37; 24.5-7, 25-26). The divine necessity of the passion, death and resurrection echoes in the necessity to slaughter the lamb for the Passo-

39. Halvor Moxnes, 'The Social Context of Luke's Community', *Int* 48 (1994), pp. 379-89.

ver feast (22.7). As noted in Chapter 4, there is a metonymy between the lamb and Jesus in this farewell meal set during Passover. The sacrifice of the other animal, the lamb, resonates in the impending death of the Lukan Jesus, so that Jesus' self-giving in death becomes a kind of sacrifice.

The farewell meal appears to displace the sacrifice of the lamb with the gift of the bread and wine. But the Lukan divine necessity that informs the self-gift of Jesus relies on several sacrifices. They are the sacrifice of the other animal, the lamb, for the feast of Passover; the sacrifice of Jesus to the oppressive might of the Roman occupiers (even as Luke downplays their culpability for Jesus' execution); and the sacrifice of the animal to a symbolic order that links animal bodies, food and Eucharist with sacrifice.[40] The kenotic self-gift of the Lukan Jesus that accompanies, as a necessity, the hospitality of the eucharistic meal is part of a community of material agency where being-for-the-other involves a sacrificial nexus that is neither wholly intentional nor just. The community of material agency that makes possible the hospitality of a meal and gives shape to the eucharistic materiality of Earth is already infused with the sacrifice of the other, not only through self-giving but also through networks of oppressive taking.

The Lukan Jesus speaks of an abstinence that precedes the expected abundance of the βασιλεία meal (22.16). This abstinence becomes part of the kenosis of his eucharistic self-giving. Applied to a theorizing of an earthy community of material agency occurring in practices of consumption, that circle around a nexus of self-giving and oppressive taking, this abstinence offers a particular tone to the kenotic hospitality of a eucharistic materiality and the ethics it calls forth from human agents.

### *Edible Matter: Consumption and Being Consumed*

In the eucharistic framework of our need to eat, poverty, hunger and malnutrition are in stark contrast to consumerism and over-consumption. As noted in Chapter 4, William Cavanaugh argues that in contemporary consumerist societies, consumption entails a kind of detachment from production, producers, and from products.[41] Products have become 'mute as to their origins'; moreover, our relationships with things 'are not made to last'.[42] Consumption is linked to pleasure 'not so much in the possession of things as in their pursuit'.[43] For Cavanaugh, 'Consumerism is an important subject for theology because it is a spiritual disposition, a way of looking at the world

40. Adams and Procter-Smith, 'Taking Life', p. 306.
41. Cavanaugh, *Being Consumed*, pp. 37-47.
42. Cavanaugh, *Being Consumed*, pp. 45-46.
43. Cavanaugh, *Being Consumed*, p. 47.

around us that is deeply formative'.[44] A distorted relation to consumption disconnects consumers from knowledge of the interdependent relationships of production in which our practices of consumption are embedded. We cannot escape this interconnectedness, but we displace the effects of our consumptive and over-consumptive habits when we systematically detach ourselves from the things we use, their producers and their manner and sites of production.

Nevertheless we need to consume to live. For Cavanaugh, we need to consider then 'what kinds of practices of consumption are conducive to an abundant life for all'.[45] When Jesus 'offers his body and blood to be consumed', Eucharist brings consumption into the sphere of the sacred and the unity of the body of Christ, engaging us in a different relationship to consumption.[46] While Eucharist could itself become a kind of product, assimilated 'into a consumerist ... spirituality', Cavanaugh argues that the 'practice of the Eucharist is resistant to such appropriation ... because the consumer of the Eucharist is taken up into a larger body, the body of Christ'.[47] Through consuming the Eucharist we are consumed into the body of Christ. We become food for others. In the Second Testament accounts of the Last Supper, Jesus offers himself as food (Mt. 26.26; Mk 14.22; Lk. 22.19; 1 Cor. 11.24) and shifts the paradigm of service by presenting himself as both host and slave (Lk. 22.27; Jn 13.1-11). Where otherwise hospitality might rely on the unseen labour of other humans and the wider Earth community, Jesus brings this labour of sustenance and service to the fore by taking it on himself. Further, in the Acts of the Apostles, Luke paints a picture of an ideal community in which eucharistic hospitality overflows into every-day generosity so that none is in need (Acts 2.44-47; see also Prov. 22.9). This eucharistic relation to consumption echoes, but also goes beyond, the embeddedness of all creatures in an interdependent Earth community where being is being-for-the-other.

Therefore, ecological-justice concerns such as the impact of food production on a wider Earth community, intensive farming practices, battery chickens, feed lots, crops and agribusiness, genetic modification, land use and water use impact on our celebration of Eucharist. They both point to a brokenness at the heart of our communion and call us to engaged communion with Earth others.[48] This is not a new communion, but a renewed recognition of, and openness to, our participation in the interconnectedness of Earth being. Part of this recognition entails the acknowledgment that the

44. Cavanaugh, *Being Consumed*, p. 35.
45. Cavanaugh, *Being Consumed*, p. 53.
46. Cavanaugh, *Being Consumed*, p. 54.
47. Cavanaugh, *Being Consumed*, p. 54.
48. Grey, 'Cosmic Communion', pp. 177-78.

brokenness of our relationships to the things we consume and the conditions of their production has become a brokenness in ourselves. As Neil Darragh argues, to use things 'in an exploitative way that does not recognise [their] continuing God-immanence is to violate both the inner being of the resource and the inner being of the user, for these are ultimately the same'.[49] Communion in this sense is inescapable.

In the Second Testament, two traditions of eucharistic language that mutually interpret each other, namely blessing and giving thanks, occur beside two traditions of mutually interpreting relationships to food, namely stories of abundance and sociality. As noted above, abundance figures in the feeding narratives of the Gospels. The abundance of the Eucharist is inseparable from Jesus' self-giving, through which, by participating in Eucharist, 'we become one with others and share their fate' (see 1 Cor. 10.16).[50] Such communion (which involves more-than-human others) is a vocation to communal sharing.[51] In the terms of the previous chapter, this vocation to communion is the visible voice of the Eucharist, a calling that arrives from the material blessing in which Eucharist subsists and which Eucharist brings into focus.

In Luke's Gospel, the abundance of the feeding narratives and the sociality of the banquet come together as an image of the βασιλεία of God. The institution of the Eucharist becomes a moment of this βασιλεία, characterized by hospitality and sacrifice, that is being-for-the-other, which Mark Brett describes as 'a kenotic hospitality'.[52] This being-for-the-other describes materiality as eucharistic, as already interconnected and interagential, in ways that have implications for our thinking of the community of agency that is a text, that is a writing in a material artefact. The sense of taste, the tongue and mouth, and the processes of digestion connect eating and speaking, perception and pleasure, and offer a sensual metaphor for corporeal engagement with the material artefact in an act of consumption.

When Ezekiel swallows the scroll (Ezek. 2.8–3.3), he is commissioned to speak (3.4). His speech will be interrupted by, and in turn interrupt, his muteness (3.26-27). Ellen Davis situates the book of Ezekiel at a crossing between prophecy as oral performance translated into writing and writing as a prophetic performance that influences succeeding oral traditions.[53] At

49. Darragh, *At Home in the Earth*, p. 154.

50. Cavanaugh, *Being Consumed*, pp. 94-5.

51. Méndez Montoya, *Theology of Food*, pp. 155-56.

52. Brett, *Decolonizing God*, p. 196. If we experience ourselves as distant from the suffering of Earth others, Brett argues, we need to overcome that distance 'through a "Eucharistic" catholicity that knits together the pain of the world'.

53. Ellen F. Davis, *Swallowing the Scroll: Textuality and the Dynamics of Discourse in Ezekiel's Prophecy* (Sheffield: Almond Press, 1989), pp. 30-39, 126.

this intersection of orality and writing, speech and text, the symbolic eating of the scroll suggests a complex relation between writing as oral communication, a visible voice, and the material artefact as a consumable thing. For Ezekiel the consumption of the material text is an ingestion and digestion of the divine word that makes possible his prophetic proclamation of that word, and in turn gives rise to the material text in which the symbol of eating the scroll is written.

This consumption of the material text also speaks to the relationship between orality and writing that, as I argued in Chapter 2, is part of a material intertextuality. Moreover, the act of consuming the material text affirms that a writing is always part of a community of more-than-human agency in which a text already relies on the consumption and labour of many more-than-human (including human) others. Several issues come together in my understanding of a text as a writing in a material artefact that consumes and is consumed within a more-than-human Earth community that has the contours of a eucharistic materiality. They are the engagement of the body, through the senses, with written language; the hermeneutic relationship between matter and our experience of it; the difference that attention to the text as a writing in a material artefact may make to both our interpretations of writings and our production and reproduction of texts.

For Michel Serres, there is a risk that opening of the mouth to language displaces the opening of the body to sense, of which taste has a particular resonance because of its primary aspect of heightened experience of the other and its overflow into speech.[54] The senses open the body to the other in a way that welcomes the prior givenness of the other and that language cannot contain. Nevertheless, in the dual aspect of the mouth that eats and speaks, a focus on the sense of taste also suggests the possibility of affirming not only the corporeal and dynamic relationship between self and other that is gustation, but also the materiality of language and texts. Underlying the consumption of the other in writing and reading are relations of hospitality and sacrifice, a kenotic hospitality of matter to writing, and of matter and writing to interpretation.

54. Serres, *Five Senses*, pp. 153-54.

# CONCLUSION:
# TOWARD A MATERIAL INTERTEXTUALITY

My focus on the text as a material thing arises in the context of an ecological sensibility that understands humans as embodied and embedded in a more-than-human Earth community. In this Earth community, human activities such as the writing and reading of biblical texts always involve engagements with more-than-human (including human) others. A text comes into being through a community of more-than-human agency. Jane Bennett writes of her own writing as a community of agency:

> The sentences of this book also emerged from the confederate agency of many striving macro- and microactants: from 'my' memories, intentions, contentions, intestinal bacteria, eyeglasses, and blood sugar, as well as from the plastic computer keyboard, the bird song from the open window, or the air or particulates in the room, to name only a few of the participants. What is at work here on the page is an animal-vegetable-mineral-sonority cluster with a particular degree and duration of power.[1]

We can approach the community of material agency that produces a text as an absent presence, a trace having the character of the semiotic. Julia Kristeva's work on intertextuality offers a model for conceptualizing a material intertextuality that sounds in particular modes of reading with an ear to the materiality of the text. This book gives ear to the materiality of the Gospel of Luke through a reading that focuses on the five senses.

When we engage a text as a writing in a specific material artefact, we come as readers to taste with our eyes and flesh the visible voice of a verbal icon. The senses are engaged as mediators of both materiality and meaning. Michel Serres suggests that it is necessary to maintain 'a distance between the senses and language, for the sake of the safety and vitality of both'.[2] Further, he cautions against reducing the given (including the sensible) to language.[3] Moreover, as Rigby also argues, writing can approach only

1. Bennett, *Vibrant Matter*, p. 23.
2. Serres, *Five Senses*, p. 192.
3. Serres, *Five Senses*, p. 187.

more or less imperfectly the things to which it pertains.[4] Nonetheless, as Serres comments, 'The world—beautiful—offers the sensible graciously.'[5] The text as a sensible, a visible voice and verbal icon gives itself to sense. This gift of the text to sense invites a reading of the text through, or in conversation with, the senses.

As a basis for reading with the senses, a text can be understood as a saturated communion between a material artefact (including its underlying material embeddedness), a writing and a reader. This saturated communion opens itself to an interpretation that is attentive to the saturation of the senses by the sensible. In this communion of more-than-human agency, interpretation is a conversation between multiple meanings and layers of meaning (the experience of texts and the reading of writings) rather than a determination of the meaning of Luke's narrative.

Building on, but departing from, Marion's understanding of a saturated phenomenon, I understand the hermeneutic relationship between matter and our experience of it to be an exchange between human bodies open to the sensible and things that are open to being sensed. As saturated, material things, both act on their interpreter prior to, and in excess of, the interpreter's making meaning from them and give themselves (or are given) to interpretation and consumption in a kind of kenotic hospitality.

This kenotic hospitality of matter arises as a quality of a eucharistic materiality and opens things to their being transformed. The interplay between matter and human experience suggests a hermeneutic community of more-than-human agency. In the production, reproduction and interpretation of texts, this community of agency opens to practices of consumption that may be more or less respectful of the kenotic hospitality of their eucharistic materiality.

In the material artefact matter gives itself, or is given, to a writing. This givenness is a call to which the reader is invited to respond. The visible voice of the material artefact may speak back to the interpreter of a writing concerning the sacrifice of the other animal, plant, ecosystem or human embedded in the enterprise of production and reproduction of texts. This speaking back may call into question the whole academic enterprise of interpretation and reproduction of writings in which we are enmeshed. It may also call us to a renewed engagement with the sensual materiality of our lives. Here we can recognize a 'communal story' that is not only corporeal but also materially more than human.[6]

4. Rigby, 'Earth, World, Text', esp. p. 437; Rigby, 'Writing after Nature'.

5. Serres, *Five Senses*, p. 215.

6. Cf. Lisa Isherwood, 'Jesus Past the Posts: An Enquiry into Post-Metaphysical Christology', in *Post-Christian Feminisms: A Critical Approach* (ed. Lisa Isherwood and Kathleen McPhillips; Aldershot: Ashgate, 2008), pp. 201-210 (210).

We can 'taste and see' that the text, as a writing in a material artefact, always touches on the death of the other. While hiding this death as an absence akin to the absence of the material artefact in writing, as a verbal icon the biblical text opens to the materiality of a visible voice. The text calls to its readers, with the potential to unsettle and transform their subjectivities. Based in the readers' prior attentiveness to the materiality of the text, this unsettling is a further impetus to engage responsively in the kenotic hospitality of Earth.

# Bibliography


Abram, David, *The Spell of the Sensuous* (New York: Vintage Books, 1997).

Adams, Carol J., and Marjorie Procter-Smith, 'Taking Life or "Taking on Life"?', in *Ecofeminism and the Sacred* (ed. Carol J. Adams; New York: Continuum, 1994), pp. 295-310.

Aichele, George, 'Electronic Culture and the Future of the Canon of Scripture or: The Hyperreal Bible', in *Redirected Travel: Alternative Journeys and Places in Biblical Studies* (ed. Roland Boer and Edgar W. Conrad; Journal for the Study of the Old Testament Supplement Series, 382; London: T. & T. Clark International, 2003), pp. 8-23.

—'Reading beyond Meaning', *Postmodern Culture* 3.3 (1993), http://muse.jhu.edu/.

—*Sign, Text, Scripture: Semiotics and the Bible* (Sheffield: Sheffield Academic Press, 1997).

Aichele, George, and Bible and Culture Collective, *The Postmodern Bible* (New Haven: Yale University Press, 1995).

Alexander, Loveday C.A., 'What If Luke Had Never Met Theophilus?', *Biblical Interpretation* 8 (2000), pp. 161-70.

Allen, Graham, *Intertextuality* (London: Routledge, 2000).

Andrejev, Vladislav, 'Art and Religion: Creativity and the Meaning of "Image" from the Perspective of the Orthodox Icon,' *Theology Today* 61 (2004), pp. 53-66.

Aristotle, *De anima (On the Soul)* (trans. Hugh Lawson-Tancred; London: Penguin Books, 1986).

—*On the Soul (De anima) with Commentaries and Glossary* (trans. Hippocrates G. Apostle; Grinnell, IA: Peripatetic Press, 1981).

Athenaeus, *Deipnosophistae*; *The Deipnosophists or Banquet of the Learned* (trans. C. D. Jonge; London: Henry G. Bohn, 1854; http://digicoll.library.wisc.edu/Literature/)

Austin-Broos, Diane J., '"Two Laws" Ontologies, Histories: Ways of Being Aranda (Aboriginal People) Today', *Australian Journal of Anthropology* 7 (1996), pp. 1-20.

Ayers, David, 'Materialism and the Book', *Poetics Today* 24 (2003), pp. 759-80.

Bakhtin, M.M., *The Dialogic Imagination: Four Essays* (trans. Caryl Emerson and Michael Holquist; Austin: University of Texas Press, 1981).

Balentine, S., '"He Unrolled the Scroll ... And He Rolled Up the Scroll and Gave It Back"', *Cross Currents* 59.2 (2009), pp. 154-75.

Barrett, C.K., *The Second Epistle to the Corinthians* (Black's New Testament Commentaries; London: A. & C. Black, 1973).

Bauer, Walter, *A Greek–English Lexicon of the New Testament and Other Early Christian Literature* (trans., revised and augmented by William F. Arndt, F. Wilbur Gingrich and Frederick W. Danker; Chicago: University of Chicago Press, 2nd edn, 1979).

Beavis, Mary Ann, 'Parable and Fable', *Catholic Biblical Quarterly* 52 (1990), pp. 473-98.

Beckett, Jeremy, 'Aboriginal Histories, Aboriginal Myths: An Introduction', *Oceania* 65.2 (1994), pp. 97-115.

Bennett, Jane, 'The Force of Things: Steps toward an Ecology of Matter', *Political Theory* 32.3 (2004), pp. 347-72.

—*Vibrant Matter: A Political Ecology of Things* (Durham, NC: Duke University Press, 2010).

Benvenisti, Meron, *City of Stone: The Hidden History of Jerusalem* (trans. Maxine Kaufan Nunn; Berkeley: University of California Press, 1996).

Berkman, John, 'The Consumption of Animals and the Catholic Tradition', in *Food for Thought: The Debate over Eating Meat* (ed. Steve F. Sapontzis; New York: Prometheus Books, 2004), pp. 198-208

Bleich, David, 'The Materiality of Reading', *New Literary History* 37 (2006), pp. 607-29.

Blomberg, Craig L., 'Interpreting the Parables of Jesus: Where Are We and Where Do We Go from Here?', *Catholic Biblical Quarterly* 53 (1991), pp. 50-76.

Boer, Roland, *Last Stop before Antarctica: The Bible and Postcolonialism in Australia* (Sheffield: Sheffield Academic Press, 2001).

Borthwick, Fiona, 'Olfaction and Taste: Invasive Odours and Disappearing Objects', *Australian Journal of Anthropology* 11.2 (2000), pp. 127-40.

Boyarin, Daniel, 'A Question of Theory or Experimentality?', *Semeia* 86 (1999), pp. 223-25.

Brawley, Robert L., *Centering on God: Method and Message in Luke–Acts* (Louisville, KY: Westminster John Knox, 1990).

—*Text to Text Pours Forth Speech: Voices of Scripture in Luke–Acts* (Bloomington: Indiana University Press, 1995).

Brett, Mark G., *Decolonizing God: The Bible in the Tides of Empire* (Sheffield: Sheffield Phoenix Press, 2008).

—'Earthing the Human in Genesis 1–3', in *The Earth Story in Genesis* (ed. Norman C. Habel and Shirley Wurst; The Earth Bible, 2; Sheffield: Sheffield Academic Press, 2000), pp. 73-86.

Brewster, Anne, 'Oodgeroo: Orator, Poet, Storyteller', *Australian Literary Studies* 16.4 (1994), pp. 92-104.

Brock, Rita Nakashima, 'Dusting the Bible on the Floor: A Hermeneutics of Wisdom', in *Searching the Scriptures: A Feminist Introduction* (ed. Elisabeth Schüssler Fiorenza; North Blackburn, Victoria: Collins Dove, 1993), pp. 64-75.

Brown, Francis, S.R. Driver and Charles A. Briggs (eds.), *A Hebrew and English Lexicon of the Old Testament: with an Appendix Containing the Biblical Aramaic* (based on the Lexicon of William Genesius; trans. Edward Robinson; Oxford: Clarendon Press, 1951).

Brown, Raymond E., *The Birth of the Messiah: A Commentary on the Infancy Narratives in Matthew and Luke* (Garden City, NY: Doubleday, 1977).

Bruteau, Beatrice, 'Eucharistic Ecology and Ecological Spirituality', *Cross Currents* 40 (1990–1991), pp. 499-514.

Bultmann, Rudolf, *The Second Letter to the Corinthians* (trans. Roy A. Harrisville; Minneapolis: Augsburg Publishing House, 1985).

Burramurra, David, with Ian McIntosh, '*Motj* and the Nature of the Sacred', *Cultural Survival Quarterly* 26.2 (2002), http://www.culturalsurvival.org/ourpublications/csq/article/motj-and-nature-sacred.

Burton, Robert, *The Language of Smell* (London: Routledge & Kegan Paul, 1976).

Butler, Judith, *Bodies That Matter: On the Discursive Limits of 'Sex'* (London: Routledge, 1993).

Byrne, Brendan, *The Hospitality of God: A Reading of Luke's Gospel* (Strathfield, New South Wales: St Pauls, 2000).

Cadwallader, Alan H., *Beyond the Word of a Woman: Recovering the Bodies of the Syrophoenician Women* (Adelaide: AFT Press, 2008).

Caputo, John D., *The Prayers and Tears of Jacques Derrida: Religion without Religion* (Indiana Series in the Philosophy of Religion; Bloomington: Indiana University Press, 1997).

Cavanaugh, William T., *Being Consumed: Economics and Christian Desire* (Grand Rapids: Eerdmans, 2008).

Charlesworth, James H. (ed.), *The Old Testament Pseudepigrapha,* I. *Apocalyptic Literature and Testaments* (Garden City, NY: Doubleday, 1983).

—*The Old Testament Pseudepigrapha,* II. *Expansions of the 'Old Testament' and Legends, Wisdom and Philosophical Literature, Prayers, Psalms and Odes, Fragments of Lost Judeo-Hellenistic Works* (Garden City, NY: Doubleday, 1985).

Chrétien, Jean-Louis, *The Call and the Response* (trans. Anne A. Davenport; New York: Fordham University Press, 2004).

Chryssavgis, John, 'The World of the Icon and Creation: An Orthodox Perspective on Ecology and Pneumatology', in *Christianity and Ecology: Seeking the Well-Being of Earth and Humans* (ed. Dieter T. Hessel and Rosemary Radford Ruether; Religions of the World and Ecology; Cambridge, MA: Harvard University Press, 2000), pp. 83-96.

Classen, Constance, David Howes and Anthony Synnott, *Aroma: The Cultural History of Smell* (London: Routledge, 1994).

Code, Lorraine, *Ecological Thinking: The Politics of Epistemic Location* (Oxford: Oxford University Press, 2006).

Coleridge, Mark, *The Birth of the Lukan Narrative: Narrative as Christology in Luke 1–2* (Sheffield: Sheffield Academic Press, 1993).

—'In Defence of the Other: Deconstruction and the Bible. [Applied to Luke's Infancy Narrative]', *Pacifica* 5 (1992), pp. 123-44.

Collange, J.-F., *Enigmes de la deuxième épître de Paul aux Corinthiens: Etude exégétique de 2 Cor. 2:14–7:4* (Cambridge: Cambridge University Press, 1972).

Coloe, Mary L., 'Anointing the Temple of God: John 12:1-8', in *Transcending Boundaries: Contemporary Readings of the New Testament* (Festschrift Francis J. Moloney; ed. Mary L. Coloe and Rekha Chennatu; Biblioteca di scienze religiose; Rome: Libreria Ateneo Salesiano, 2005), pp. 105-18.

—'Welcome into the Household of God: The Foot Washing in John 13', *Catholic Biblical Quarterly* 66 (2004), pp. 400-415.

Cosgrove, Charles H., 'The Divine Δεῖ in Luke–Acts', *Novum Testamentum* 26 (1984), pp. 168-90.

Coward, Rosalind, and John Ellis, *Language and Materialism: Developments in Semiology and the Theory of the Subject* (London: Routledge and Kegan Paul, 1977).

Croft, Brenda L., *Michael Riley, Sights Unseen* (Canberra: National Gallery of Australia, 2006).

Curkpatrick, Stephen, 'Parable Metonymy and Luke's Kerygmatic Framing', *Journal for the Study of the New Testament* 25 (2003), pp. 289-307.

Darragh, Neil, *At Home in the Earth: Seeking an Earth-Centred Spirituality* (Ponsonby, Auckland: Accent Publications, 2000).

Davis, Ellen F., *Swallowing the Scroll: Textuality and the Dynamics of Discourse in Ezekiel's Prophecy* (Sheffield: Almond Press, 1989).

Deist, Ferdinand, *The Material Culture of the Bible: An Introduction* (ed. Robert P. Carroll; Sheffield: Sheffield Academic Press, 2000).

Derrida, Jacques, *Adieu to Emmanuel Levinas* (trans. Pascale-Anne Brault and Michael Naas; Meridian; Crossing Aesthetics; Stanford, CA: Stanford University Press, 1999).

—*The Gift of Death* (trans. David Wills; Religion and Postmodernism; Chicago: University of Chicago Press, 1995).

—*Given Time,* I. *Counterfeit Money* (trans. Peggy Kamuf; Chicago: University of Chicago Press, 1992).

—'*Le toucher*', *Paragraph* 16.2 (1993), pp. 122-57.

— *Le toucher, Jean-Luc Nancy* (Paris: Galilée, 2000).

—*On the Name* (trans. John P. Leavey, David Wood, Jr, and Ian McLeod; Stanford, CA: Stanford University Press, 1995).

—*On Touching—Jean-Luc Nancy* (trans. Christine Irizarry; Meridian; Crossing Aesthetics; Stanford, CA: Stanford University Press, 2005).

—*Paper Machine* (trans. Rachel Bowlby; Cultural Memory in the Present; Stanford, CA: Stanford University Press, 2005).

Derrida, Jacques, and Anne Dufourmantelle, *Of Hospitality* (trans. Rachel Bowlby; Cultural Memory in the Present; Stanford, CA: Stanford University Press, 2000).

Dillard, Annie, 'Teaching a Stone to Talk', in *This Sacred Earth: Religion, Nature, Environment* (ed. Roger S. Gottlieb; London: Routledge, 1996), pp. 32-36.

Diprose, Rosalyn, *The Bodies of Women: Ethics, Embodiment and Sexual Difference* (London: Routledge, 1994).

—'The Hand That Writes Community in Blood', *Cultural Studies Review* (*Affective Community*) 9 (2003), pp. 35-50.

Diringer, David, *The Book before Printing: Ancient, Medieval and Oriental* (New York: Dover Publications, 1982).

Dodd, C.H., *The Parables of the Kingdom* (New York: Charles Scribner's Sons, 1961).

Donne, John, 'Meditation XVII. *Nunc lento sonitu dicunt, morieris.*' *Devotions upon Emergent Occasions* (1624) http://www.luminarium.org/sevenlit/donne/meditation 17.php.

Dowling, Elizabeth V., *Taking away the Pound: Women, Theology and the Parable of the Pounds in the Gospel of Luke* (Library of New Testament Studies, 324; London: T. & T. Clark, 2007).

Du Bois, Page. *Sowing the Body: Psychoanalysis and Ancient Representations of Women* (Chicago: University of Chicago Press, 1991).

Edelstein, Marilyn, 'Metaphor, Meta-Narrative, and Mater-Narrative in Kristeva's "Stabat Mater"', in *Body/Text in Julia Kristeva: Religion, Women, and Psychoanalysis* (ed. David Crownfield; Albany: State University of New York Press, 1992), pp. 27-52.

Edwards, Denis, 'Celebrating Eucharist in a Time of Global Climate Change', *Pacifica* 19 (2006), pp. 1-15.

Elledge, C.D., *The Bible and the Dead Sea Scrolls* (SBL Archaeology and Biblical Studies, 14; Atlanta: Society of Biblical Literature, 2005).

Ellis, E. Earle, *The Gospel of Luke* (New Century Bible Commentary; Grand Rapids: Eerdmans, 1981).

Elvey, Anne, 'Ashes and Dust: On (Not) Speaking about God Ecologically', *Concilium* 3 (2009), pp. 33-42.

—'Can There Be a Forgiveness That Makes a Difference Ecologically? An Eco-Materialist Account of Forgiveness as Freedom (Ἄφεσις) in the Gospel of Luke', *Pacifica* 22 (2009), pp. 148-70.

—'Desiring the "Peaceable Kingdom"? Use/Respect Dualism, the Enigma of Predation and Human Relationships to Other Animals', *PAN: Philosophy, Activism, Nature* 3 (2005), pp. 31-40.

—'Earth as Intertext: " ... the stones would shout out ..." (Luke 19:40)', *Council of Societies for the Study of Religion Bulletin* 35.2 (April 2006), pp. 27-29.

—'Earthing the Text? On the Status of the Biblical Text in Ecological Perspective', *Australian Biblical Review* 52 (2004), pp. 64-79.

—*An Ecological Feminist Reading of the Gospel of Luke: A Gestational Paradigm* (Studies in Women and Religion, 45; Lewiston, NY: Edwin Mellen Press, 2005).

—'Legacies of Violence toward the Other: Toward a Consideration of the Outsider within the Lukan Narrative', *Colloquium: The Australian and New Zealand Theological Review* 34 (2002), pp. 21-34.

—'Material Elements: The Matter of Women, the Matter of Earth, the Matter of God', in *Post-Christian Feminisms: A Critical Approach* (ed. Lisa Isherwood and Kathleen McPhillips; Aldershot: Ashgate, 2008), pp. 53-69.

—'The Material Given: Bodies, Pregnant Bodies and Earth', *Australian Feminist Studies* 18.4 (2003), pp. 199-209.

—'To Bear the Other: Toward a Passionate Compassion (An Ecological Feminist Reading of Luke 10:25-37)', *Sea Changes: Journal of Women Scholars of Religion and Theology* 1 (2001), http://www.wsrt.com.au/seachanges/volume1/elveyframes.html.

—'Touching (on) Death: On "Being toward" the Other in the Gospel of Luke', *The Bible and Critical Theory* 2.2 (2006), pp. 15.1–15.17. DOI: 10.2104/bc060015

—'Women, Authority and the Bible: Ecological Feminist Considerations', *Interface* (forthcoming).

Felstiner, John, '"O Taste and See": The Question of Content in American Jewish Poetry', *Jewish Social Studies* 5.1/2 (1998–99), pp. 111-23.

Fincke, Jeannette C., 'The Nineveh Tablet Collection', http://www.fincke.uni-hd.de/nineveh/babylonian/letter.htm.

Fisher, David, 'Kristeva's Chora and the Subject of Postmodern Ethics', in *Body/Text in Julia Kristeva: Religion, Women, and Psychoanalysis* (ed. David Crownfield; Albany: State University of New York Press, 1992), pp. 91-106.

Fitzmyer, Joseph A., *The Gospel according to Luke I–IX: Introduction, Translation, and Notes* (Anchor Bible; New York: Doubleday, 1981).

—*The Gospel according to Luke X–XXIV: Introduction, Translation, and Notes* (Anchor Bible; New York: Doubleday, 1985).

Frymer-Kensky, Tikva, *In the Wake of the Goddesses: Women, Culture and the Biblical Transformation of Pagan Myth* (New York: Free Press, 1992).

Gadamer, Hans-Georg, *Truth and Method* (trans. Joel Weinsheimer and Donald G. Marshall; London: Continuum, 2nd rev. edn, 2004).

Gamble, Harry Y., 'Bible and Book', in *In the Beginning: Bibles before the Year 1000* (ed. Michelle Brown; Washington, DC: Freer Gallery of Art and Arthur M. Sackler Gallery Smithsonian Institution, 2006), pp. 15-35.

Gatta, John, 'The Transfiguration of Christ and Cosmos: A Focal Point of Literary Imagination', *Sewanee Theological Review* 49 (2006), pp. 484-506.

Gilbert, Gary, 'Luke–Acts and the Negotiation of Authority and Identity in the Roman World', in *The Multivalence of Biblical Texts and Theological Meanings* (ed. Christine Helmer, Charlene T. Higbe and Brenna Moore; Atlanta: Society of Biblical Literature, 2006), pp. 83-104.

Gowler, D.B., *Host, Guest, Enemy and Friend: Portraits of the Pharisees in Luke and Acts* (New York: Peter Lang, 1991).

Graham, William A., *Beyond the Written Word: Oral Aspects of Scripture in the History of Religion* (Cambridge: Cambridge University Press, 1987).

Gray, Robert, *Certain Things* (Port Melbourne: William Heinemann Australia, 1993).

Green, Joel, *The Gospel of Luke* (New International Commentary on the New Testament; Grand Rapids: Eerdmans, 1997).

Grey, Mary, 'Cosmic Communion: A Contemporary Reflection on the Eucharistic Vision of Teilhard de Chardin', *Ecotheology* 10.2 (2005), pp. 165-80.

Grosz, Elizabeth, *Jacques Lacan: A Feminist Introduction* (St Leonards, New South Wales: Allen & Unwin, 1990).

—*Sexual Subversions: Three French Feminists* (Sydney: Allen & Unwin, 1989).

—*Volatile Bodies: Toward a Corporeal Feminism* (St Leonards, New South Wales: Allen & Unwin, 1994).

Guyer, Paul, *Kant* (London: Routledge, 2006).

Habel, Norman C., 'Geophany: The Earth Story in Genesis 1', in *The Earth Story in Genesis* (ed. Norman C. Habel and Shirley Wurst; The Earth Bible, 1; Sheffield: Sheffield Academic Press, 2000), pp. 34-48.

—'Introducing the Earth Bible', in *Readings from the Perspective of Earth* (ed. Norman C. Habel; The Earth Bible, 1; Sheffield: Sheffield Academic Press, 2000), pp. 25-37.

—'Introducing Ecological Hermeneutics', in *Exploring Ecological Hermeneutics* (ed. Norman C. Habel and Peter L. Trudinger; SBL Symposium Series, 46; Atlanta: Society of Biblical Literature, 2008), pp. 1-8.

—Review of *An Ecological Feminist Reading of the Gospel of Luke: A Gestational Paradigm* (Lewiston, NY: Edwin Mellen Press, 2005), by Anne Elvey, in *Australian Religion Studies Review* 21 (2008), pp. 116-17.

Habel, Norman C. (ed.), *The Earth Story in the Psalms and the Prophets* (The Earth Bible, 4; Sheffield: Sheffield Academic Press, 2001).

—*Readings from the Perspective of Earth* (The Earth Bible, 1; Sheffield: Sheffield Academic Press, 2000).

Habel, Norman C., and Vicky Balabanski (eds.), *The Earth Story in the New Testament* (The Earth Bible, 5; London: Sheffield Academic Press, 2002).

Habel, Norman C., and Peter L. Trudinger (eds.), *Exploring Ecological Hermeneutics* (SBL Symposium Series, 46; Atlanta: Society of Biblical Literature, 2008).

Habel, Norman C., and Shirley Wurst (eds.), *The Earth Story in Genesis* (The Earth Bible, 2; Sheffield: Sheffield Academic Press 2000).

—*The Earth Story in Wisdom Traditions* (The Earth Bible, 3; Sheffield: Sheffield Academic Press, 2001).

Hafemann, Scott J., *Suffering and Ministry in the Spirit: Paul's Defense of his Ministry in II Corinthians 2:14–3:3* (Grand Rapids: Eerdmanns, 1990).

Hamm, Dennis M., 'The Tamid Service in Luke–Acts: The Cultic Background behind Luke's Theology', *Catholic Biblical Quarterly* 65 (2003), pp. 215-31.

Harris, Murray J., *Second Epistle to the Corinthians* (New International Greek Testament Commentary; Grand Rapids: Eerdmans, 2005).

Hart, Kevin, 'Forgotten Sociality' [under the heading Personal Well-Being and Social Conscience], in *Discerning the Australian Social Conscience: From the Jesuit Lenten Series* (ed. Frank Brennan; Richmond, Victoria: Jesuit Publications, 1999), pp. 53-71.

—'Horizons and Folds: Elizabeth Presa', *Contretemps* 2 (2001), pp. 171-75.

—'Poetry and Revelation: Hopkins, Counter-Experience and *Reductio*', *Pacifica* 18 (2005), pp. 259-80.

Hartsock, Chad, *Sight and Blindness in Luke–Acts: The Use of Physical Features in Characterization* (Leiden: E.J. Brill, 2008).

Harvey, Susan Ashbrook, *Scenting Salvation: Ancient Christianity and the Olfactory Imagination* (Transformation of the Classical Heritage, 42; Berkeley: University of California Press, 2006).

Heidegger, Martin, *The Fundamental Concept of Metaphysics* (trans. William McNeill and Nicholas Walker; Bloomington: Indiana University Press, 1995).

Heil, John Paul, *The Meal Scenes in Luke–Acts: An Audience-Oriented Approach* (Atlanta: Society of Biblical Literature, 1999).

—*The Transfiguration of Jesus: Narrative Meaning and Function of Mark 9:2-8, Matt 17:1-8 and Luke 9:28-36* (Analecta Biblica, 144; Rome: Biblical Institute Press, 2000).

Horner, Robyn, 'The Face as Icon: A Phenomenology of the Invisible', *Australasian Catholic Record* 82 (2005), pp. 19-28.

—'Translator's Introduction', in *In Excess: Studies of Saturated Phenomena,* by Jean-Luc Marion (New York: Fordham University Press, 2002), pp. ix-xx.

Horrell, David G., Cherryl Hunt and Christopher Southgate, 'Appeals to the Bible in Ecotheology and Environmental Ethics: A Typology of Hermeneutical Stances', *Studies in Christian Ethics* 21.2 (2008), pp. 219-38.

Horrell, David G., and Dominic Coad, '"The Stones Would Cry Out" (Luke 19.40): A Lukan Contribution to a Hermeneutics of Creation's Praise', *Scottish Journal of Theology* 64 (2011), pp. 29-44.

Humphrey, Edith M., *And I Turned to See the Voice: The Rhetoric of Vision in the New Testament* (Grand Rapids: Baker Academic, 2007).

Hurtado, Larry W., *The Earliest Christian Artifacts: Manuscripts and Christian Origins* (Grand Rapids: Eerdmans, 2006).

Idhe, Don, *Listening and Voice: Phenomenologies of Sound* (Albany: State University of New York Press, 2nd edn, 2007).

Irigaray, Luce, *Divine Women* (trans. S. Muecke; Local Consumption Papers, 8; Sydney: Local Consumption, 1986).

—*An Ethics of Sexual Difference* (trans. Carolyn Burke and Gillian C. Gill; Ithaca, NY: Cornell University Press, 1993).

—*Je, Tu, Nous: Toward a Culture of Difference* (trans. Alison Martin; London: Routledge, 1993).

—*Sexes and Genealogies* (trans. Gillian C. Gill; New York: Columbia University Press, 1993).

Irwin, William, 'Against Intertextuality', *Philosophy and Literature* 28 (2004), pp. 227-42.

Isherwood, Lisa, 'Jesus Past the Posts: An Enquiry into Post-Metaphysical Christology', in *Post-Christian Feminisms: A Critical Approach* (ed. Lisa Isherwood and Kathleen McPhillips; Aldershot: Ashgate, 2008), pp. 201-10.

Jagersma, H., *A History of Israel from Alexander the Great to Bar Kochba* (trans. John Bowden; London: SCM Press, 1985).

Jantzen, Grace M., *Becoming Divine: Towards a Feminist Philosophy of Religion* (Bloomington: Indiana University Press, 1999).

Johns, Adrian, *The Nature of the Book: Print and Knowledge in the Making* (Chicago: University of Chicago Press, 1998).

Jones, Owain, and Paul Cloke, 'Non-Human Agencies: Trees in Place and Time', in *Material Agency: Toward a Non-Anthropocentric Approach* (ed. Carl Knappett and Lambros Malafouris; New York: Springer, 2008), pp. 79-96.

Kahl, Brigitte, 'Reading Luke against Luke: Non-Uniformity of Text, Hermeneutics of Conspiracy and the "Scriptural Principle" in Luke 1', in *A Feminist Companion to Luke* (ed. Amy-Jill Levine with Marianne Blickenstaff; Feminist Companion to the New Testament and Early Christian Writings, 3; London: Sheffield Academic Press, 2002), pp. 70-88.

Kamuf, Peggy, 'Introduction', *Paragraph* 16.2 (1993), pp. 103-107.

Karris, Robert, 'The Gospel according to Luke', in *The New Jerome Biblical Commentary* (ed. Raymond E. Brown, Joseph A. Fitzmyer and Roland E. Murphy; London: Geoffrey Chapman, 1991), pp. 675-721.

Kartsonis, Anna, 'The Responding Icon', in *Heaven on Earth: Art and the Church in Byzantium* (ed. Linda Safran; University Park: Pennsylvania State University Press, 1998), pp. 58-80.

Keenan, Dennis King, 'Irigaray and the Sacrifice of the Sacrifice of Woman', *Hypatia* 19.4 (2004), pp. 167-83.

Kelber, Werner H., 'Oral Tradition in Bible and New Testament Studies', *Oral Tradition* 18 (2003), pp. 40-42.

Keller, Catherine, *Apocalypse Now and Then: A Feminist Guide to the End of the World* (Boston: Beacon Press, 1996).

—*Face of the Deep: A Theology of Becoming* (London: Routledge, 2003).

Kessler, Herbert L., 'The Book as Icon', in *In the Beginning: Bibles before the Year 1000* (ed. Michelle Brown; Washington, DC: Freer Gallery of Art and Arthur M. Sackler Gallery Smithsonian Institution, 2006), pp. 77-103.

Kingsbury, Jack Dean, *Conflict in Luke: Jesus, Authorities, Disciples* (Minneapolis: Fortress Press, 1991).

Kinman, Brent, 'Lucan Eschatology and the Missing Fig Tree', *Journal of Biblical Literature* 113 (1994), pp. 669-78.

Kirk, Alan, Review of *Oral and Manuscript Culture in the Bible: Studies on the Media Texture of the New Testament—Explorative Hermeneutics* (Stellenbosch: Sun Press, 2007), by J.A. (Bobby) Loubser, in *Review of Biblical Literature* (April 2008), http://www.bookreviews.org/pdf/5924_6288.pdf.

Kitchen, Merrill, 'The Good News of Restoration: Reading Luke–Acts Then and Now', *Pacifica* 23 (2010), pp. 157-72.

Kittel, Gerhard, and Gerhard Friedrich (eds.), *The Theological Dictionary of the New Testament, Abridged in One Volume* (Grand Rapids: Eerdmans, 1985).

Knappett, Carl, 'The Neglected Networks of Material Agency: Artefacts, Pictures and Texts', in *Material Agency: Toward a Non-Anthropocentric Approach* (ed. Carl Knappett and Lambros Malafouris; New York: Springer, 2008), pp. 139-56.

Kort, Wesley A., *'Take Read': Scripture, Textuality, and Cultural Practice* (University Park: Pennsylvania State University Press, 1996).

Kristeva, Julia, 'From One Identity to an Other', in *The Portable Kristeva* (ed. Kelly Oliver; New York: Columbia University Press, 2002), pp. 93-115.

—'"*Nous Deux*" or a (Hi)Story of Intertextuality', *Romanic Review* 93 (2002), pp. 7-13.

—'Reading the Bible', in *New Maladies of the Soul* (trans. Ross Guberman; European Perspectives; New York: Columbia University Press, 1995), pp. 115-26.

—*Revolution in Poetic Language* (trans. Margaret Waller; New York: Columbia University Press, 1984).

—'Stabat Mater', trans. Léon S. Roudiez, in *The Kristeva Reader* (ed. Toril Moi; Oxford: Basil Blackwell, 1986), pp. 160-86.

—'The System and the Speaking Subject', in *The Kristeva Reader* (ed. Toril Moi; Oxford: Basil Blackwell, 1986), pp. 24-33

—'Word, Dialogue and Novel', trans. Alice Jardine, Thomas Gora and Léon S. Roudiez, in *The Kristeva Reader* (ed. Toril Moi; Oxford: Basil Blackwell, 1986), pp. 34-61.

Kruse, Colin, *2 Corinthians* (Tyndale New Testament Commentaries; Leicester: Inter-Varsity Press, 1987).

Kuhn, Karl A., 'Beginning the Witness: The αὐτόπται καὶ ὑπηρέται of Luke's Infancy Narrative', *New Testament Studies* 49 (2003), pp. 237-55.

Lakoff, George, and Rafael E. Núñez, *Where Mathematics Comes from: How the Embodied Mind Brings Mathematics into Being* (New York: Basic Books, 2000).

Lambrecht, Jan, *Second Corinthians* (Sacra Pagina; Collegeville, MN: Liturgical Press, 1999).

LaVerdiere, Eugene, *The Eucharist in the New Testament and the Early Church* (Collegeville, MN: Liturgical Press, 1996).

Law, John, and Annemarie Mol, 'The Actor–Enacted: Cumbrian Sheep in 2001', in *Material Agency: Toward a Non-Anthropocentric Approach* (ed. Carl Knappett and Lambros Malafouris; New York: Springer, 2008), pp. 57-77.

Lee, Dorothy, *Flesh and Glory: Symbolism, Gender and Theology in the Gospel of John* (New York: Crossroad, 2002).

—'The Gospel of John and the Five Senses', *Journal of Biblical Literature* 129 (2010), pp. 115-27.

—'Touching the Sacred Text: The Bible as Icon in Feminist Reading', *Pacifica* 11 (1998), pp. 249-64.

—*Transfiguration* (New Century Theology; London: Continuum, 2004).

Lewy, Zeev, 'Short Communication: Geological and Religious Factors for Subsurface Quarrying That Formed the Zedekiah Cave in Jerusalem', *Israel Geoarchaeology: An International Journal* 21.2 (2006), pp. 187-96.

Liddell, Henry George, and Robert Scott, *A Greek–English Lexicon* (revised and augmented throughout by Sir Henry Stuart Jones, with the assistance of Roderick McKenzie; Oxford: Clarendon Press, 1940; http://www.perseus.tufts.edu).

Lieu, Judith, *The Gospel of Luke* (Epworth Commentaries; Peterborough: Epworth Press, 1997).

Longenecker, Bruce W., 'Lukan Aversion to Humps and Hollows: The Case of Acts 11.27–12.25', *New Testament Studies* 50 (2004), pp. 185-204.

Louth, Andrew, 'The Theology of the Word Made Flesh', in *The Bible as Book: The Manuscript Tradition* (ed. John L. Sharpe and Kimberly Van Kampen; London: British Library, 1998), pp. 223-28.

Loya, Melissa Tubbs, '"Therefore the Earth Mourns": The Grievance of Earth in Hosea 4:1-3', in *Exploring Ecological Hermeneutics* (ed. Norman C. Habel and Peter Trudinger; SBL Symposium Series, 46; Atlanta: Society of Biblical Literature, 2008), pp. 53-62.

Lucretius, *De rerum natura* (*On the Nature of Things*) (trans. William Ellery Leonard; The Internet Classics Archive; http://classics.mit.edu/Carus/nature_things.html).

—*Sensation and Sex* (trans. R.E. Latham; London: Penguin, 2005).

Mackinlay, Shane, *Interpreting Excess: Jean-Luc Marion, Saturated Phenomena, and Hermeneutics* (Perspectives in Continental Philosophy; New York: Fordham University Press, 2009).

Magowan, Fiona, 'The Joy of Mourning: Resacralising "the Sacred" in the Music of Yolngu Christianity and an Aboriginal Theology', *Anthropological Forum* 9 (1999), pp. 11-36.

Malafouris, Lambros, 'At the Potter's Wheel: An Argument for Material Agency', in *Material Agency: Toward a Non-Anthropocentric Approach* (ed. Carl Knappett and Lambros Malafouris; New York: Springer, 2008), pp. 19-36.

Malina, Bruce J., *The New Testament World: Insights from Cultural Anthropology* (Louisville, KY: Westminster John Knox, 3rd, rev. and exp. edn, 2001).

Marion, Jean-Luc, 'The Banality of Saturation', in *Counter-Experiences: Reading Jean-Luc Marion* (ed. Kevin Hart; Notre Dame, IN: University of Notre Dame Press, 2007), pp. 383-418.

—*In Excess: Studies of Saturated Phenomena* (trans. Robyn Horner and Vincent Berraud; Perspectives in Continental Philosophy, 27; New York: Fordham University Press, 2002).

—'The Saturated Phenomenon', *Philosophy Today* 40 (1996), pp. 103-24.

—'They Recognized Him; and He Became Invisible to Them', *Modern Theology* 18.2 (2002), pp. 145-52.

Marshall, I. Howard, *The Gospel of Luke: A Commentary on the Greek Text* (New International Greek Testament Commentary; Grand Rapids: Eerdmans, 1978).

Martin, Thomas W., 'What Makes Glory Glorious? Reading Luke's Account of the Transfiguration over against Triumphalism', *Journal for the Study of the New Testament* 29 (2006), pp. 3-26.

Matera, Frank J., *II Corinthians: A Commentary* (New Testament Library; Louisville, KY: Westminster John Knox Press, 2003).

McCance, Dawne, '*L'écriture limite*: Kristeva's Postmodern Feminist Ethics', *Hypatia* 11.2 (1996), pp. 141-60.

McCant, Jerry W., *2 Corinthians* (Readings: A New Biblical Commentary; Sheffield: Sheffield Academic Press, 1999).

McFague, Sallie, *Super, Natural Christians: How We Should Love Nature* (London: SCM Press, 1997).

McGann, Jerome J., *The Textual Condition* (Princeton, NJ: Princeton University Press, 1991).

McIntosh, Ian, 'Anthropology, Self Determination and Aboriginal Belief in the Christian God', *Oceania* 67.4 (1997), pp. 273-88.

McKendrick, Scot, and Kathleen Doyle, *Bible Manuscripts: 1400 Years of Scribes and Scripture* (London: British Library, 2007).

Méndez Montoya, Angel F., *The Theology of Food: Eating and the Eucharist* (Malden, MA: Wiley–Blackwell, 2009).

Merchant, Carolyn, *The Death of Nature: Women, Ecology and the Scientific Revolution* (originally published 1980; republished with new preface; San Francisco: Harper & Row, 1990).

Merleau-Ponty, Maurice, *Phenomenology of Perception* (trans. Colin Smith; London: Routledge Classics, 2002).

Metzger, Bruce M., *A Textual Commentary on the Greek New Testament* (Stuttgart: United Bible Societies, corrected edn, 1975).

Mews, Constant J. 'The World as Text: The Bible and the Book of Nature in Twelfth-Century Theology', in *Scripture and Pluralism: Reading the Bible in the Religiously Plural Worlds of the Middle Ages and Renaissance, Studies in the History of Christian Traditions* (ed. Thomas J. Heffernan and Thomas E. Burman; Leiden: E.J. Brill, 2005), pp. 95-122.

Moi, Toril, *Sexual/Textual Politics: Feminist Literary Theory* (London: Routledge, 1985).

Moore, Stephen D., 'Illuminating the Gospels without the Benefit of Colour: A Plea for Concrete Criticism', *Journal of the American Academy of Religion* 60 (1992), pp. 257-79.

Morgan, Janet, *Earth's Cry: Prophetic Ministry in a More-than-Human World* (DMin Studs dissertation; Melbourne College of Divinity, 2010).

Morgan, Monica, 'Colonising Religion', *Chain Reaction* Summer (2005–2006), pp. 36-37.

Morton, Timothy, *Ecology without Nature: Rethinking Environmental Aesthetics* (Cambridge, MA: Harvard University Press, 2007).

Moxnes, Halvor, 'The Social Context of Luke's Community', *Interpretation* 48 (1994), pp. 379-89.

Mulder, Anne-Claire, *Divine Flesh, Embodied Word: Incarnation as a Hermeneutical Key to a Feminist Theologian's Reading of Luce Irigaray's Work* (Amsterdam: Amsterdam University Press, 2006).

Murphy-O'Connor, Jerome, 'The Second Letter to the Corinthians', in *The New Jerome Biblical Commentary* (ed. Joseph A. Fitzmyer, Raymond E. Brown and Roland E. Murphy; London: Geoffrey Chapman, 1991), pp. 816-29.

Muzj, Maria Giovanna, *Transfiguration: Introduction to the Contemplation of Icons* (Boston: St Paul Books & Media, 1991).

Nancy, Jean-Luc, *Being Singular Plural* (trans. Robert D. Richardson and Anne E. O'Byrne; Meridian; Crossing Aesthetics; Stanford, CA: Stanford University Press, 2000).

—'Corpus', in *The Birth to Presence* (trans. Brian Holmes, *et al.*; Meridian; Crossing Aesthetics; Stanford, CA: Stanford University Press, 1993), pp. 189-207.

—*Corpus* (trans. Richard A. Rand; Perspectives in Continental Philosophy; New York: Fordham University Press, 2008).

—*The Ground of the Image* (trans. Jeff Fort; Perspectives in Continental Philosophy; New York: Fordham University Press, 2005).

—*Listening* (trans. Charlotte Mandell; New York: Fordham University Press, 2007).

—*On the Commerce of Thinking: Of Books and Bookstores* (trans. David Wills; New York: Fordham University Press, 2009).

—*The Sense of the World* (trans. Jeffrey S. Librett; Minneapolis: University of Minnesota Press, 1997).

Neale, David A. *'None but the Sinners': Religious Categories in the Gospel of Luke* (Journal for the Study of the New Testament Supplement Series, 58; Sheffield: JSOT Press, 1991).

Nes, Solrunn, *The Uncreated Light: An Iconographical Study of the Transfiguration in the Eastern Church* (Grand Rapids: Eerdmans, 2007).

Neyrey, Jerome H., 'Clean/Unclean, Pure/Polluted and Holy/Profane: The Idea and System of Purity', in *The Social Sciences and New Testament Interpretation* (ed. Richard Rohrbaugh; Peabody, MA: Hendrickson, 1996), pp. 80-104.

Nikolchina, Miglena, *Matricide in Language: Writing Theory in Kristeva and Woolf* (New York: Other Press, 2004).

Nutu, Ela, *Incarnate Word, Inscribed Flesh: John's Prologue and the Postmodern* (The Bible in the Modern World, 6; Sheffield: Sheffield Phoenix Press, 2007).

Oliver, Kelly, *Reading Kristeva: Unraveling the Double-Bind* (Bloomington: Indiana University Press, 1993).

Ong, Walter J., *Orality and Literacy* (London: Routledge, 2002).

Pattel-Gray, Anne, 'Dreaming: An Aboriginal Interpretation of the Bible', in *Text and Experience: Towards a Cultural Exegesis of the Bible* (ed. Daniel L. Smith-Christopher; Sheffield: Sheffield Academic Press, 1995), pp. 247-59.

Pattie, Thomas S., 'The Creation of the Great Codices', in *The Bible as Book: The Manuscript Tradition* (ed. John L. Sharpe III and Kimberly Van Kampen; London: British Library, 1998), pp. 61-72.

Payne, Michael, *Reading Theory: An Introduction to Lacan, Derrida, and Kristeva* (Oxford: Basil Blackwell, 1993).

Payton, James R., Jr, 'John of Damascus on Human Cognition: An Element in his Apologetic for Icons', *Church History* 65 (1996), pp. 173-83.

Pedersen, Olaf, *The Book of Nature* (Rome: Vatican Observatory Publications, 1992).

Pelikan, Jaroslav, *Imago Dei: The Byzantine Apologia for Icons* (A.W. Mellon Lectures in the Fine Arts 1987; Princeton, NJ: Princeton University Press, 1990).

Perkins, Pheme, 'If Jerusalem Stood: The Destruction of Jerusalem and Christian Anti-Judaism', *Biblical Interpretation* 8 (2000), pp. 194-204.

Philo, *De vita Mosis* (*On the Life of Moses*), in *Philo: In Ten Volumes,* VI (trans. F.H. Colson; Loeb Classical Library; London: William Heinemann, 1935).

Pike, Elizabeth, 'The Power in the Story: Advent Leads Us to Christmas', *Madonna* (November–December 2001), pp. 27-28.

Pliny the Elder, *Natural History: A Selection* (trans. John F. Healy; with an introduction and notes; London: Penguin, 1991).

Plumwood, Val, *Environmental Culture: The Ecological Crisis of Reason* (Environmental Philosophies; London: Routledge, 2002).

—*Feminism and the Mastery of Nature* (Feminism for Today; London: Routledge, 1993).

—'Journey to the Heart of Stone', in *Culture, Creativity and Environment: New Environmental Criticism* (ed. Fiona Becket and Terry Gifford; Amsterdam: Rodopi, 2007), pp. 17-36.

—'Nature as Agency and the Prospects for a Progressive Naturalism', *Capitalism Nature Socialism* 12.4 (2001), pp. 3-32.

—'Tasteless: Towards a Food-Based Approach to Death', *PAN: Philosophy, Activism, Nature* 5 (2008), pp. 63-68.

Polybius, *Historiae* (ed. Theodorus Büttner-Wobst after L. Dindorf; Leipzig: Teubner, 1893); *Histories* (trans. Evelyn S. Shuckburgh; London, New York: Macmillan, 1889; reprinted, Bloomington, 1962; http://www.perseus.tufts.edu).

Prevelakis, Nicolas, 'Iconography: Its Historical, Theological and Philosophical Background', *Ekistics* 70.418/419 (2003), pp. 47-51.

Price, Jonathan J., *Jerusalem under Siege: The Collapse of the Jewish State 66–70 C.E.* (Leiden: E.J. Brill, 1992).

Primavesi, Anne, *Gaia's Gift: Earth, Ourselves and God after Copernicus* (London: Routledge, 2003).

—*Sacred Gaia: Holistic Theology and Earth System Science* (London: Routledge, 2000).

Purvis, Sally B., 'Mothers, Neighbours and Strangers: Another Look at Agape', *Journal of Feminist Studies in Religion* 7 (1991), pp. 19-34.

Quast, Kevin, *Reading the Corinthian Correspondence: An Introduction* (New York: Paulist Press, 1994).

Reasoner, Mark, 'The Theme of Acts: Institutional History or Divine Necessity in History?', *Journal of Biblical Literature* 118 (1999), pp. 635-59.

Reid, Barbara E., *Choosing the Better Part? Women in the Gospel of Luke* (Collegeville, MN: Liturgical Press, 1996).

—'"Do You See This Woman?" A Liberative Look at Luke 7.36-50 and Strategies for Reading Other Lukan Stories against the Grain', in *A Feminist Companion to Luke* (ed. Amy-Jill Levine with Marianne Blickenstaff; London: Sheffield Academic Press, 2002), pp. 106-20.

Rhoads, David, 'Who Will Speak for the Sparrow? Eco-Justice Criticism of the New Testament', in *Literary Encounters with the Reign of God* (Festschrift Robert Tannehill; ed. Sharon H. Ringe and H.C. Paul Kim; Harrisburg, PA: Trinity Press International, 2004), pp. 64-86.

Rigby, Kate, 'Earth, World, Text: On the (Im)Possibility of Ecopoiesis', *New Literary History* 35 (2004), pp. 427-42.

—'Introduction', *Religion and Literature* 40 (2008), pp. 1-8.

—'Writing after Nature', *Australian Humanities Review* 39–40 (2006), http://www.australianhumanitiesreview.org/archive/Issue-September-2006/rigby.html.

Ringe, Sharon H., *Luke* (Westminster Bible Companion; Louisville, KY: Westminster John Knox, 1995).

Robbins, Jill, *Prodigal Son/Elder Brother: Interpretation and Alterity in Augustine, Petrarch, Kafka, Levinas* (Chicago: University of Chicago Press, 1991).

Robbins, Vernon, 'Historical, Rhetorical, Literary, Linguistic, Cultural, and Artistic Intertextuality—A Response', *Semeia* 80 (1997), pp. 291-303.

Roberts, David Andrew, '"Language to Save the Innocent": Reverend L. Threlkeld's Linguistic Mission', *Journal of the Royal Australian Historical Society* 94.2 (2008), pp. 107-25.

Rose, Deborah Bird, *Reports from a Wild Country: Ethics for Decolonisation* (Sydney: University of New South Wales Press, 2004).

Ruether, Rosemary Radford, 'Ecological Theology: Roots in Tradition, Liturgical and Ethical Practice for Today', *Dialog: A Journal of Theology* 42.3 (2003), pp. 226-34.

—*Gaia and God: An Ecofeminist Theology of Earth Healing* (San Francisco: HarperCollins, 1992).

Salleh, Ariel, *Ecofeminism as Politics: Nature, Marx and the Postmodern* (London: Zed Books, 1997).

Sanders, Jack T., *The Jews in Luke–Acts* (Philadelphia: Fortress Press, 1987).

Savage, Timothy B., *Power through Weakness: Paul's Understanding of the Christian Ministry in 2 Corinthians* (Society for New Testament Studies Monograph Series; Cambridge: Cambridge University Press, 1996).

Scaer, Peter J., *The Lukan Passion and the Praiseworthy Death* (New Testament Monographs, 10; Sheffield: Sheffield Phoenix Press, 2005).

Schniedewind, William M., *How the Bible Became a Book: The Textualization of Ancient Israel* (Cambridge: Cambridge University Press, 2004).

Schüssler Fiorenza, Elisabeth, *But She Said: Feminist Practices of Biblical Interpretation* (Boston: Beacon Press, 1992).

Schwartz, Regina M., *The Curse of Cain: The Violent Legacy of Monotheism* (Chicago: University of Chicago Press, 1997).

Seim, Turid Karlsen, *The Double Message: Patterns of Gender in Luke and Acts* (Nashville: Abingdon Press, 1994).

Serres, Michel, *The Five Senses: A Philosophy of Mingled Bodies,* I (trans. Margaret Sankey and Peter Cowley; London: Continuum, 2008).

Sink, Susan, *The Saint John's Bible: An Introduction* (Collegeville, MN: Liturgical Press, 2007).

Skye, Lee Miena, *Kerygmatics of the New Millennium: A Study of Australian Aboriginal Women's Christology* (Delhi: ISPCK, 2007).

Smith, Dennis Edwin, *From Symposium to Eucharist: The Banquet in the Early Christian World* (Minneapolis: Fortress Press, 2003).

Squires, John T., *The Plan of God in Luke–Acts* (Cambridge: Cambridge University Press, 1993).

Staubli, Thomas, and Silvia Schroer, *Body Symbolism in the Bible* (trans. Linda M. Maloney; Collegeville, MN: Liturgical Press, 2001).

Sterling, Gregory E., '*Mors Philosophi*: The Death of Jesus in Luke', *Harvard Theological Review* 94 (2001), pp. 383-402.

Svenbro, Jesper, *Three-Toed Gull: Selected Poems* (trans. John Matthias and Lars-Håkan Svensson; Evanston, IL: Northwestern University Press, 2003).

Syrotinski, Michael, 'Introduction: *Hors d'oeuvre*', in *Sensual Reading: New Approaches to Reading in its Relation to the Senses* (ed. Michael Syrotinski and Ian Maclachlan; London: Associated Universities Presses, 2001), pp. 7-12.

Talbert, Charles H., *Reading Corinthians: A Literary and Theological Commentary on 1 and 2 Corinthians* (New York: Crossroad, 1987).

—*Reading Luke: A Literary and Theological Commentary on the Third Gospel* (New York: Crossroad, 1988).

Tannehill, Robert C., 'Israel in Luke–Acts: A Tragic Story', *Journal of Biblical Literature* 104 (1985), pp. 69-85.

—*Luke* (Abingdon New Testament Commentaries; Nashville: Abingdon Press, 1996).

—*The Narrative Unity of Luke–Acts: A Literary Interpretation,* I. *The Gospel according to Luke* (Foundations and Facets: New Testament; Philadelphia: Fortress Press, 1986).

— *The Narrative Unity of Luke–Acts: A Literary Interpretation,* II. *The Acts of the Apostles* (Minneapolis: Fortress Press, 1994).

Teilhard de Chardin, Pierre, *Hymn of the Universe* (trans. Gerald Vann; London: Collins, 1965).

Thrall, Margaret E., *The Second Epistle to the Corinthians*, I (International Critical Commentary; London: T. & T. Clark, 2004).

Threkeld, L.E. *An Awabakal–English Lexicon to the Gospel by St Luke* (Sydney: Charles Potter, Government Printer, 1892).

— *The Gospel by St Luke Translated into the Language of the Awabakal* (Sydney: Charles Potter, Government Printer, 1891).

Tilborg, Sjef van, and Patrick Chatelion Counet, *Jesus' Appearances and Disappearances in Luke 24* (Leiden: E. J. Brill, 2000).

Tilley, Christopher, *The Materiality of Stone: Explorations in Landscape Phenomenology* (Oxford: Berg, 2004).

Toorn, Karel van der, 'The Iconic Book: Analogies between the Babylonian Cult of Images and the Veneration of the Torah', in *The Image and the Book: Iconic Cults, Aniconism, and the Rise of Book Religion in Israel and the Ancient Near East* (ed. Karel van der Toorn; Leuven: Peeters, 1997), pp. 229-48.

Tredinnick, Mark, *The Blue Plateau: A Landscape Memoir* (St Lucia: University of Queensland Press, 2009).

Tsagalis, Christos C., 'Style and Construction, Sound and Rhythm: Thetis' Supplication to Zeus (Iliad 1.493-516)', *Arethusa* 34 (2001), pp. 1-29.

Wainwright, Elaine M., 'Anointing/Washing Feet: John 12:1-8 and its Intertexts within a Socio-Rhetorical Reading', in *'I Sowed Fruits into Hearts' (Odes Sol. 17:13)* (Festschrift Professor Michael Lattke; ed. Majella Franzmann, Pauline Allen and Rick Strelan; Early Christian Studies, 12; Sydney: St Paul's Publications, 2007), pp. 203-20.

—'Rachel Weeping for her Children: Intertextuality and the Biblical Testaments—A Feminist Approach', in *A Feminist Companion to Reading the Bible: Approaches, Methods and Strategies* (ed. Athalya Brenner and Carole Fontaine; Sheffield: Sheffield Academic Press, 1997), pp. 452-69.

—*Shall We Look for Another? A Feminist Rereading of the Matthean Jesus* (Maryknoll, NY: Orbis Books, 1998).

—'Unbound Hair and Ointmented Feet: An Ecofeminist Reading of Luke 7.36-50', in *Exchanges of Grace* (Festschrift Ann Loades; ed. Natalie K. Watson and Stephen Burns; London: SCM Press, 2008), pp. 178-89.

—*Women Healing/Healing Women: The Genderization of Healing in Early Christianity* (London: Equinox, 2006).

Walling, Jane. 'Reading (in) Proust: With the Senses, beyond the Senses', in *Sensual Reading: New Approaches to Reading in its Relation to the Senses* (ed. Michael Syrotinski and Ian Maclachlan; London: Associated Universities Presses, 2001), pp. 271-91.

Walsh, Brian J., Marianne B. Karsh and Nik Ansell, 'Trees, Forestry, and the Responsiveness of Creation', in *This Sacred Earth: Religion, Nature, Environment* (ed. Roger S. Gottlieb; New York: Routledge, 1996), pp. 423-35.

Watson, Lyall, *Jacobson's Organ and the Remarkable Nature of Smell* (New York: Norton, 2000).

Watson, Nigel, *The Second Epistle to the Corinthians* (London: Epworth Press, 1993).

Weissenrieder, Annette, 'The Plague of Uncleanness? The Ancient Illness Construct "Issue of Blood" in Luke 8:43-48', in *The Social Setting of Jesus and the Gospels* (ed. Wolfgang Stegemann, Bruce J. Malina and Gerd Theissen; Minneapolis: Fortress Press, 2002), pp. 207-22.

West, Gerald, 'Redirecting the Direction of Travel: Discerning Signs of a Neo-Indigenous Southern African Biblical Hermeneutics', in *Redirected Travel: Alternative Journeys and Places in Biblical Studies* (ed. Roland Boer and Edgar W. Conrad, Journal for the Study of the Old Testament Supplement Series, 382; London: T. & T. Clark International, 2003), pp. 201-25.

Westphal, Merold, 'Transfiguration as Saturated Phenomenon', *Journal of Philosophy and Scripture* 1 (2003), pp. 26-34.

White, Lynn, 'The Historical Roots of our Ecological Crisis', in *This Sacred Earth: Religion, Nature, Environment* (ed. Roger S. Gottlieb; New York: Routledge, 1996), pp. 184-93.

Wills, David, 'Translator's Foreword: Thinking Singular Plural', in *On the Commerce of Thinking: Of Books and Bookstores,* by Jean-Luc Nancy (New York: Fordham University Press, 2009), pp. xiii-xx.

Wright, Judith, *Collected Poems* (Pymble, NSW: Angus & Robertson, 1994).

Würthwein, Ernst, *The Text of the Old Testament: An Introduction to the Biblica Hebraica* (trans. Erroll F. Rhodes; Grand Rapids: Eerdmans, 2nd edn, 1995).

# Index of References

# Index of Authors

www.ingramcontent.com/pod-product-compliance
Lightning Source LLC
LaVergne TN
LVHW011758200926
848484LV00003B/738

* 9 7 8 1 9 0 7 5 3 4 1 6 4 *